Clinical Review of Surgery

ABSITE & Board Preparation

Also from Catalyst Publishers

Question and Answer Review of Surgery
High-Yield Review of Surgery
Slide Review of Surgery
Flash Card Review of Surgery
Clinical Review of Vascular Surgery
Clinical Review of Medicine

Clinical Review for the USMLE Step 1
Clinical Review for the USMLE Step 2
Clinical Review for the USMLE Step 3

Clinical Review of Surgery

ABSITE & Board Preparation

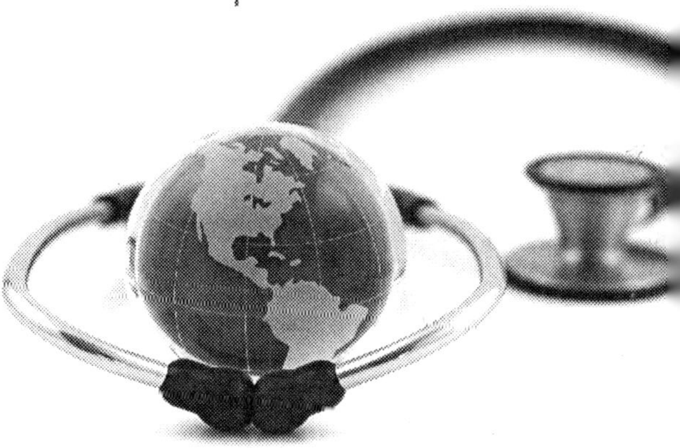

EDITORS

SAPAN S. DESAI MD, PhD

DANNY O. JACOBS MD, MPH

CATALYST PUBLISHERS

Clinical Review of Surgery | ABSITE & Board Preparation

Edited by Sapan S. Desai, M.D., Ph.D. & Danny O. Jacobs, M.D., M.P.H.

www.ClinicalReview.com | www.CatalystPublishers.com | www.Surgisphere.com

Prepared in the United States of America

Third Edition

Cataloging-In-Publication Data

Surgisphere Corporation
Clinical Review of Surgery, ABSITE & Board Preparation

1. Surgery	2. Medicine
I. Surgisphere Corporation	II. Clinical Review of Surgery
ISBN 9780980210378	C6168
617 SUR	2008901178

01 / 10 9 8 7 6 5 4 3 2
First published in 2003.

SURGISPHERE

For Niketa, Krish, and Eashan, the
ones who define my life.
SSD

Many thanks for the extraordinary dedication of time and effort made by the faculty and residents who have contributed to this text. Special thanks to Drs. Niketa Desai, Jeff Hoehner, Charles Murphy, Scott Pruitt, John Scarborough, Randall Scheri, Cynthia Shortell, and Mark Williams. With appreciation and admiration for the people we work with, our friends, and most importantly, our families.

SSD & DOJ

CONTRIBUTORS

Tara Brennan, M.D.
Ophthalmology Resident
Department of Ophthalmology
University of Illinois, Chicago, IL

Johnny T. Chang, M.D.
Plastic Surgery Resident
Department of Surgery
Brown University, Providence, RI

Melissa E. Danko, M.D.
General Surgery Resident
Department of Surgery
Duke University, Durham, NC

Niketa Desai, Pharm.D.
Registered Pharmacist
Department of Pharmacology
Long Island University, Brooklyn, NY

Sapan S. Desai, M.D., Ph.D.
General Surgery Resident
Department of Surgery
Duke University, Durham, NC

Amahuaro Edebiri, M.D.
Professor and Chair
Department of Obstetrics & Gynecology
Bayero University, Kano, Nigeria

William Eward, D.V.M., M.D.
Orthopaedic Surgery Resident
Department of Surgery
Duke University, Durham, NC

Jeff C. Hoehner, M.D., Ph.D.
Assistant Professor
Pediatric Surgery
Department of Surgery
Duke University, Durham, NC

Prateek Kumar Gupta, M.D.
General Surgery Resident
Department of Surgery
Creighton University, Omaha, NE

Danny O. Jacobs, M.D., M.P.H
David C. Sabiston, Jr. Professor & Chair
Surgeon-in-Chief
Department of Surgery
Duke University, Durham, NC

Issam Koleilat, M.D.
General Surgery Resident
Department of Surgery
Albany Medical Center, Albany, NY

Keri Lunsford, M.D., Ph.D.
General Surgery Resident
Department of Surgery
Duke University, Durham, NC

Jerimiah Mason, M.D.
General Surgery Resident
Department of Surgery
Baptist Medical Center, Birmingham, AL

Stephanie Mayer, M.D.
Orthopaedic Surgery Resident
Department of Surgery
Duke University, Durham, NC

Daniel Murariu, M.D.
General Surgery Resident
Department of Surgery
University of Hawaii, Honolulu, HI

Charles Murphy, M.D.
Assistant Professor
Trauma and Critical Care Surgery
Department of Surgery
Duke University, Durham, NC

Leontine Narcisse, M.D., Ph.D.
Surgery Fellow
Department of Surgery
Westchester Medical Center,
Westchester, NY

Luigi Pascarella, M.D.
General Surgery Resident
Department of Surgery
Duke University, Durham, NC

Scott K. Pruitt, M.D., Ph.D.
Associate Professor
Surgical Oncology
Department of Surgery
Duke University, Durham, NC

John Scarborough, M.D.
Assistant Professor
Trauma and Critical Care Surgery
Department of Surgery
Duke University, Durham, NC

Randall Scheri, M.D.
Assistant Professor
Endocrine Surgery
Department of Surgery
Duke University, Durham, NC

Cynthia K. Shortell, M.D.
Professor and Chief
Vascular Surgery
Department of Surgery
Duke University, Durham, NC

Suzanne Stewart, M.D.
Urology Resident
Department of Surgery
Duke University, Durham, NC

Elisabeth T. Tracy, M.D.
General Surgery Resident
Department of Surgery
Duke University, Durham, NC

Immanuel Turner, M.D.
General Surgery Resident
Department of Surgery
Duke University, Durham, NC

Jackie Garonzik Wang, M.D.
General Surgery Resident
Department of Surgery
Johns Hopkins, Baltimore, MD

Tamarah J. Westmoreland, M.D., Ph.D.
General Surgery Chief Resident
Department of Surgery
Duke University, Durham, NC

Judson B. Williams, M.D.
General Surgery Resident
Department of Surgery
Duke University, Durham, NC

Mark D. Williams, M.D.
Professor and Program Director
General Surgery
Department of Surgery
St. Elizabeth, Youngstown, OH

Jocelyn Wittstein, M.D.
Orthopaedic Surgery Chief Resident
Department of Surgery
Duke University, Durham, NC

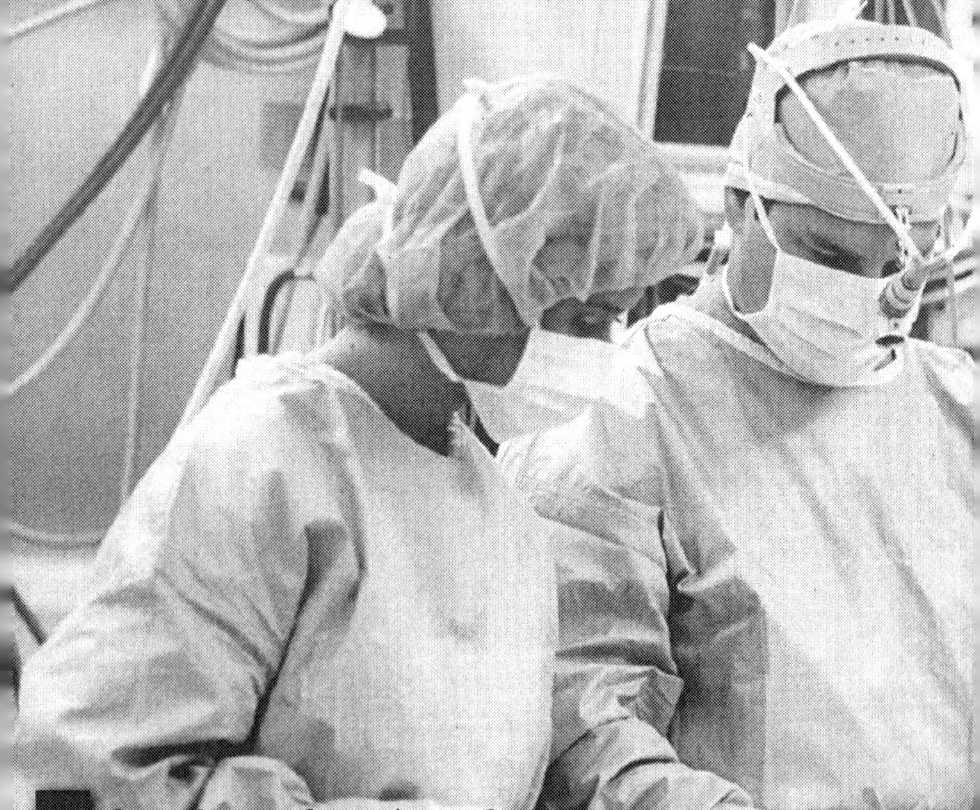

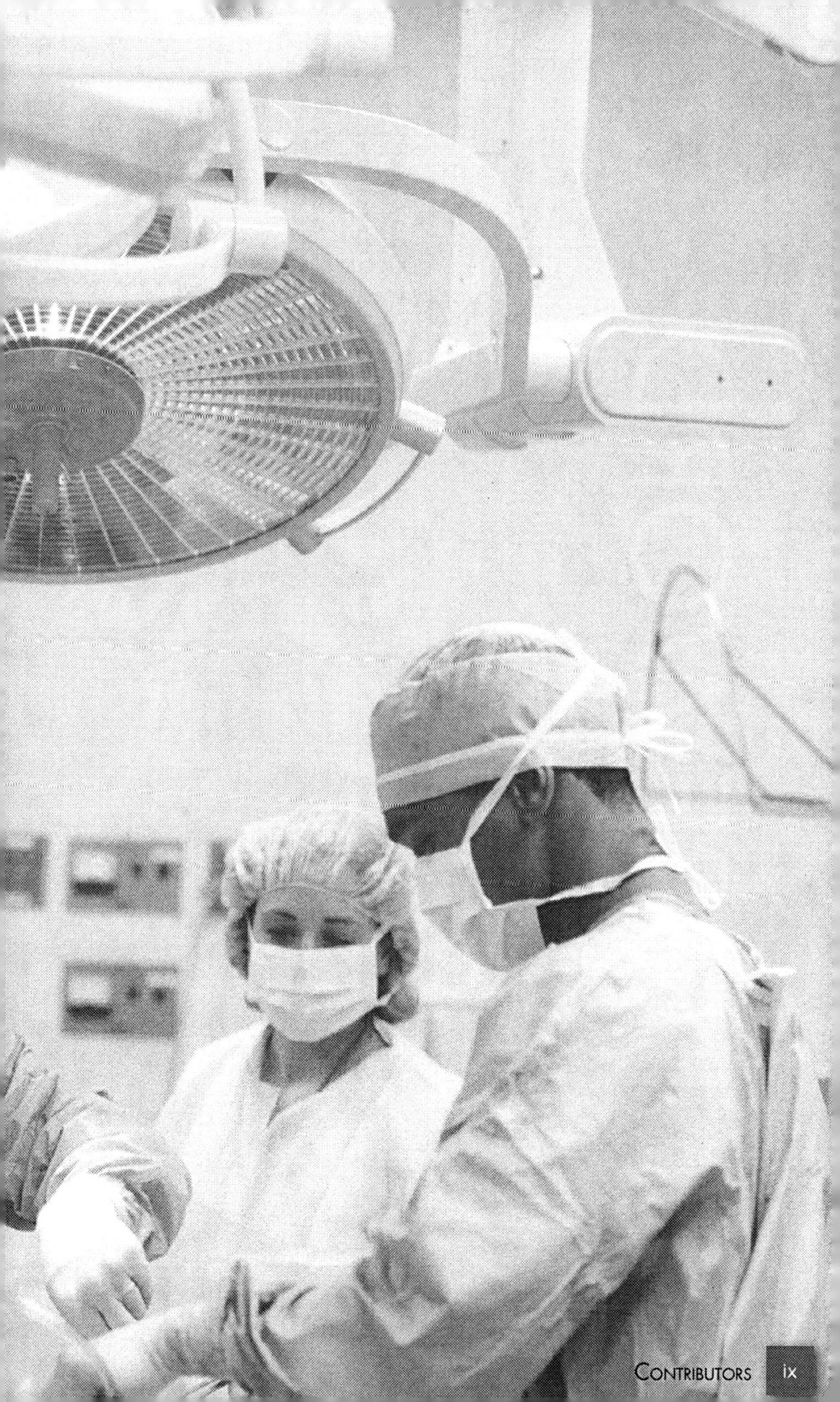

FOREWORD

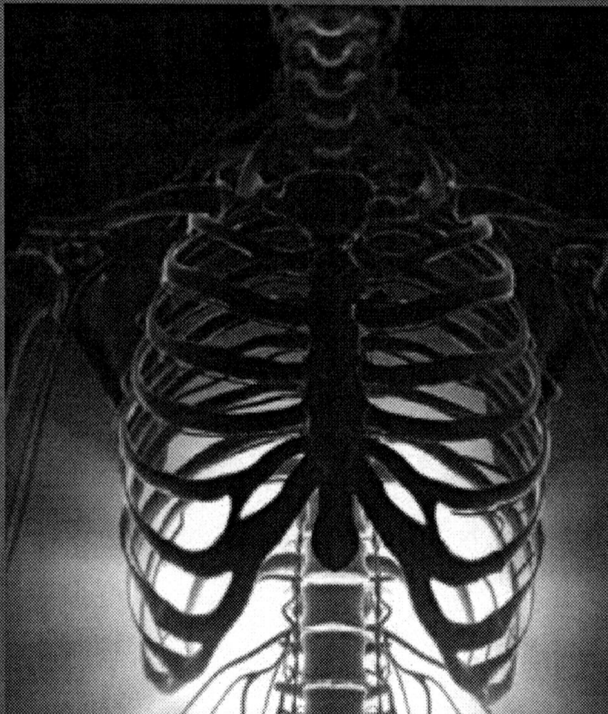

Equally doubtful for the anatomists is a gland called pancreas. They pretend that it is created as a support for the stomach.

Gabriele Fallopius
Observationes anatomicae, 1561

SURGISPHERE

FOREWORD

Danny O. Jacobs, M.D., M.P.H.

This Clinical Review of Surgery is now in its third edition. Through the hard work of the editors and authors, this peer-reviewed textbook is recognized as an extremely valuable resource for program directors and their residents throughout the United States of America—and increasingly throughout the world. Their effort to include relevant, timely and clearly written source material for surgical trainees is substantial. The standard surgical textbooks, of course, contain vital information and should be visited regularly. Nevertheless, I believe it is accurate to comment that it is often too difficult for many trainees to determine precisely what information needs to be retained to provide the best care rendered to patients. It is knowledge of these fundamentals that is required to be the best physician and surgeon—and it is this knowledge that is tested by the ABSITE and surgery qualifying examination. These challenges occur at a time when the scientific foundation of modern surgical practice is expanding exponentially.

So, what is the trainee to do when the pace of training has increased so significantly, when the amount of information that must be read and understood is so vast, and when the nature of surgical training has changed to meet the expectations and demand of the new millennium? He or she looks for tools that can be used to help focus their educational efforts. This peer-reviewed Clinical Review of Surgery is one such tool. Its material closely mirrors the content of the qualifying examination administered by the American Board of Surgery as well as the material that is tested by the yearly ABSITE. Every effort is made to organize the text so that it can be read or reviewed quickly and efficiently. Standard nomenclature is used to focus the reader to information that is essential or complex enough to require in depth review. The reader is pointed to resource material that is available online. Important drugs that are commonly used in practice are highlighted. Review questions are provided along with detailed answers.

The busy resident now has a companion text that nicely complements the standard tomes, integrates with a rich variety of online resources at the companion website, and which summarizes and highlights information essential for the best surgical care—all this in a book that fits in a coat pocket.

Danny O. Jacobs M.D., M.P.H.
Chair of Surgery
David C. Sabiston, Jr. Professor
Duke University Hospitals and School of Medicine

CONTENTS

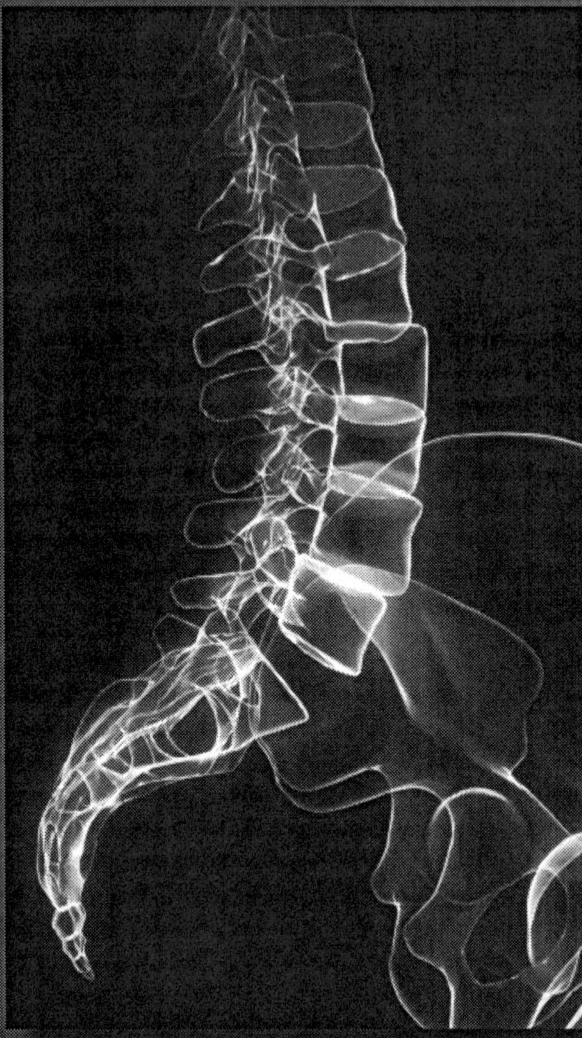

I will pass over the other arts in silence and direct my words for a while to that which is responsible for the health of mankind; certainly of all the arts that human genius has discovered, this is by far the most useful, indispensible, difficult, and laborious.

Andreas Vesalius
De Humani Corporus Fabrica, 1543

SURGISPHERE

CONTENTS

INTRODUCTION

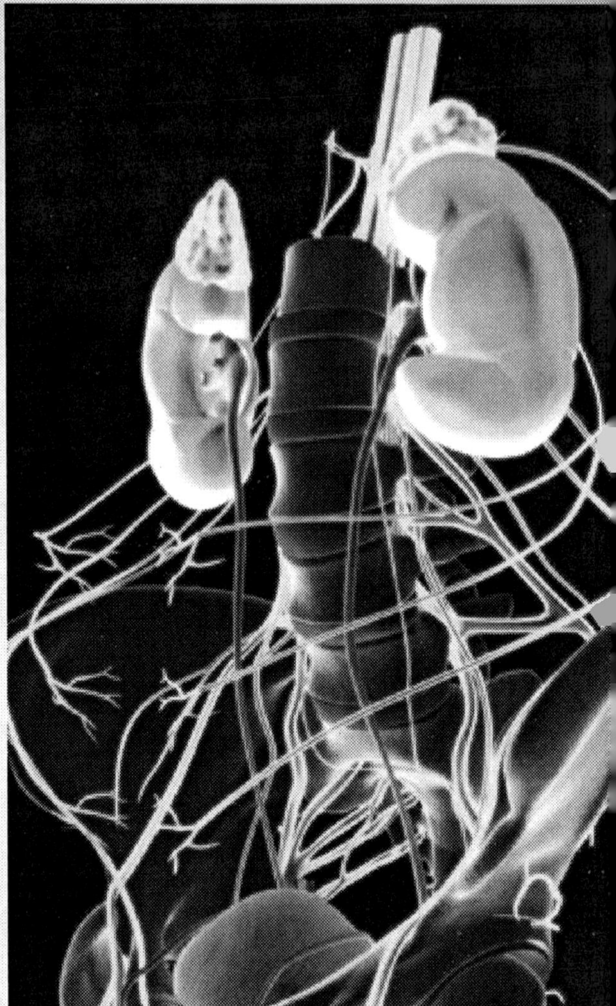

The matter is already quite difficult enough, and I have no wish to make it even more obscure.

Andreas Vesalius
De Humani Corporus Fabrica, 1543

INTRODUCTION

Sapan S. Desai, M.D., Ph.D.

I. OVERVIEW

This peer-reviewed textbook and its accompanying multidisciplinary review course were created to improve the quality of surgical education and thereby improve the quality of care our patients receive. While there can be no substitute for studying key reference textbooks and participating in thousands of operations, there are precious moments during training that can be used to quickly refresh and reinforce key topics in surgery. The focus of this integrated review program is to provide a unique comprehensive review of topics commonly tested on the ABSITE, the surgery qualifying examination, and in the modern practice of surgery.

The overall organization of this textbook reflects the content outline of the surgery qualifying examination produced by the American Board of Surgery to ensure that every subject area is given due consideration. Thousands of surgery residents from nearly every training program across the country have used these resources in recent years to improve their scores and better prepare for the challenges ahead. Surgery training programs have implemented our educational resources as a cornerstone of their didactic programs and use it to advance resident education.

Those who have completed our review course have reported significant improvements in ABSITE scores and clinical performance. Program directors have noted higher pass rates on the surgery qualifying exam and oral boards. This unique solution to the challenges of resident education has changed the way we learn and improved the depth and breadth of our clinical knowledge.

II. THIRD EDITION

Since the publication of the first edition in 2003, we have actively sought feedback from our readers on what we did well and what we could do better. After listening to your thoughts, we have made a number of improvements to our textbook and online review course. This textbook has been extensively reviewed, rewritten, and edited by residents and faculty from leading surgery training programs. Entire sections have been completely rewritten and emphasis has been placed on topics that are commonly tested on the surgery board examination and the ABSITE. Hundreds of new topics covering all areas of surgical care and management have been added throughout the textbook.

We are pleased to bring you this third edition – the culmination of intense effort from residents and surgeons from leading surgery programs around the country. As always, we are delighted to hear your thoughts. Contact us anytime.

III. Examination Topics

The surgery qualifying examination and the ABSITE cover a broad array of disciplines that span both basic science and clinical surgery. Questions are derived from nearly every basic science subject and field of surgery, with the junior version of the ABSITE focusing on mostly basic science questions. Topics include Head and Neck Surgery, Breast Surgery, Gastrointestinal Surgery, Hepatopancreatobiliary Surgery, Vascular Surgery, Endocrine Surgery, Trauma Surgery, Surgical Critical Care, Transplant Surgery, Pediatric Surgery, Thoracic Surgery, Gynecology, Urology, Orthopedic Surgery, Plastic Surgery, Surgical Oncology, Anesthesia, and Medical Ethics.[1] The ABSITE covers all of these subjects.[2]

Within each of these clinical disciplines, questions are derived from both basic science and clinical topics. Of the 225 questions on the ABSITE, 60% of the questions are derived from basic science topics for the junior ABSITE and 20% of the questions are derived from basic science topics for the senior ABSITE. Table 1 shows the breakdown of questions for both versions of the ABSITE.

[1] This information is based on the annual publication by the American Board of Surgery. It is derived from http://home.absurgery.org/xfer/GS-QE.pdf

[2] The ABSITE covers roughly the same information presented on the qualifying exam, hence the reason why it is predictive of performance on this exam. This information is extrapolated from http://home.absurgery.org/default.jsp?certabsite

TABLE 1. Breakdown of the ABSITE by post-graduate year

	Junior ABSITE (PGY 1 and 2)	Senior ABSITE (PGY 3+)
Basic Science	60% (135)	20% (45)
Clinical Medicine	40% (90)	80% (180)
Total	100% (225)	100% (225)

The breakdown of topics on the ABSITE is presented in Table 2.

TABLE 2. Breakdown of the ABSITE by category

	Junior ABSITE	Senior ABSITE
General Surgery and Surgical Critical Care	66.6%	25%
Gastrointestinal Tract	10%	25%
Cardiothoracic Surgery	7.8%	16.7%
Head and Neck Surgery, Gynecology, and Orthopedic Surgery	7.8%	16.7%
Endocrine Surgery, Hepatopancreatobiliary Surgery, Surgical Oncology, and Breast Surgery	7.8%	16.7%

Table 3 yields an estimate of the number of questions per subject area.

TABLE 3. Breakdown of the ABSITE by number of questions

	Junior ABSITE		Senior ABSITE	
General Surgery and Surgical Critical Care	Basic Science	90	Basic Science	10
	Clinical Surgery	60	Clinical Surgery	45
Gastrointestinal	Basic Science	15	Basic Science	10
	Clinical Surgery	9	Clinical Surgery	45
Cardiothoracic	Basic Science	11	Basic Science	8
	Clinical Surgery	6	Clinical Surgery	30
Head and Neck, Gynecology, and Orthopedics	Basic Science	11	Basic Science	8
	Clinical Surgery	6	Clinical Surgery	30
Endocrine, Hepatopancreatobiliary, Surgical Oncology, and Breast	Basic Science	11	Basic Science	8
	Clinical Surgery	6	Clinical Surgery	30

Every subject area is important and worth the time taken to review in detail.[3]

[3] Extrapolation based on analysis of resident exams and score outcomes from the 2007, 2008, and 2009 ABSITE exams.

IV. Textbook Organization

This textbook and its corresponding online review program cover all of the major topics that appear on the surgery qualifying exam and the ABSITE. High-yield topics are covered with an emphasis on understanding the key information. Every attempt is made to highlight the tested material. All of the surgical disciplines are covered and the appropriate emphasis is placed on basic science topics and clinical surgery topics. While all of the topics that appear in the outline for the surgery qualifying examination are covered, for the sake of clarity, the topics have been rearranged to improve the flow of the material.

Within each surgical discipline, topics are organized into one of six areas including Congenital and Structural Disorders, Metabolic and Degenerative Disorders, Inflammatory and Infectious Disorders, Vascular Disorders, Trauma, and Cancer. Where appropriate, a review of the relevant basic science is presented in a General Concepts section. The majority of the basic science topics are presented in the first chapter of the book, Surgical Principles. Following each section are pertinent questions to help you further your knowledge in additional areas while practicing what you have learned.

V. Study Plan

How you study for the ABSITE depends on how much time you have available. Motivated residents who prepare in advance will benefit the most from the online review program and the enormous library of information available on the website. Regardless of how much time you have available, this entire review program is designed to be done piecemeal using the short periods of time you have available on call nights and in between cases. Each topic is designed to be covered in just a few minutes, and many residents report making good progress on the question bank by doing a few questions in between cases each day. Those who are on night float rotations or taking call report making good progress on the high-yield slide reviews.

This third edition textbook has been revised and formatted to fit in your pocket. Carry it with you and access it whenever you have a few minutes to go over material. Reference it before cases and whenever you havetime to read about your patients. Pairing interesting patients or cases with the reading material will greatly enhance your retention.

While each individual study plan will be different, there are a few trends that we have noticed with high scorers:

1. Use this book in conjunction with the online questions and your existing reference books
2. Do at least a dozen questions and read through several topics every night
3. Review the high-yield slide presentations a week in advance of your exam
4. Take note of your strengths and weaknesses and focus on them accordingly
5. Keep your notes and review material from year to year

Whether you are preparing for the ABSITE or the surgery qualifying exam, we recommend going through this resource in its entirety. Topics that have appeared on recent exams or more than once are marked by stars. In addition, topics that the reviewers have deemed to be particularly worthwhile are highlighted. It is important to reiterate that the purpose of this book is to help you become a better doctor and surgeon – your score on this exam should reflect your mastery of basic science and clinical surgery, and their application to the modern practice of surgery.

VI. Nomenclature

Everything in this book is high-yield for surgery, but some things are more high-yield than others. Our faculty and resident panel has gone through this textbook in detail and highlighted all of the most worthwhile topics for you. Two conventions are used: special icons in the margins point out important material, while concepts we feel to be important appear in **bold**. The icons used in this book are explained on the next page.

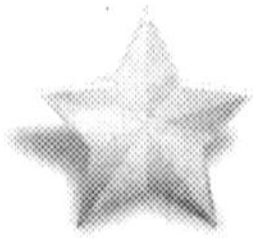

Essential topic for the modern practice of surgery. Commonly tested on both written and oral exams.

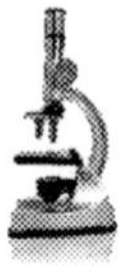

High-yield basic science topic.

Important drug used in routine practice.

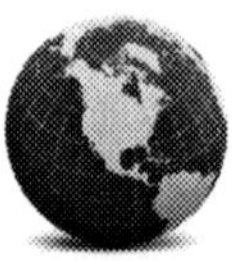

Additional high-yield resources available online.

VII. FEEDBACK

If you have comments or suggestions to help us perfect our learning resources, we would love to hear from you. Our mission is to improve the quality of surgical education and thereby enhance the care we provide to our patients. Talk to us and find out how you can make a difference. Contact us anytime using the e-mail address below, or visit us online.

- Support@ClinicalReview.com
- www.ClinicalReview.com

Sapan S. Desai M.D., Ph.D.

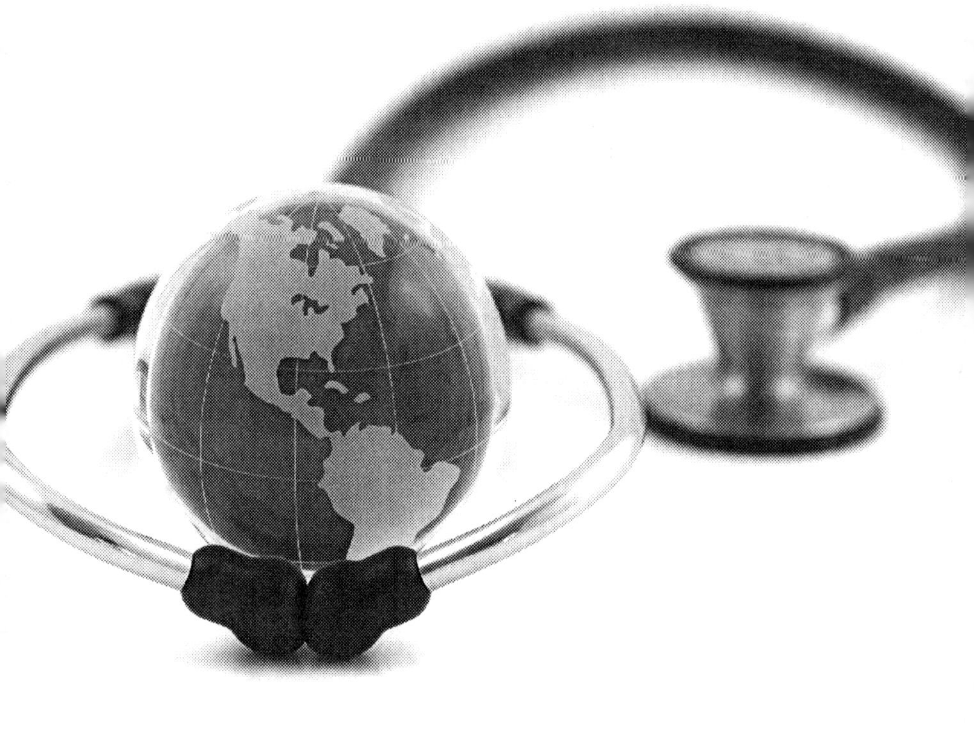

SURGICAL PRINCIPLES

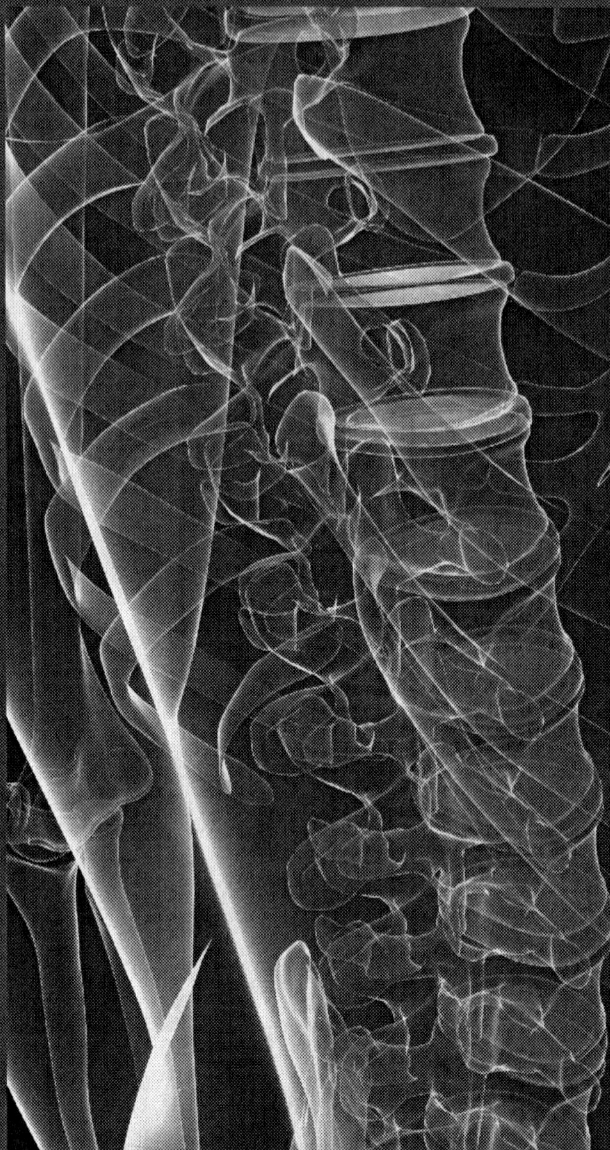

I dressed him, God cured him.

Ambroise Pare
Field Surgeon and "Father of Surgery", 1545

SURGISPHERE

SURGICAL PRINCIPLES

Tara Brennan, M.D., Leontine Narcisse, M.D., Ph.D.,
Jerimiah Mason, M.D., and Scott K. Pruitt, M.D., Ph.D.

I. Biostatistics

I.A. Statistical Tests

The sample size of a medical study is the total number of patients enrolled in that particular study, and is typically denoted n. All else being equal, the larger the sample size, the more powerful the study, and the more precise the conclusions drawn concerning the various properties of the group(s) being studied.

The standard deviation of a study is a measure of the variability of the population being studied, denoted as σ. A low standard deviation indicates that the data points being considered tend to be similar in value, and close to the mean of the sample, while a high standard deviation indicates that the data points are dispersed over a large range of values.

The standard error of the mean is given by the formula:

$$SEM = SD \div \sqrt{n}.$$

As n increases, the standard error of the mean, or the variability of the study, decreases.

I.B. Prevalence

Prevalence is a measure of the number of cases of a particular disease or condition in a population at a particular point in time. It is calculated by dividing the number of people with the disease or condition at a particular time by the number of individuals examined. For example, if there have been two cases of swine flu identified among the two hundred people examined in the University Emergency Department with flu symptoms over the past two weeks, the prevalence of diagnosed swine flu among patients with flu-like symptoms examined in the University Emergency Department over the past two weeks is $\frac{1}{200} = 0.005 = 0.5\%$.

I.C. Incidence

Incidence is a measure of the rate of occurrence of new cases of a disease or condition, and is calculated as the number of new cases of a disease or condition in a specified period of time (usually a year) divided by the size of the population under consideration (who were initially disease-free). For example, in 2006, an estimated 56,300 new cases of HIV were identified, which was substantially higher than estimates in previous years (however, note that more effective and widely-implemented disease detection systems may overestimate increases in the incidence of certain disease processes, as likely occurred with this figure from the CDC).

I.D. Sensitivity

The sensitivity of a test measures the proportion of actual positives (actual positives meaning people with a disease who test positive for that disease) among the total number of people testing positive for a particular disease (this includes both the truly disease positive people as well as the people testing falsely positive for a disease).

Sensitive tests can be used as screening tests because they have a low false negative rate (that is, they will miss very few people who have a disease). High sensitivity tests are like very fine sand sifters: very few non-sand particles (or individuals with disease) get past its filter. With a highly sensitive test, you can trust that a negative result is a true negative (i.e. rules out a disease). However, positive test results need to be confirmed with a more specific test, as the price of a low false negative rate is a higher false positive rate.

		Disease +	Disease -	
Test	+	TP	FP	TP / (TP+FP)
	-	FN	TN	TN / (TN+FN)
		TP / (TP+FN)	TN / (TN+FP)	

I.E. Specificity

The specificity of a test measures the proportion of negative test results that are truly negative. Highly specific tests have low false positive rates (that is, you can be pretty sure you are positive for a particular disease if you test positive using a highly specific test). They are used to confirm positive test results obtained from an initial screening test.

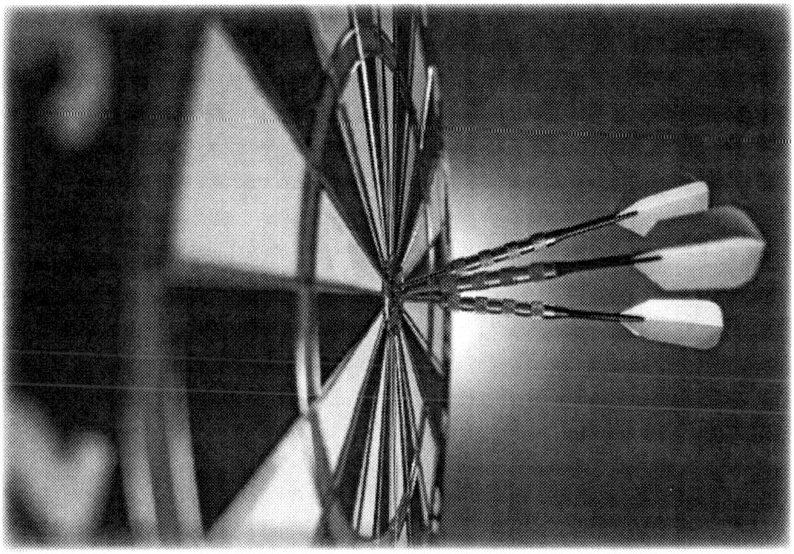

I.F. Positive Predictive Value

The positive predictive value (PPV) of a test is the proportion of people with a positive test result who are truly positive for disease. Tests with higher specificity rates (and thus lower false positive rates) have higher positive predictive values: positive results of these tests, therefore, are more meaningful. Note that the PPV of a test also depends on the prevalence of a disease in a given population: tests for disease in a particular population with a higher prevalence of the disease being tested have a higher PPV because a positive test result is more likely to be true in this population. Note also that the PPV (or the post-test probability) is always used in conjunction with the pretest probability in determining the likelihood that a particular patient has a disease.

I.G. Negative Predictive Value

The negative predictive value (NPV) of a test is the proportion of patients with a negative test result who are truly negative for disease (that is, the chance that a negative test result means you are actually disease-free). Tests with higher sensitivity rates (and thus lower false negative rates) have higher negative predictive values: negative results of these tests, therefore, are more meaningful. Note that this is the opposite of the explanation of PPV, above. Accordingly, the NPV of a test, like the PPV of a test, depends on the disease prevalence within a population (negative test results in a population with a low prevalence of the disease being tested are more meaningful). Note also that the NPV, like the PPV, is used in conjunction with pretest probability and clinical suspicion in evaluating whether a patient is truly disease-free.

I.H. Odds Ratio

The odds ratio is used in retrospective studies to determine the particular effect of a risk factor on disease. The odds ratio is a measure of the strength of association between two data values (i.e. a particular risk factor and disease). The odds ratio is calculated using a table similar to that for sensitivity and specificity (see above).

I.I. Relative Risk

Relative risk (RR), as it applies to medicine, is the risk that a particular exposure will lead to disease relative to the risk incurred by the non-exposed. RR is used in cohort or other prospective studies. For example, if the probability of smokers developing lung cancer was 25%, and the probability of non-smokers developing lung cancer was 1%, then the relative risk of developing lung cancer as a smoker would be twenty-five (smokers would be 25 times as likely as nonsmokers to develop lung cancer).

I.J. Attributable Risk

A variation of relative risk, attributable or absolute risk is used to determine the difference in the number of people incurring disease in two groups--those exposed and those unexposed to a particular risk factor. Attributable risk is more relevant to decision making in risk management than relative risk because it takes into account how likely a person is to acquire a particular disease by taking into account how common it is in the first place. For example, if one were to be given the choice of doubling their risk of death from lung cancer or oral cancer, informed people would opt for the latter because, while the relative risk of dying is the same (two), the attributable risk is lower for oral cancer because it is a rare disease.

I.K. Gaussian Distribution

A normal, or Gaussian, distribution is a bell-shaped distribution with its highest point at the mean, and with three distinct standard deviations: the first standard deviation contains 68% of all values of the bell curve (34% on each side of the mean), the second contains 95.5%, and the third contains 99.7%.

I.L. Mean, Median, and Mode

In a perfectly normal distribution, Mean = Median = Mode. The mean is the mathematical average of all the values in a given distribution, and is the highest point of a bell curve. The median is the number separating the higher half of the sample from the lower half when the values are arranged in ascending order (if there is an even number of values, the median is computed by taking the mean of the two middle values). The mode is the value that occurs the most frequently in a data set, and can be quite unique from the values of the median and the mode in strongly skewed distributions.

I.M. Other Distributions

In statistics, skew is a measure of the asymmetry of a particular probability distribution, and results in differing values among the mean, median, and mode of a distribution. The skew is named for the side of the distribution with the tail. The tail is on the side of the curve with fewer data points. For example, a negatively-skewed (or left-skewed) distribution has a tail on the left side of the curve (the left side of a normal x-y axis graph) because, while most of the data points (and the mode

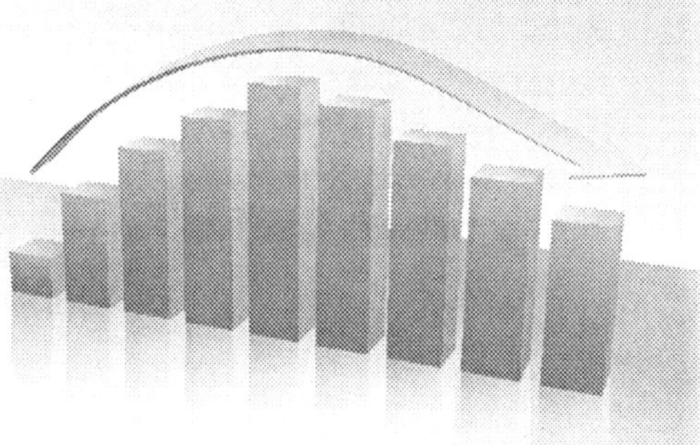

and median) are on the right side of the curve, the mean is skewed to the left, or negatively, because of some outlying data points on the left side (the tail side) of the distribution. In this way, in a negatively-skewed distribution, the mean < median < mode.

Right- or positive-skewed distributions, in contrast, have their tails on the right side of their distributions, and their mean values are shifted to the right relative to the median and mode due to outlying data points on the right (mean > median > mode).

A bimodal distribution is a probability distribution with two distinct modes, one median, and one mean. The age of incidence of Hodgkin's lymphoma is a disease process with a bimodal distribution, with one peak among young adults (aged 15 to 35) and one peak among adults over 55 years old.

I.N. Hypothesis Testing

The null hypothesis (H0) in evaluating a particular treatment is always that the treatment being evaluated will have no effect. For example, in comparing the scores of four and five year olds on a particular test, the null hypothesis would be that the mean score for each group would be the same (H0: mean score among the four year olds = mean score among the five year olds). If a difference is detected, one can reject the null hypothesis.

While the null hypothesis assumes no difference between/among groups, the alternative hypothesis is often that there is a difference--that a particular treatment has the desired effect. The alternative hypothesis is accepted if it meets a particular statistical criterion (often $p < 0.05$ on a T-test).

1. Type I Error

Type I (α) error occurs when one incorrectly rejects the null hypothesis. Or, in other words, when one concludes, incorrectly, that the treatment being tested had an effect on the outcome being measured. Type I error is also known as a "false positive" effect. Repeating a study is one way to determine whether or not a Type I error has occurred. Decreasing the p value (< 0.05 is typically acceptable) is also an important step, as this decreases the likelihood of making a Type I error as well.

2. Type II Error

Type II (ß) error occurs when one incorrectly fails to reject the null hypothesis. Or, in other words, when one fails to see a treatment effect that is, in fact, present. Type II error is also known as a "false negative" effect, or "the error of excessive skepticism". Type II error can be avoided by increasing the power of a study (by increasing the sample size -- it is easier to detect a difference, or a treatment effect, between a control group and a treatment group if there are a large number of subjects being studied).

3. Power

Power reflects the probability that a test will detect true differences between/among groups being evaluated. As power increases, therefore, the chances of a Type II error (failing to see a treatment effect that is, indeed, present) decrease. Power is directly proportional to sample size: increasing sample size increases power. Additionally, power is dependent on the fidelity of the measuring tools being used, as an improved ability to measure differences increases the power of a study.

4. Correlation

Correlations are easily depicted using a two-dimensional graph with the X-axis representing the independent variable, and Y-axis representing the dependent variable (changes with changes in the variable on the X-axis), and with a best-fit line connecting data points. A correlation coefficient of 0 means that there is no direct or indirect correlation between two variables. A correlation coefficient between 0 and 1 means a direct correlation exists – as one variable increases, so does the other variable. Conversely, a negative correlation (a coefficient between 0 and -1) implies the existence of an inverse relationship between two variables.

5. T-Test

A T-test is used to determine whether two quantified variables are sufficiently different based on their standard deviations and the variability of their distributions. T-tests compute the so-called signal to noise ratio, and are appropriate for comparing the means of two groups.

6. ANOVA

ANOVA, or analysis of variance, is used to determine whether three or more variables are sufficiently different. ANOVA is similar to a T-test, with the exception that ANOVA is used to compare more than 2 groups of data.

7. Chi-Square

The chi-square distribution is used to determine whether any number of groups are different, but does so using qualitative terms such as "yes" and "no".

8. Precision and Accuracy

Precision is a measure of the reliability of an instrument, and the degree to which further measurements will show the same or similar results. Precision can be gauged by the spread of the values in a distribution, as specified by the standard deviation. Precision is often referred to as the reproducibility of a test result (i.e. a precise, finely calibrated machine will always produce the same result).

Accuracy is the difference between the true value and the mean of the underlying process that generates the data. The degree of accuracy of a test measures the ability to obtain a result that closely resembles the true result. Validity is the key element in gauging test accuracy. For example, a test that always positively diagnoses people with a disease would have a very high accuracy rate. The dartboard on page 11 is an example of a highly accurate (i.e. close to the bulls eye) and precise (all darts in the same place) player.

1.0. Study Design

1. Prospective Cohort Study

Cohort studies involve subjects selected for a particular characteristic hypothesized to cause or play a role in a particular disease process. In cohort studies, subjects identified to have a particular risk factor for disease are followed over time to determine if they do, in fact, develop disease more often than those in the control cohort. Cohort studies are considered prospective studies because they select patients with a hypothesized risk factor but without the disease process in question, and then follow them over a certain period of time to observe the effect of this risk factor (or exposure). One drawback of this design is that studies involving longer periods of time are likely to lose more patients to follow-up than other study designs. One example of a cohort study is one that sought to determine the effect of cholecystectomy on bowel habits: fifty-one patients undergoing cholecystectomy were evaluated before, one month after, and 3 months after surgery to detect changes such as abdominal pain, flatulence, and dyspepsia.

2. Retrospective Case-Control Trial

Case-control studies begin with the presence or absence of a particular outcome and look backward to try and detect possible causes or risk factors (lacking in the control group) that may have played a role in the development of the outcome. They are considered retrospective studies because they involve looking back in time to try and figure out the factors responsible for a particular disease process. One example of a case-control study involved comparing patients who developed an infection following laminectomy to those who did not following the same procedure, and finding that those patients with longer hospital stays and higher readmission rates were more likely to acquire an infection at the surgical site. Case-control studies are especially useful when attempting to analyze risk factors for rare diseases. However, they are susceptible to recall bias, as patients with knowledge of their disease are more likely to recall having been exposed to a particular risk factor.

3. Randomized Controlled Trial

The randomized controlled trial (RCT) is regarded as the best research design because it provides the strongest evidence that a particular factor caused an effect. The randomization component of assigning patients to either the intervention or control groups minimizes selection bias; and the placebo control component helps to ensure that the trial is double-blinded, which minimizes investigator and patient bias and reduces measurement bias. Furthermore, the more centers from which patients are drawn for the study, the better as it reduces measurement bias from a narrow sample. Crossover control, in which the patient receives treatment for half of the trial and placebo for the other half, may also be used to reduce measurement bias. In order for a RCT to be properly evaluated, the sample size must be known.

In the Physicians' Health Study, a RCT that investigated the role of aspirin in CVD, participants were randomly assigned to receive either aspirin or a placebo and followed over 60 months for evidence of myocardial infarction. The investigators found that fewer physicians in the aspirin group experienced myocardial infarction than those in the placebo group, which has since significantly shaped how we prevent adverse cardiovascular events. The major obstacle to this study design is the high costs associated with its execution.

4. Meta-Analysis

Meta-analysis uses advanced statistical methods to compare similar published studies by pooling their numbers together and attempting to see whether this increased power (due to the pooled sample size) is sufficient to identify statistically significant conclusions. This study design is helpful when research on a particular topic or disease process has small sample sizes or have drawn different conclusions. One important limitation is that it relies on work done by other investigators, which may not always be accurate, precise, or comparable to the data gained from the other pooled studies.

5. Bias

- Late-look bias re-examination of the collected data after the study has been unblinded.
- Lead time bias earlier examination of patients with a particular disease lead to earlier diagnosis, giving the false impression that the patient will live longer (i.e. screening mammography detecting invasive ductal carcinoma at an earlier stage than would be detected if the patient waited until she was symptomatic).
- Measurement bias an investigator familiar with the study favors measurements biased toward the conclusion s/he expects.
- Recall bias patients informed about their disease are more likely to recall risk factors than uninformed patients.
- Sampling bias the sample used in the study is not representative of the population and so conclusions may not be relevant.
- Selection bias occurs when patients are not randomized into either the experimental group or the control group. This lack of randomization

introduces confounding factors into the interpretation of the results of the study, as patients more motivated to pursue treatment may select to be included in the experimental group, and perhaps would be more likely to notice and report effects of the treatment.

II. Preventive Health Care

II.A. Primary Prevention

Primary prevention is an effort to prevent the development of disease. Many health promotion initiatives are primary prevention measures. Examples include education (on how to prevent the spread of STD's, for example) and vaccinations (i.e. to prevent the resurgence of polio).

II.B. Secondary Prevention

Secondary prevention aims to reduce progression of disease. Efforts in this area of healthcare focus on early disease detection in order to prevent emergence of symptoms and to optimize health outcomes for patients with a particular disease. One example of a secondary prevention initiative is blood glucose screening to detect diabetes among at-risk patients, and initiation of early treatment among those identified with the disease in order to improve long-term health outcomes. Another example is the Pap smear--this screening exam identifies patients with cervical dysplasia for early intervention in order to prevent disease progression to cervical cancer.

II.C. Tertiary Prevention

Tertiary prevention describes efforts to reduce the negative impact an existing disease has on a patient's life. Treatment for heart disease, for example, aims to reduce debilitating symptoms (like angina or dyspnea) as well as prevent further disease-related complications (like progression of dyspnea or myocardial infarction).

II.D. Routine Screening

Routine screening tests should be carried out at every visit to a physician. Generally, young adults should undergo physical exams every 3-5 years, blood pressure and weight measurements every 2 years, cholesterol measurement every 5 years, glaucoma screening at least once, and a Pap smear in women every 1-3 years. The screening guidelines in middle-aged adults should continue with the screening recommendations for young adults with the addition of fasting blood sugars measured every 3 years, mammography yearly for women, and colonoscopy every 10 years. Those over 65 should receive yearly physical exams, periodic hearing tests, and vision screening yearly. A digital rectal exam should be done yearly after age 50 with tests for occult bleeding.

III. Medical Ethics

III.A. Autonomy

Autonomy as it applies to medical ethics refers to a patient's right to self-determination with respect to decisions related to their healthcare. It recognizes that, at times, patients' preferences may be at odds with the well-researched and -intended recommendations of a physician, and encourages physicians to honor the patient's right to request or refuse medical care whenever possible.

This principle has become increasingly important in recent years, as patient-centered healthcare has overridden the prior, traditional, more paternalistic model of medical practice and modified the doctor-patient relationship. This autonomy is the basis for informed consent and advanced directives. And it can sometimes come into conflict with Beneficence when patients disagree with recommendations physicians feel are in the patient's best interest (see page 21). To enjoy this Autonomy, however, one must have a certain level of well-being--medically, psychologically, and otherwise. Many diseases that affect this wellbeing, therefore, may complicate a patient's right to Autonomy, and surrogate decision-makers may be required in these cases.

Autonomy is usually tested on the exam by testing the limits of when it is appropriate to listen to a patient and follow their requests or when ancillary measures must be taken, such as receiving parental permission or obtaining a court order in order to take action. For example, minors have autonomy in treatment for sexually transmitted diseases. No parental consent is required, and minors have the right to refuse care for their illness. Minors also have autonomy in treatment for substance abuse, birth control, and prenatal care. However, parental permission must be obtained before conducting an abortion (although there is some variation by state).

III.B. Beneficence

Beneficence is a related concept that refers to physicians taking actions to serve the patient's best interest. The physician must act as a fiduciary for the patient. However, at times, patients' desires are at conflict with physician recommendations. In these cases, patient Autonomy supersedes physician Beneficence in Western medicine. It is both legally and ethically difficult to institute treatment for a patient against his or her will. An exception to this is when the patient poses a danger to themselves or to others.

III.C. Noncompliance

In situations in which the patient is noncompliant with medical recommendations, such as not taking a prescribed medication, the best course of action for the physician is to identify the basic issue hindering compliance (i.e. socioeconomic barriers to care, poor medical literacy, or miscommunication between the physician and patient). The best way to proceed in these cases is to communicate with the patient to discover the barrier to compliance, and to improve trust within the context of the physician-patient relationship.

III.D. Confidentiality

Information flow among healthcare team members, patients, and family members should adhere to HIPPA guidelines. Accordingly, the healthcare issues of a patient should not be discussed with anybody not immediately involved in his or her care. With permission from the patient, information can be provided to family members. According to HIPPA guidelines, discussions involving these sensitive matters should take place in a private place that protects the privacy of the information.

III.E. Exceptions To Confidentiality

Respect for patient confidentiality, however, has some exceptions. Patient information may be disclosed in situations in which there is potential for harm to others if the information is kept private (this is required by law). An example of this is warning a person against whom a patient has expressed plans to hurt or kill. Confidentiality is also waived in situations in which the patient poses a danger to him or herself. In these cases, the physician may make decisions to protect the patient or others as necessary.

Other exceptions to maintaining confidentiality include the need to inform people at risk of contracting an infectious disease from a patient who has not revealed their health conditions (i.e. STDs), and informing appropriate officials in cases of suspected child or elder abuse. Appropriate authorities also need to be notified about patients whose inability to properly operate a motor vehicle or heavy machinery in their vocation may pose a risk to others.

III.F. Demanding Patients

Patients may occasionally make demands on physicians that are both uncomfortable and unethical. Patients seeking procedures that are not medically indicated, or refusing to undergo a procedure deemed medically necessary, deserve a discussion with the physician. Understanding the patient's thinking is the key to resolving these types of problems. Unnecessary procedures should not be performed in the interest of nonmaleficence (primum non nocere). For example, patients with Body Dysmorphic Disorder, who repeatedly seek cosmetic surgery aimed to correct a perceived disfigurement but can ultimately harm the patient, deserve treatment aimed at alleviating underlying issues of psychological insecurity (and not another rhinoplasty). Physician-assisted suicide is another uncomfortable request often made to physicians. Physician-assisted suicide is illegal; however physicians are permitted to administer narcotics that have the potential to decrease a patient's lifespan if doing so will treat a suffering patient's pain.

III.G. Angry Patients

There are a variety of reasons for patients to become frustrated or angry in the healthcare setting. Anger over the amount of time waiting to see a physician should be handled by apologizing to the patient for the inconvenience. In these cases, the physician is not obligated (and should not attempt) to explain the reasons for the delay. A patient upset with another physician or the level of care he/she has received elsewhere should be handled carefully. It is not professionally appropriate to discuss this situation with the patient; instead, the patient should be encouraged to speak directly with the individual that caused his/her grievance. In cases where the patient is upset with a member of your staff, the patient should be told that you will personally speak with that individual and address the patient's concerns.

III.H. Patient-Physician Relationships

There may come a time when a patient expresses a romantic interest in you. While standards may vary a bit from place to place (and are often left up to the discretion of the physician but are never advisable from a legal standpoint), for the purposes of the exam, romantic relationships are never appropriate between a physician and a patient. In this situation, direct, close-ended questions should be used, and the presence of a chaperone may be indicated.

III.I. Informed Consent

Informed consent for a particular medical action can be said to have been given by a patient if the patient does so in the context of having a clear understanding of the facts, implications, and future consequences of a particular action (i.e. surgery or other invasive treatment). They must be educated regarding the risks and benefits of the procedure, alternatives to the procedure, and the consequences of not having the procedure. In order to achieve informed consent, therefore, a patient must be an adult, have adequate reasoning skills, and have been informed of all relevant facts before consenting. Informed consent is traditionally in the written form and can serve as a legal document. Situations in which achieving informed consent from a patient is impossible include cases involving patients with severe mental retardation, mental illness, intoxication, or dementia. In these situations, another person is usually deemed a surrogate decision maker on the patient's behalf. In cases when an unconscious patient needs medical treatment, and there is no one available to give informed consent, physicians have an obligation to give whatever care necessary to save a patient's life.

III.J. Exceptions To Informed Consent

Informed consent is not practically obtained in a number of circumstances. Informed consent does not need to be obtained in cases where emergency treatment is required to alleviate a life-threatening condition and there is no time to discuss the benefits and alternatives; in cases where therapeutic privilege is instituted, in which information must be withheld from the patient to prevent even greater harm than would occur with the therapy (but make this decision very carefully, as therapeutic privilege is often successfully challenged in a court); when the patient lacks the cognitive or physical ability to competently make an informed decision; and in cases where the patient signs a waiver to obtaining informed consent. It is important to note that family members cannot require a physician to withhold information from the patient regarding their illness. In this case, the appropriate course of action is to discuss the situation in a private room with the family members, and determine whether informing the patient would be so distressing that it would be detrimental to their care.

III.K. Competency

Establishing whether or not a patient is "competent" to make their own decisions related to their healthcare is done by considering the following factors: the patient's ability to communicate his or her desires and decisions to the physician, the stability of the patient's decision over time, the consistency of a particular decision to other healthcare decisions made by the patient in the past, and any psychosocial issues that may complicate a patient's ability to make an informed decision,

III.L. Oral Advanced Directives

Advanced directives are a guide to providing treatment to a patient when he or she is otherwise unable to make a choice due to an intervening medical illness. In this case, a patient's prior oral directives take precedence, especially if the patient was able to make an informed, clear choice and communicate this lucidly to the physician ahead of time. The decision is considered valid if it is repeated over time.

Written advanced directives are used in cases where an oral directive was not established. There are two major types of written advanced directives, including living wills and durable power of attorney. Living wills direct the physician to employ only certain life-saving measures and dictate if and when they can be withheld or withdrawn. Living wills take precedence only when there is no prior oral directive. Living wills are not flexible and are being replaced with durable power of attorney in many cases.

III.M. Durable Power of Attorney

Durable power of attorney is the designation of a surrogate, usually a spouse or other family member, to make judgments on behalf of the patient regarding medical decisions. The legality of durable power of attorney is predicated on the designated person making a decision similar to what the patient would choose if she were competent. A durable power of attorney incorporates elements of a living will in that the patient can designate that certain measures be taken in various clinical situations. Written advanced directives can be revoked at any time by the patient.

III.N. Malpractice

Malpractice lawsuits often take place in civil court. The burden of proof is lower than in a criminal court. Civil court convictions require demonstration of breach of duty such that healthcare obligations to a patient are not met, and that the patient suffers harm from the breach of duty. The most common cause of malpractice lawsuits is poor physician communication.

IV. Cell Biology

IV.A. Fluid Balance

1. ECF and ICF

Water makes up 60% of the lean body mass of the human body, and is distributed between two compartments: the extracellular fluid (ECF) and the intracellular fluid (ICF). The ICF contains ⅔ of the body's water, and the ECF contains the remaining ⅓. The ECF is characterized by high concentrations of sodium and calcium, with chloride constituting the major anion. The ICF, by contrast, is high in potassium and magnesium, with phosphate as the major anion. Glucose is high in the ECF, while proteins are more abundant in the ICF. Relative concentrations of these substances in the ECF and ICF are tabulated below.

Table 1. ECF and ICF solute concentrations

Substance	ECF	ICF
Na^+	140 mmol/L	10 mmol/L
K^+	4 mmol/L	140 mmol/L
Cl^-	100 mmol/L	4 mmol/L
HCO_3^-	30 mmol/L	10 mmol/L
Ca^{2+}	2.5 mmol/L	0 mmol/L
Mg^{2+}	1.5 mmol/L	30 mmol/L
PO_4	2 mmol/L	60 mmol/L
Protein	2 g/dL	16 g/dL

2. Crystalloids

Parenteral fluids are classified according to their molecular weight and oncotic pressure. Colloids are those with high molecular weight and oncotic pressure, and include albumin, blood products, and synthetics like hetastarch and dextran. Crystalloids are those with low molecular weight and oncotic pressure, and include the following:

Table 2. Crystalloid Composition

Fluid	Glucose (g/L)	Na^+	Cl^-	K^+	Ca^{2+}	HCO_3^-
Lactated Ringers (LR)	-	130	110	4	3	27 (via lactate)
Normal Saline (NS) (0.9% NaCl)	-	154	154	-	-	-
D5W (5% dextrose in water)	50	-	-	-	-	-
D5 ½NS + 20 KCl	50	77	97	20	-	-

IV.B. Cell Cycle

1. Control Points

The transitions allowing the cell to pass from a growth phase to the DNA replication and mitotic phases are governed by specific prolific cell signals and braking mechanisms designed to prevent aberrant and inaccurate cell replication and division. Enzymes called cyclin-dependent kinases (CDKs) are responsible for cell cycle progression; enzymes called CDK inhibitors (CDKIs) inhibit cell cycling. Cyclin A/CDK2 is responsible for the G1-S transition propelling the cell into DNA synthesis, and cyclin A/CDK1 and cyclin B/CDK1 drive the progression of the cell into the mitotic phase.

In M phase the nuclear and cytoplasmic material divide to make two identical daughter cells, each with diploid chromosome complements.

The G1 phase may be extended or even permanent in some cells; these cells are called "resting cells" in a special G1 state called G0.

G2 follows the S phase and resembles G1 in terms of cellular activity, but the cell is tetraploid during this phase.

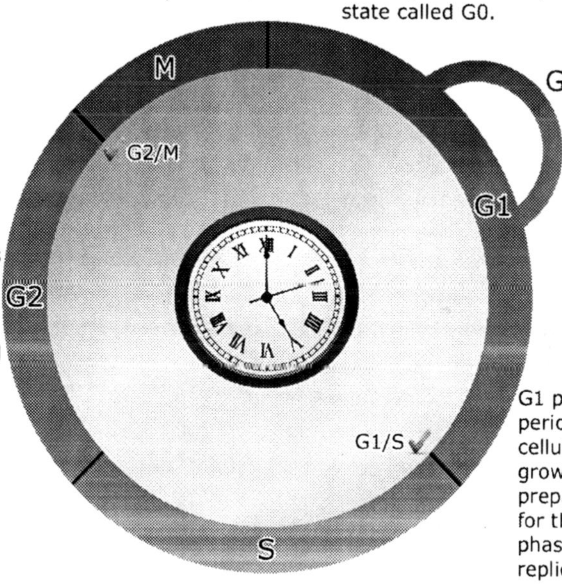

G1 phase is a period of cellular growth in preparation for the S phase of DNA replication.

The S phase is the DNA synthesis and chromosomal replication phase, and is shorter than the G1 phase.

Cyclins are essential for CDK activities, and their expression fluctuates throughout the cell cycle in response to stimulation from mitogenic factors and/or inhibition from developmental and environmental factors. Accelerated proliferation, premature cell cycle progression, or inappropriate cell division (when the S phase resulted in damaged DNA replication, for example) can result in gained oncogenic functions and/or lost tumor suppressive functions that can result in malignant transformation of cells.

In addition to cell cycle control, programmed cell death plays an important role in maintaining tissue homeostasis. Apoptosis is activated by a plethora of physiologic stimuli in order to remove unwanted or damaged cells from tissue. These stimuli include death receptor signals from Fas or TNF, growth factor deprivation, DNA damage, and stress signals, all of which activate a cascade of proteinases called caspases and result in the destruction of the cell. Apoptosis, like the cell cycle, is highly controlled by both positive and negative regulators, and disruptions in this process can result in neoplastic transformation.

2. Signal Transduction

Cell signaling pathways allow cells to sense changes in their external environment, and adapt accordingly through modification of their nuclear activity. Cell signaling begins at the cell surface and, after initiating a signaling cascade involving a variety of intracellular proteins, ends up in the nucleus, where transcriptional and translational modifications are made so that the cell may better meet the demands of the extracellular environment.

The binding of extracellular ligands (which may include proteins, peptides, or fatty acids, to name a few) to an extracellular receptor initiates a series of biochemical events known as signal transduction. Through a variety of protein-protein interactions and transfers of high energy phosphate groups (ATP to ADP, and so on), various cellular responses are achieved. Signal transduction also involves catalytic activities that modify key signaling proteins; these signals ultimately reach the transcriptional apparatus in the nucleus, where alteration of DNA binding and transcription factors results in the promotion or termination of gene activity in response to environmental stimuli.

Signaling pathways are classified according to the type of signaling receptor involved in a particular transduction cascade. Hydrophobic signaling molecules like steroids, thyroid hormones, and vitamin D can diffuse across lipophilic plasma membranes to directly influence cytoplasmic targets. In contrast, most hydrophilic signaling molecules are confined to the ECF, and thus must interact with transmembrane protein receptors and rely on intracellular signal transduction to effect transcriptional regulation and biologic action. The three main classes of cell surface receptors are transmitter-gated ion channels, seven transmembrane domain G-protein coupled receptors, and enzyme-linked receptors.

IV.C. Genetics

1. Gene Expression And Regulation

a) DNA Repair

Cellular events resulting in DNA damage can occur up to a million times per cell per day. This damage is due to both the byproducts of normal metabolism (like oxidative free radicals) as well as exposure to deleterious environmental factors (including UVR, X-rays, man-made aromatic chemicals, viruses, and toxins). DNA damage manifests in many forms: free radical damage can result in the alkylation, oxidation, hydrolysis, and mismatch of bases, while the damage from exogenous agents can result in inaccurate base pairing, crosslinking between DNA strands, or DNA strand breakage. These endogenous and exogenous mutagens can have disastrous effects if they happen to disrupt critical functions of the cell, or tumor suppressive activity, which are then passed on to all future products of cell replication. Thus, the process of DNA repair within cells is critical in order to avoid mutations that either disrupt cell function and/or promote tumorigenesis.

b) DNA Repair Disorders

Patients with ataxia-telangiectasia have a defective AT gene, which is a tumor suppressor gene located on chromosome 11. When intact, the AT gene detects damaged DNA, and, in particular, double-stranded breaks in DNA, tagging affected cells for cell cycle arrest and apoptosis. These patients have a high predisposition to developing malignancies, and are hypersensitive to ionizing radiation, which induces double-stranded breaks in DNA.

Bloom syndrome is a rare autosomal recessive disease caused by mutations in the BLM gene, which codes for a member of the DNA helicase family involved in DNA synthesis and repair. Bloom syndrome is characterized by a high frequency of DNA mutations, and affected patients therefore have a correspondingly high risk of developing cancer, leukemias, lymphomas, and carcinomas throughout their lifetimes.

Fanconi anemia is an autosomal recessive disease characterized by bone marrow failure, skeletal anomalies, and hypersensitivity to DNA damaging agents. Fanconi anemia is a result of defects in genes thought to be involved in responding to cellular oxidative stress, and in DNA repair.

Trichothiodystrophy (TTD) is an autosomal recessive disease characterized by growth and mental retardation and brittle hair. TTD is caused by defective synthesis of high sulfur matrix proteins, and many affected patients also have abnormalities in nucleotide excision repair (NER) of UV-damaged DNA.

Xeroderma pigmentosa (XP) is an autosomal recessive disease involving mutations in NER enzymes and is characterized by premature aging and multiple cutaneous malignancies. UVR leads to damage in susceptible persons, triggering early senescence and skin CA.

2. RNA

a) Messenger RNA

The mature mRNA that exits the nucleus and is destined to serve as a template for protein synthesis is significantly different than the one originally transcribed from the DNA template. Within the nucleus, several posttranscriptional modifications occur in order to prepare the mRNA as a template for translation. Non-coding introns are removed from the mRNA, and the remaining coding exons are spliced together to form the mature mRNA.

Alternative splicing of nonconsecutive exons may also be done, allowing the creation of a variety of mature mRNA products, and, thus, proteins, from one mRNA transcript. Next, a 5' methyl cap is added to the mRNA to permit binding to ribosomes in the cytoplasm of the cell. A 3' polyadenylated ("poly-A") tail is then added to prevent early breakdown of the mRNA transcript by exonucleases, lending stability to the transcript. The poly-A tail also facilitates exit of the mRNA from the nucleus. This mature mRNA then exits the nucleus and is translated into protein by ribosomes anchored to the rough endoplasmic reticulum (rER).

b) Transfer RNA

tRNA is a small RNA molecule (usually around 90 nucleotides) that transfers amino acids to growing polypeptide chains in the process of translation of mRNA into proteins. Its 3' end carries an amino acid, and, upstream, its anticodon region recognizes a complementary codon sequence on an mRNA that codes for the amino acid it carries. Each mRNA codon calls for the tRNA to deliver only one amino acid to the growing polypeptide chain (a so-called "unambiguous code"). Due to distinct initiation and termination sequences, there is only one reading frame in which the three-nucleotide codons are read (a so-called "comma less" sequence).

c) Ribosomal RNA

rRNA plays an integral role in the process of translation. As the central component of the ribosome, rRNA interacts with the amino acid bearing tRNAs, and provides peptidyl transferase activity to execute the lengthening of the polypeptide chain.

Eukaryotic rRNA is made in the nucleolus and is composed of two subunits: a large subunit (contains 3 rRNA species: 5S, 5.8S, and 28S) and a small subunit (18S). In the process of translation, tRNA is sandwiched between these subunits as the ribosome catalyzes the formation of a peptide bond between the incoming amino acid and the amino acid added previously to the growing polypeptide chain.

d) Small Nuclear RNA

snRNA (small nuclear RNA) is a term used to describe functional RNA molecules that are not translated into proteins after being transcribed from DNA, but instead serve as critical actors in the processes of transcription and translation. snRNA is used for RNA splicing and methylation, maintaining telomere integrity, and regulating transcription factors. RNA polymerase II, which transcribes mRNA from DNA templates, is also a type of snRNA. snRNAs are referred to as "snurps" when complexed with small nuclear ribonucleoproteins, including the spliceosome, which excises introns in the development of the mature mRNA transcript.

3. Protein Processing

a) Post-Translational Modification

Post-translational modification (PTM) refers to changes made to proteins after the process of translation. PTMs occur in the rER and Golgi apparatus, and may include the addition of functional groups or other peptides, structural changes like covalent linkages or cleavages, or changes in the chemical nature of the amino acids.

b) Types Of Modification

- Acetylation to N-terminus
- Biotinylation on lysine residues
- Glutamylation on glutamic acid residues
- Glycosylation on C-terminal
- Glycosylation on asparagine, hydroxylysine, serine, or threonine
- Phosphorylation on serine, tyrosine, threonine, or histidine groups
- Sulfonylation to tyrosine
- Disulfide bridges added to cysteine groups
- Ubiquitination affects the stability, function, and intracellular localization of a wide variety of proteins, and also plays a role in labeling proteins destined for proteasomal degradation.

The ubiquitination system plays a key role in a variety of cellular processes, including DNA transcription and repair, antigen processing, the immune/inflammatory response, neural and muscular degeneration, cell division, and apoptosis, to name a few. Disruption in the ubiquitination system has been linked with a number of genetic disorders, including Angelman syndrome and Von Hippel-Lindau syndrome.

In Angelman syndrome, the UBE3A gene on the maternally-inherited chromosome 15 encoding an ubiquitin ligase enzyme is disrupted, resulting in a neurodevelopmental disorder that has become a classic case of genetic imprinting. Von Hippel-Lindau syndrome is another genetic disorder caused by a disruption in an ubiquitin gene call the VHL tumor suppressor gene. In addition, antibodies to ubiquitin are used to identify inclusion bodies in the brains of patients with Parkinson's disease (Lewy bodies) and Pick's disease (Pick bodies). These ubiquitin antibodies also localize Mallory bodies in the livers of patients with alcoholic hepatitis, and neurofibrillary tangles in the brains of patients with Alzheimer's disease.

V. Surgical Infections

V.A. Common Iatrogenic Infections

Urinary tract infection is the most common infection in the hospital and in diabetics. The most common cause of a UTI is from E. coli. For community-acquired infections Klebsiella and S. saprophyticus are significant causes. For hospital-acquired infections Proteus, Klebsiella, Serratia, and Pseudomonas are major contributors. The most common cause of bacteremia is from central line placement and is typically from S. aureus.

V.B. Surgical Prophylaxis

Cefazolin or cefuroxime is preferred as antibiotic prophylaxis for most clean general surgery procedures. Upper GI procedures or hepatobiliary procedures receive ciprofloxacin and metronidazole. Large bowel resections can be prepared with erythromycin with ceftizoxime, bisacodyl, and polyethylene glycol; however, this is controversial and some centers will do a limited bowel prep or no prep at all. Appendectomy receives either ceftizoxime or cefotetan, and metronidazole. Vancomycin is used with pancreas or kidney procedures.

Antibiotics must be given within 60 minutes before incision for maximal effectiveness. If vancomycin or a fluoroquinolone is used, they should be infused 1-2 hours prior to incision. Antibiotic prophylaxis should end within 24 hours after surgery; empiric treatment should continue for contaminated cases.

V.C. Wound Contamination

1. Etiology

The most important considerations for wound infection are the type of operation and how contaminated the field becomes as a result of surgery. Adequate skin preparation is essential in order to limit the initial bacterial inoculation into the incisional plane. Wound infections become more common with operations over two hours and with extensive tissue damage, such as with coagulation of dermal or fascial planes instead of incising them. Seromas and hematomas increase the risk of infection. Patient factors include advanced age, chronic illness, cardiovascular instability, malnutrition (especially an albumin < 2.5), and immunosuppression.

The most common cause of postoperative wound infection in non-gastrointestinal and non-biliary procedures is due to skin flora: Staphylococcus and Streptococcus spp. With GI and biliary procedures, gram negative and anaerobic organisms are more common.

TABLE 3. Classification of Wound Contamination

Classification of Wound Contamination		
Clean	1-5% infection rate	Elective operation with incision under ideal conditions. No entry into GI or respiratory tract.
Clean-Contaminated	8% infection rate	Elective operation with incision under ideal conditions. Controlled entry into GI or respiratory tract with no gross spillage or infection.
Contaminated	18% infection rate	Emergency operations with entry into GI, respiratory, or urinary tract with gross spillage or infection. Trauma operations.
Dirty	40% infection rate	Wounds with frank pus, old trauma wounds, or grossly contaminated tissues. Open, contaminated fractures are an example.

2. Treatment

Contaminated wounds have a bacterial count less than 100,000 and are able to mount a response to infection. Once the host response is overwhelmed and bacteria proliferate, the wound is infected. Contaminated wounds are débrided thoroughly during surgery with satisfactory hemostasis to prevent hematoma formation.

Halsteadian principles should be followed: tissues should be approximated, closure should be tension-free, and no open spaces should remain by closing tissues in layers. Copious irrigation is done to ensure removal of foreign bodies and detritus; pulse irrigation is especially effective. If these criteria cannot be met, the fascia should be closed and the overlying tissues permitted to close by secondary intention. The use of a wound V.A.C. device has shown to reduce the time needed for this type of wound closure. The rate of infection of such open wounds is less than 15%, and even lower with V.A.C. therapy.

V.D. Tetanus

Tetanus is caused by neurotoxin release by C. tetani, leading to a 30% mortality rate if not treated early. Tetanus infection must be especially considered in the presence of dirty wounds contaminated by soil or feces, puncture wounds, burns, and frostbite. For clean, minor wounds, children under 7 should be treated with DPT (Diphtheriae, Pertussis, and Tetanus) vaccination. Children over 7 can be treated with the Td (tetanus toxoid) vaccination. Adults should receive a Td if the most recent vaccination is over 10 years ago. All dirty or major wounds receive a Td unless the full immunization schedule has been followed and the most recent vaccination is less than 5 years ago.

V.E. Microbiology

1. Bacteria

Table 4. Common Bacterial Infections

Please see page 36 for this table.

2. Encapsulated Organisms

Encapsulated organisms that cause infection following splenectomy are S. pneumoniae, N. meningitidis, H. influenzae B (HIB), and K. pneumoniae. Pneumococcal, meningococcal, and HIB vaccines are indicated in all post-splenectomy patients. Overwhelming postsplenectomy infection is a rapid, devastating cause of sepsis. It is most common in children, but the incidence decreases with age. The incidence is also lower following a trauma-related splenectomy than for an elective splenectomy. Vaccinations should be given at least two weeks prior to surgery or prior to discharge home.

3. Exotoxins

Exotoxin production occurs with Clostridial spp., which can lead to necrotizing fasciitis within six hours of surgery. C. perfringens produces several

Text continued on page 38

	Etiology	Features	Pathophysiology
Gram Positive Cocci - Staphylococcus	Staphylococcus aureus		Most common bacteria found in surgical site.
	Staphylococcus epidermidis		Causes endocarditis, prosthetic joint infections, vascular graft infections, and bacteremia from intravascular devices.
Gram Positive Cocci - Streptococcus	Streptococcus pneumoniae	IgA protease permits colonization on mucosal surfaces. Encapsulated.	Complement activation.
	Streptococcus pyogenes	Exotoxin	• Erythrogenic toxin (superantigen), necrotizing fasciitis (other causes include C. perfringens and Vibrio). • Superantigen SSA expression may lead to systemic symptoms.
Gram Negative Cocci	Neisseria meningitidis		Common cause of meningitis.
Gram Positive Rods	Actinomyces israelii	Non-spore forming	
	Clostridium difficile	Spore forming	Caused by clindamycin, neomycin, and broad-spectrum antibiotics.
	Clostridium perfringens	Spore forming	Lecithinase with gas production.

Presentation	Treatment
Ventilator associated pneumonia (VAP), toxic shock syndrome, and osteomyelitis	• MSSA: Methicillin. • MRSA: Vancomycin, clindamycin, TMP-SMX, linezolid, daptomycin.
	• Remove or replace intravascular device • Antibiotics are the same for S. aureus
Community acquired pneumonia (#1 cause in adults), meningitis, and otitis media.	Penicillins, cephalosporins, vancomycin.
Cellulitis, necrotizing fasciitis, toxic shock syndrome, rheumatic fever, and pharyngitis.	• Penicillin and clindamycin. • Prompt surgical debridement.
Meningitis, Waterhouse-Friderichsen syndrome.	Vaccination. Ceftriaxone.
Oral and facial abscess. IUD infection.	Penicillin.
Pseudomembranous colitis.	Metronidazole (PO>IV), vancomycin (PO).
Necrotizing fasciitis.	Surgical debridement, penicillin and clindamycin.

Category	Organism	Type	Notes
Gram Negative Rods	Pseudomonas aeruginosa	Aerobe	Eschar formation in burn patients with secondary infection.
	Helicobacter pylori	Facultative Anaerobe	Uses urease to breakdown mucus layer cause ulcers in stomach and duodenum.
	Bacteroides fragilis	Anaerobe	Normal bowel flora and most common organism.
	Enterobacter	Enterobacteriaceae	
	Escherichia coli	Enterobacteriaceae	Endotoxin (lipopolysaccharide lipid A).
	Klebsiella pneumoniae	Enterobacteriaceae	
	Proteus mirabilis	Enterobacteriaceae	Ammonium magnesium phosphate stones.
	Salmonella enteritidis	Enterobacteriaceae	Invasive.
Atypical Bacteria	Mycobacterium tuberculosis		Found in the apex of the lung due to the highest PO_2.

toxins, including a necrotizing, hemolytic lecithinase (alpha toxin), a hemolysin (theta toxin), a collagenase (kappa toxin), a hyaluronidase (mu toxin), and a deoxyribonuclease (nu toxin). Immediate surgical debridement is required, and death may ensue even with aggressive therapy.

C. difficile produces an exotoxin that leads to pseudomembranous colitis and profuse, foul-smelling diarrhea. Metronidazole or vancomycin is given orally with infection. Cholestyramine can be given to bind toxin. Antidiarrheals are to be avoided as these can increase the severity of symptoms.

Burn patients, pneumonia in cystic fibrosis, otitis externa, and UTIs.	Piperacillin/tazobactam, ciprofloxacin, imipenem (double coverage often recommended).
Gastritis, gastric and duodenal ulcer formation.	Triple therapy (PPI, clarithromycin, amoxicillin); if this fails, then change antibiotics to bismuth, metronidazole, and tetracycline.
Most common anaerobe in surgical infections.	Clindamycin, metronidazole, carbapenems.
• Bacteremia, lower respiratory tract infection. • Most common cause of liver abscess in a patient with diverticulitis.	Imipenem, cefepime, ciprofloxacin.
UTI (most common), bacteremia in biliary tract (most common).	Augmentin, imipenem, ciprofloxacin.
• Pneumonia with currant jelly sputum, especially in alcoholics. • Cholecystitis (uncommon).	Cephalosporins, gentamicin, piperacillin/tazobactam.
Struvite stones in UTI.	• Cephalosporins, gentamicin, imipenem. • Surgical stone removal.
Food poisoning from poultry leading to bloody diarrhea.	TMP-SMX for systemic disease; otherwise supportive care only.
Tuberculosis.	Rifampin, isoniazid, streptomycin, pyrazinamide, ethambutol.

Surgical Principles

C. tetani produces a neurotoxin that leads to rigidity and muscular spasms, culminating in asphyxiation and death. Treatment is wound debridement and penicillin. C. botulinum produces a neurotoxin leading to GI symptoms, diplopia, and flaccid paralysis.

4. Endotoxins

Bacterial lipopolysaccharides (LPS) are formed from the outer membrane of gram negative bacteria. This endotoxin leads to septic shock when released in significant amounts. The O-antigen is the major source of antigenicity and consists of polysaccharides. LPS induces septic shock by activating TNF and IL-1, leading to cascade activation of IL-6, IL-8, GM-CSF, and other immunomodulators.

5. Toxic Shock Syndrome

a) Etiology and Pathophysiology

Toxic shock syndrome (TSS) is an erythema with systemic manifestations due to S. aureus. The formation of a superantigen known as TSS toxin-1 (TSST-1) leads to cytokine release and shock.

b) Presentation and Diagnosis

TSS presents with fever, hypotension, and distal extremity desquamation. A scarlatiniform eruption, cherry red tongue, and hyperemia of mucous membranes are common. Multiorgan dysfunction syndrome may occur with advanced disease. Diagnosis is made by culture.

c) Treatment

Supportive therapy is used with TSS, including IVF, pressors, antibiotics, and surgical drainage. Silver sulfadiazine cream is contraindicated; mupirocin ointment is used instead.

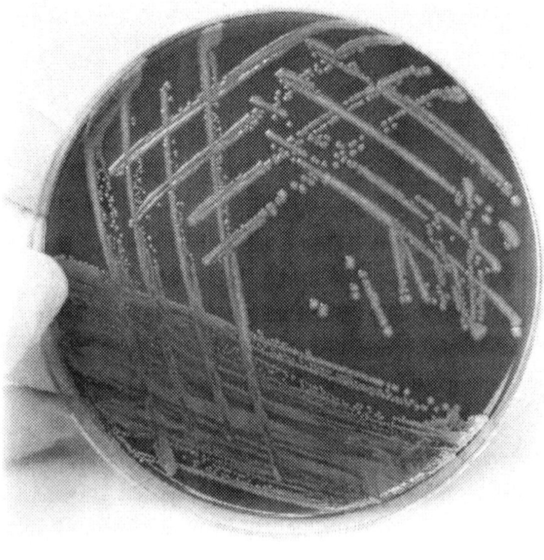

V.F. Fungology

Table 5. Common Fungal Infections

Etiology	Pathophysiology	Presentation	Treatment
Candida albicans	Water soluble toxin leads to pain.	Oral thrush, infectious esophagitis, fungemia in patients with intravascular devices.	Nystatin, ketoconazole, or fluconazole for topical therapy. Fluconazole for esophageal infections. Amphotericin B for systemic infection.
Aspergillus fumigatus	Allergic reaction to a septate, monomorphic, hyphae mold.	Lung cavitary lesions with fungus balls & disseminated cutaneous infection.	Amphotericin B.
Coccidioidomycosis		Flu-like illness and erythema nodosum in kids and travelers.	Fluconazole, amphotericin B.
Cryptococcus neoformans	From pigeon droppings. Latex agglutination test.	Meningitis or acute pulmonary infection in immunocompromised.	Amphotericin B.
Pneumocystis carinii	Yeast.	Diffuse pneumonia in immunocompromised.	Pentamidine, TMP-SMX, dapsone.

V.G. Pharmacology

1. Pharmacokinetics

Most drugs are cleared by first-order kinetics, in which the rate of elimination of drug from the plasma is directly proportional to the drug concentration. First-order elimination proceeds as exponential decay with a fixed ratio of drug eliminated per unit of time. The half-life of a drug in this model is inversely related to the elimination constant: the higher the rate of elimination, the shorter the half-life. Note that approximately four half-lives are required to achieve 95% clearance of drug from the plasma. Note, also, that four half-lives is also about the same amount of time required to reach a drug's "steady state" plasma concentration, which is achieved via maintenance dosing that takes into account the rate of elimination of a drug.

In a few cases, including ethanol, phenytoin, and salicylate, the rate of clearance of drug from the plasma compartment follows a zero-order kinetics model. In these cases, a constant amount of drug is eliminated from the plasma per unit time, independent of its concentration in the plasma. This model of elimination has also been called saturation kinetics, because it reflects those cases in which the elimination of a particular drug is controlled by elimination enzymes that become saturated once a drug reaches a certain level. Once this level is exceeded, the amount of the drug in the body will, in principle, increase indefinitely if its administration continues.

For example, ethanol's clearance from the plasma is constant at about 4 mmol/L per hour regardless of its plasma concentration. This is because its rate of oxidation by alcohol dehydrogenase reaches a maximum at low plasma concentrations of ethanol because of a limited availability of the enzyme's cofactor, NAD^+. Therefore, once this low plasma concentration is achieved, only 4 mmol/L of ethanol will be eliminated from the plasma per hour, regardless of the amount of ethanol being consumed (which is why it is fairly easy to become intoxicated).

2. Pharmacodynamics

The majority of drugs exert their effects by interacting with cellular membranes, proteins, and receptors to promote or interfere with ligand-receptor binding and signal transduction. Drugs can interact with receptors in a variety of ways, including as a competitive antagonist, noncompetitive antagonist, or partial agonist.

3. Competitive Antagonist

A competitive antagonist binds to a receptor but does not activate it. By competing with agonists for receptor sites, a lower frequency of receptors will be activated.

4. Partial Agonist

A partial agonist binds to and activates a given receptor, but with only partial efficacy (relative to the efficacy of a full agonist). Thus, in competing with full agonists for receptor binding, partial agonists decrease the efficacy of a particular medication.

5. Noncompetitive Antagonist

A noncompetitive antagonist (also known as an allosteric antagonist) reduces the activity of a particular receptor, but does so by binding to site that is distinctly separate from the agonist binding site.

The therapeutic index of a drug examines the relationship between the dose required to achieve the desired effect and the dose that would produce untoward side effects. The narrower the margin, the more likely it is that a negative side effect will be experienced by a patient.

6. Common Antibiotics

a) General Concepts

Penicillins bind to PBPs with subsequent inhibition of the transpeptidase step leading to cell lysis. It will not affect organisms that do not have a cell wall. Resistance to penicillins comes from beta-lactamases that cleave the penicillins to make them impotent. Resistance to cephalosporins comes from beta-lactamases that cleave the penicillins to make them impotent. R-factor resistance with aminoglycosides, tetracyclines, and chloramphenical leads to drug inactivation by acetyltransferase and decreased uptake.

Aminoglycosides may also be modified through acetylation, adenylation, or phosphorylation of the compound, or may be excreted unchanged by kidney. Resistance to macrolides is occurs through rRNA methylation leading to prevention of binding to 50S unit. Resistance to fluoroquinolones occurs through mutations in DNA gyrase. Drug penetration may also change. Resistance to TMP/SMX is by modification of DHP synthase, increased synthesis of PABA, or decreased uptake of drug. Resistance to vancomycin comes from mutation of D-ala D-ala to D-ala D-lac and is plasmid-mediated.

Table 6. Common Antibiotics

The table for common antibiotics is discussed on page 44.

Text continued on page 48

	DRUG	INDICATIONS	MECHANISM OF ACTION
Penicillins	Penicillin G	GPC, GPR, GNC, spirochetes	Prevents synthesis of cell wall. Bactericidal.
	Amoxicillin	GPC, GPR, GNR, E. coli, H. influenzae, Proteus.	Prevents synthesis of cell wall. Bactericidal.
	Piperacillin	• Extended spectrum. • Pseudomonas, GNR.	Prevents synthesis of cell wall. Bactericidal.
Cephalosporins	Cefazolin (First generation)	GPC, E. coli, Klebsiella, Proteus.	Prevents synthesis of cell wall. Bactericidal.
	Cefoxitin (Second generation)	GPC, E. coli, Enterobacter, H. influenzae, Klebsiella, Neisseria spp., Proteus, Serratia.	Prevents synthesis of cell wall. Bactericidal.
	Ceftriaxone (Third generation)	Gram-negatives. Meningitis, resistant organisms, serious infections. Broad range. Low activity vs. gram positives.	Prevents synthesis of cell wall. Bactericidal. Broadest range.
Monobactams and Carbapenems	Aztreonam	GNR, Klebsiella, Pseudomonas, Serratia.	• Prevents synthesis of cell wall. Bactericidal. • Improved activity with aminoglycosides
	Imipenem	GPC, GNR, Anaerobes, Enterobacter.	Beta-lactamase resistant cell wall synthesis inhibitor. Bactericidal.

SURGISPHERE

COMPLICATIONS	CONTRAINDICATIONS	NOTES
Hypersensitivity (anaphylaxis), hemolytic anemia	Do not use in bacteria with beta-lactamases or w/ known hypersensitivity	Especially effective against Neisseria spp., C. perfringens, and Treponema Used for syphilis.
As above plus pseudomembranous colitis. Seizures at high doses.	Do not use if hypersensitivity to penicillins.	Use with clavulanic acid or sulbactam to block beta-lactamases. Wide spectrum. Oral.
Hypersensitivity, hemolytic anemia, platelet dysfunction.	Do not use if hypersensitivity to penicillins. Sodium loading.	Often combined with a beta-lactamase inhibitor, such as tazobactam.
Hypersensitivity (rash). 10% penicillin cross hypersensitivity	• Aminoglycosides (nephrotoxicity). • Alcohol (disulfiram reaction).	• Less susceptible to beta-lactamases. • Often used as surgical prophylaxis.
Hypersensitivity (rash).	• Avoid with aminoglycosides (nephrotoxicity). • Avoid with alcohol (disulfiram reaction).	• Less susceptible to beta-lactamases. • Broader range compared to first generation.
Hypersensitivity (rash).	• Avoid with aminoglycosides (nephrotoxicity). • Avoid with alcohol (disulfiram reaction).	Cross blood-brain barrier. Ceftazidime is especially good against Pseudomonas.
GI Sx.	No effect against anaerobes or gram-positive bacteria.	No cross-sensitivity with penicillins. Especially recommended in renal disease.
GI Sx. Rash. CNS toxicity leading to seizures at high doses. Nephrotoxic. Eosinophilia.	Renal disease.	Imipenem is always given with cilastatin to avoid inactivation in kidney. Synthetic.

	DRUG	INDICATIONS	MECHANISM OF ACTION
Aminoglycosides	Gentamicin	• Severe gram-negative infections. • Aerobes, Pseudomonas.	• 30S inhibitor. • Bacteriostatic. • Cause mRNA misreading by preventing formation of initiation complex – bactericidal.
Tetracyclines	Doxycycline	B. burgdorferi, Chlamydia, Mycoplasma, Rickettsia, V. cholerae.	• 30S inhibitor prevents tRNA attachment. • Bacteriostatic.
Macrolides	Azithromycin	Pneumonia and URTI. GPC, Mycoplasma, Legionella, Neisseria.	50S inhibitor prevents translocation and inhibits protein synthesis. Bacteriostatic.
Fluoroquinolones	Ciprofloxacin	GNR, Pseudomonas, Neisseria spp., Gram-positives (MRSA), UTI .	Prevents action of topoisomerase II. Bactericidal.
Trimethoprim	Trimethoprim and sulfamethoxazole	Gram-positives, Gram-negatives, Chlamydia, UTI.	• Inhibits DHP synthase by PABA metabolites. • Bacteriostatic. • TMP prevents the use of bacterial DHFR
Other Antibiotics	Metronidazole	Protozoa, anaerobes, Bacteroides, Clostridium.	Formation of toxic products. Bactericidal.
	Vancomycin	Serious infections, resistant gram-positive bacteria, S. aureus (MRSA), C. difficile.	Prevents cell wall formation through D-ala D-ala binding and sequestration.
	Clindamycin	Anaerobic infections, B. fragilis, C. perfringens.	50S inhibitor. Bacteriostatic.

COMPLICATIONS	CONTRAINDICATIONS	NOTES
Nephrotoxic. Ototoxic. Cause NMJ blockade after surgery. Possible superinfection.	• Do not use with cephalosporins. • Do not use with loop diuretics. • Renal clearance – avoid in renal disease.	• Require O_2 for use – no effect against anaerobes. • Given IV.
GI Sx. Tooth discoloration and stunted growth in children. Fanconi syndrome. Photosensitivity. Possible superinfection.	• Avoid in renal patients. Avoid in children. • Do not use with dairy products or antacids.	Do not use in CNS infections.
GI Sx. Hepatitis. Eosinophilia. Skin rashes.	Avoid in hepatic patients. Macrolides are excreted in bile.	
GI Sx. Tendon rupture.	• Avoid in pregnancy and children due to cartilage damage. • Avoid in renal patients.	• Broad spectrum except against anaerobes and some GPC. • Renal secretion.
• Allergic reactions. • Nephrotoxicity, rash, anemia, megaloblastic anemia, pancytopenia, BMS.	G6PD deficiency, avoid in infants, use with care with other drugs. Avoid in pregnancy.	• Penetrate CNS. • Give with folate.
GI Sx.	Avoid with alcohol due to disulfiram reaction.	Used for numerous STDs.
Nephrotoxic. Ototoxic (deafness). DVTs. Red man syndrome.	Renal disease.	Avoid red man syndrome with antihistamines and gradual administration.
Pseudomembranous colitis.	Renal and hepatic clearance.	PO. Treat pseudomembranous colitis with flagyl.

V.H. Common Antifungals

Table 7. Antifungals

DRUG	INDICATIONS	MECHANISM OF ACTION	COMPLICATIONS	NOTES
Amphotericin B	Systemic fungal infections.	Sequesters ergosterol and has detergent-like effect on cell wall. Fungicidal at high doses.	• F/C. • Hypotension. • Nephrotoxic. • Arrhythmias.	Does not cross BBB. Must be given intrathecally for meningitis.
Nystatin	Candida.	Sequesters ergosterol, disrupts cell wall.		Oral candidiasis. Topical only.
Fluconazole	Systemic fungal infections.	Block formation of ergosterol by lanosterol. Fungistatic.	Gynecomastia, hepatitis, F/C.	Good absorption and CNS penetration.

V.I. Common Antivirals

Table 8. Antivirals

DRUG	INDICATIONS	MECHANISM OF ACTION	COMPLICATIONS	NOTES
Acyclovir	HSV VZV EBV	Inhibits viral DNA polymerase, guanine analog.	Tremor, nephrotoxicity.	Also treated with vidarabine (adenosine analog).
Ganciclovir	CMV in IC EBV in IC	Inhibits viral DNA polymerase.	Pancytopenia, especially with WBCs.	Like ACV.

VI. Hematology

VI.A. Coagulation

1. Platelets

Platelets are critical components to the coagulation system. There are three important steps in which platelets are involved at the beginning of the coagulation cascade: platelet adhesion, platelet activation ("degranulation"), and platelet aggregation. In the first step, activation of receptors on platelet membranes allows for attachment to endothelial cells of injured blood vessel walls. Their membranes also contain phospholipids that are required for the formation of an integral protease of the coagulation cascade-prothrombinase. In the second step, platelets "degranulate" in response to thrombin, ADP, platelet-activating factor, or collagen (the latter occurring when collagen underlying the endothelial cells and basement membrane of blood vessel walls is exposed after blood vessel wall injury). Platelet degranulation releases ADP and coagulation-activating proteins like platelet factor 4. In the third step, platelets aggregate to form a firm platelet plug at the site of blood vessel injury.

2. Coagulation Factors

The coagulation factors form the other major component of the coagulation system. They are plasma proteins that circulate in the bloodstream in their inactive forms, and are activated to become serine proteases. In turn, these proteases activate other factors which become active proteolytic enzymes, thereby amplifying the actions of the coagulation cascade in order to form the end result of the whole process: a complex of cross-linked fibrin molecules and platelets that prevent hemorrhage after blood vessel injury. Most of the coagulation factors are made by the liver, with the exception of factors XIII (from platelets) and VIII (from endothelial cells). Factors II, VII, IX, X, as well as proteins C and S are gamma-carboxylase dependent clotting factors that depend on vitamin K for activity (the anticoagulant warfarin interferes with this by blocking vitamin K recycling during this process).

3. Coagulation Cascade

The coagulation cascade is a highly complex and regulated interaction of proteins which involves both procoagulant and anti-coagulant activities. The most critical step of the process, however, is the activation of factor X (into factor Xa) and the subsequent formation of the Xa-Va-Ca^{2+}-PL complex known as prothrombinase. The prothrombinase complex then activates thrombin (II into IIa), which cleaves fibrinogen into fibrin monomers and activates factor XIII (into XIIIa). XIIIa then catalyzes the cross-linking of the fibrin monomers, which results in the end product of the coagulation cascade: a cross-linked fibrin complex covering the site of injury in the blood vessel wall.

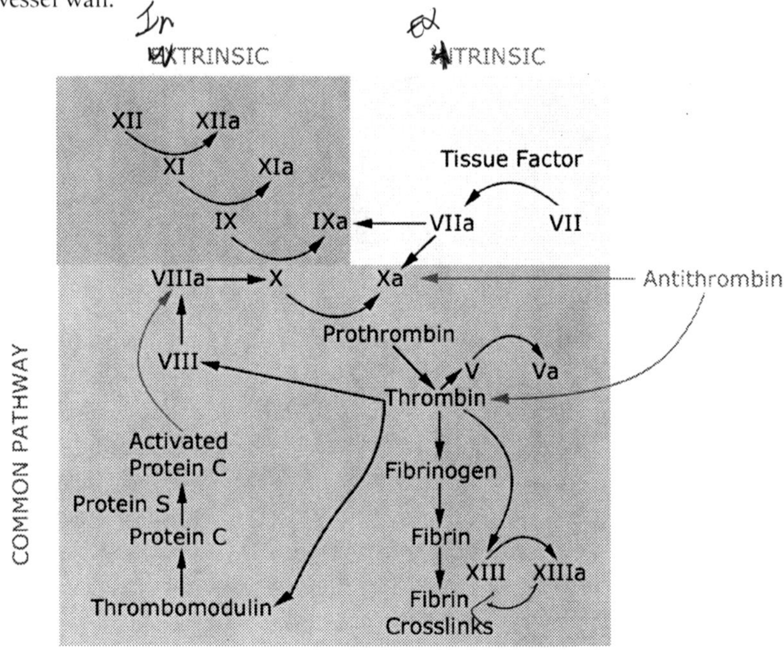

4. Factor X

Factor X is activated by two pathways. The first pathway involves the release of thromboplastin (also called "tissue factor") upon exposure of subendothelial collagen in blood vessel walls (this is known as the "extrinsic" pathway). Tissue factor then activates factor VII to form a TF-VIIa complex, which both directly and indirectly activates factor X (the latter through the activation of factor IX, which combines with factor VIIIa to activate factor X in the formation of the Xa-Va-Ca^{2+}-PL prothrombinase complex). The other pathway that leads to the activation of Factor X begins, again, with the exposure of subendothelial collagen in blood vessel walls (this is known as the "intrinsic", or contact, pathway). In the presence of collagen, protease factor XII is activated by high-molecular-weight kininogen and kallikrein. XIIa, then, goes on to activate factor XI, which, in its active form, converts IX to IXa. Then, as in the former pathway, IXa works with VIIIa to convert factor X to its active form.

The activation of factor X was mentioned before as the most crucial step in the coagulation cascade. The regulation of factor X is also a crucial step in the tight control, and termination of, the clotting cascade. The pro-coagulant activity of factor X is terminated almost as soon as it has begun by tissue factor pathway inhibitor (TFPI), which binds to and inhibits the activity of factor Xa, itself, as well as the upstream pro-coagulant factor VIIa. In this way, continued downstream procoagulant activity may only be sustained in the face of continued blood vessel injury, thus preventing uncontrolled clotting within blood vessels.

5. Tests of Coagulation Factors

There are several general tests of clotting factors commonly used to measure overall function of the coagulation cascade. The activated partial thromboplastin time test (PTT) measures the intrinsic pathway, and will be increased in deficiencies of factors VII, IX, XI, XII, von Willebrand fibrinogen. PTT testing is used to monitor heparin efficacy in patients on heparin drips. The prothrombin time test (PT) measures the extrinsic pathway and will be ab normal in deficiencies of factors II, V, VII, X and fibrinogen. Because of variations in PT level reporting, the international normalized ratio (INR) was developed to allow comparison of levels across laboratories. PT/INR testing is used to monitor vitamin K and warfarin efficacy.

6. Thrombolytics

Two other complex systems help to control coagulation: the first is the thrombolytic system, which involves plasmin and tissue plasminogen activator (tPA), and the second involves a group of inhibitors of the coagulation factors, including antithrombin III, protein C, and protein S.

The thrombolytic system dissolves fibrin clots using the serine protease plasmin. Plasmin is formed from its inactive precursor, plasminogen, by tPA. Interestingly, plasmin is also activated by thrombin, which thereby limits its own clot-forming ability (recall that thrombin, aka factor IIa, is responsible for activating fibrin and XIIIa, which work together to form the cross-linked fibrin complex known as the final blood clot in the coagulation cascade).

The second anticoagulant system is made up of antithrombin III and proteins C and S. Antithrombin III directly inhibits serine proteases in the clotting cascade, and its activity is enhanced up to 2000-fold by heparin. Protein C is activated by thrombin (again, another self-limiting reaction in the clotting cascade), and works with its cofactor, protein S, to inactivate factor Va (a component of the "prothrombinase" complex that activates prothrombin into thrombin).

7. Hypercoagulable States

Hypercoagulable states may result from a variety of inherited or acquired conditions that increase the chances of developing inappropriate blood clots in the arterial or venous systems. Common inherited hypercoagulable disorders include factor V Leiden and the prothrombin mutation 20210A; less common examples include protein C, protein S, and antithrombin III deficiencies. Acquired states of hypercoagulability include malignancy, recent surgery or trauma, obesity, liver or renal disease, and use of certain medications (one example is a female smoker over 35 years old taking oral contraceptives).

8. Factor V Leiden

Factor V Leiden is a common hereditary hypercoagulability disorder: in North America, it is found in about 5% of Caucasians, but is less common among Hispanics and African Americans. It is inherited in an autosomal dominant fashion, and demonstrates incomplete penetrance. Factor V Leiden represents a variant of factor V that is less susceptible to inactivation by activated protein C than the normal variant (recall that protein C is one of the natural "brakes" on the coagulation cascade). Patients with this mutation are more prone to develop the consequences of hypercoagulation because their factor V spends more time as an active component of the "prothrombinase" complex, which acts in concert with factor X to activate thrombin in the coagulation cascade. Common consequences of this condition are deep venous/pulmonary thromboses (up to 30% of patients presenting with DVT or PE have this condition, according to some studies), and increased risk of miscarriage and stillbirth among affected women. Arterial thromboses are much less common clinical manifestations.

9. Hyperhomocysteinemia

Many relatively recent studies have linked elevated homocysteine levels in the circulation with increased risk for arterial disease, including cardiovascular, cerebrovascular, and peripheral vascular disease. Others have cited elevated risk for venous thromboembolism. Hyperhomocysteinemia can occur as a result of inherited mutations in three enzymes responsible for its degradation: methylenetetrahydrofolate reductase (MTHFR), cystathionine beta-synthase (CBS), and methionine synthase (MS). These enzymes require vitamin B12 and folate as cofactors; therefore, deficiencies in these vitamins may also increase levels of homocysteine in the blood. Beyond supplementation with vitamin B12 and folate, no long-term anticoagulation therapy has been recommended for this condition at this time. Patients with hyperhomocysteinemia who develop a clinically significant blood clot, therefore, are treated according to the guidelines for treating DVT/PE among the general population.

10. Von Willebrand Disease

Von Willebrand disease is one of the most common inherited disorders of bleeding in humans, and occurs with a worldwide frequency of about 1%. vWD is a disease involving dysfunction in both platelet adhesion and aggregation (because vWF is involved in platelet adhesion to the subendothelial matrix, and in aggregation by binding to activated GpIIb/IIIa receptors). vWD also interferes with the clotting cascade since vWF stabilizes factor VIII by binding to it, and a deficiency of vWF therefore results in a secondary decrease in factor VIII. There are more than 20 variants of vWD that have been described with a variety of inheritance patterns, but most are transmitted in an autosomal dominant fashion. There is a large degree of variance in both penetrance and expressivity, so the clinical expression of this disease is also correspondingly variable: patients may be asymptomatic, or may present with bleeding from mucous membranes, excessive bleeding from wounds, or menorrhagia in the setting of a prolonged bleeding time (and PTT). Since this disease is represents a qualitative (and not quantitative) defect in platelets, the platelet count is normal in these patients. The plasma level of active vWF (measured as the ristocetin cofactor activity level) is reduced.

11. Hemophilia A

Hemophilia A is a disorder of impaired blood clotting resulting from an X-linked recessive inherited defect in factor VIII (or impaired conversion of factor VIII into its active form). Severe cases (i.e. patients with less than 1% of normal activity of factor VIII) may be diagnosed in infancy--i.e. infants born with multiple hemarthroses or who bleed profusely upon circumcision. Other, less severe cases (i.e. among patients with between 2 and 50% activity of factor VIII) may be not be diagnosed until later in life, and may be discovered among patients who get occasional hemarthroses, or who bleed profusely following a dental or surgical procedure. The diagnosis may also be suspected among patients with a prolonged PTT. Treatment of hemophilia A involves infusion of recombinant factor VIII. Excessive bleeding in these patients may require treatment with cryoprecipitate (contains factor VIII, fibrinogen, vWF, and factor XIII) or lyophilized factor VIII.

12. Hemophilia B

Hemophilia B, also known as Christmas disease, results from a deficiency of factor IX, and presents similarly to hemophilia A. It, too, is an X-linked recessive disease, and results in a prolonged PTT; however, it occurs only about one-sixth as frequently as hemophilia A.

13. Antithrombin III Deficiency

A defect in antithrombin III leads to a disinhibition of coagulation and permissive activation of factors IX and X, and thrombin. The result is arterial and venous thrombosis. Initial therapy is heparinization, followed by lifelong anticoagulation.

14. Factor XI Deficiency

Factor XI deficiency is an uncommon disorder that has few clinical effects. This autosomal dominant disorder can be corrected with FFP on a PRN basis.

VI.B. Platelet Disorders

1. Immune Thrombocytopenic Purpura

a) Etiology and Pathophysiology

ITP is a bleeding diathesis that presents with thrombocytopenia, purpura, and petechiae. Autoantibodies against platelets lead to decreased platelet longevity. Concurrent lupus, leukemia, or myelodysplastic syndrome may be present; the disorder may also follow infection by EBV, VZV, CMV, rubella virus, hepatitis, HIV, or other infection. Medications that can lead to sensitization include quinine, cephalosporins, rifampin, gold salts, NSAIDs, antihypertensives, diuretics, and abciximab. Heparin-induced thrombocytopenia (HIT) may also lead to ITP.

b) Presentation and Diagnosis

ITP may lead to morbidity through intracranial hemorrhage or bleeding in other parts of the body. Diagnosis is confirmed by CBC and large platelets found in peripheral blood smears. Antiplatelet antibodies may also be present. A positive Coombs test is common; a negative Coombs test implies non-immunogenic causes such as TTP.

c) Treatment

ITP is treated with corticosteroids, IVIG, and platelet transfusions. Splenectomy results in remission in 70% of cases. Platelets should be given only after the spleen has been removed or the splenic artery is clamped. IVIG should be given prior to splenectomy to permit a transient rise in platelets.

2. Glanzmann Thrombasthenia

Glanzmann's thrombasthenia is an autosomal recessive bleeding disorder caused by defective platelet aggregation. It involves a deficiency or dysfunction in glycoprotein IIb/IIIa, which normally aggregates platelets together by binding fibrinogen and vWF in the presence of ADP, collagen, epinephrine, or thrombin.

3. Uremia

One consequence of the accumulation of nitrogenous waste products in the circulation is platelet dysfunction. This acquired defect in platelet function is most commonly seen in patients with renal failure. In this condition, while the quantity of platelets in the circulation is adequate, their function, through a variety of incompletely understood abnormalities, is inadequate for normal coagulation. DDAVP stimulates platelet function.

4. HIT

Thrombocytopenia can result from immune-mediated destruction of platelets triggered by drugs, among which quinine, quinidine, sulfa-containing antibiotics, and heparin are commonly offending agents. Heparin-induced thrombocytopenia (HIT) is an especially important entity because of the degree to which heparin is used to prevent consequences of coagulopathy in the hospital, and because of the severe consequences that HIT can have if not quickly recognized and treated. HIT occurs in approximately 5% of patients receiving heparin.

Among these, most develop type I, which occurs rapidly after initiation of therapy and has little clinical consequences. In contrast, type II HIT is more severe. It usually occurs within 5 to 14 days of initiating heparin therapy, and can lead to life-threatening venous and arterial thromboses. This occurs because heparin binds to and modifies the conformation of platelet factor 4 and renders it susceptible to immune recognition. If antibodies to PF4 are created and immune complexes are formed, platelets are activated, promoting thrombosis even in the setting of marked thrombocytopenia.

5. DIC

Disseminated intravascular coagulation (DIC) is an acquired consumption of clotting factors and platelets that result in both diffuse microthrombus formation and hemorrhage with an often poor and sometimes fatal prognosis. This "consumptive coagulopathy" may be triggered by many causes, including sepsis (especially gram negative sepsis), malignancy, a variety of obstetric complications, extensive burns, and major trauma.

These inciting processes have in common either substantial endothelial injury and/or the release of thromboplastic substances into the circulation, both of which result in the uncontrolled activation of the coagulation system (by both the extrinsic and intrinsic pathways). This results in the consumption of platelets, fibrin, and clotting factors as microthrombi are formed throughout the body, resulting in tissue hypoxia and infarction. The brain, heart, lungs, liver, kidneys, adrenals, and spleen are often affected.

Once the clotting factors have been consumed, and the fibrinolytic system has been activated to counter the activation of the coagulation system, and widespread hemorrhage ensues.

Diagnosis of DIC is confirmed in the laboratory, upon demonstrating low platelets and fibrinogen, as well as the presence of fibrin degradation products (d-dimers) in the bloodstream; a microangiopathic hemolytic anemia may also be seen upon examination of a peripheral blood smear.

Treatment is directed at the underlying disease. Other treatment methods include the use of heparin (controversial) to slow the consumption of clotting factors and fresh frozen plasma and/or platelet concentrate to replace clotting factor deficits.

VI.C. Blood Product Supplementation

1. Whole Blood

Whole blood is the product of one unit of donated blood (contains plasma, red blood cells, and platelets) plus anticoagulant/preservative. While whole blood can be used to resuscitate a patient who has lost significant amounts of blood volume, it is no longer routinely used because the transfusion of red blood cells, themselves, usually suffices. Additionally, there is a heightened risk of disease transmission when whole blood is used.

2. Packed Red Blood Cells

Packed red blood cells (PRBCs) are used to correct low hemoglobin levels in anemic patients. One unit of PRBCs will typically increase the hemoglobin by 1 gm/dL and the hematocrit by 3-4%. PRBCs begin as whole blood from which platelets and plasma are removed. They may also be leukoreduced and irradiated for immunocompromised patients.

3. Plasma

Plasma is the liquid component of blood composed of water, proteins, glucose, clotting factors, minerals, hormones, and CO_2. It is isolated from the cellular component of blood by centrifugation.

4. Fresh Frozen Plasma

Fresh frozen plasma (FFP) is the fluid portion of human blood collected and frozen after centrifugation. It contains all coagulation factors in normal concentrations, and is free of red blood cells, leukocytes, and platelets (and thus does not carry a risk of CMW transmission). It is used to treat deficiencies of coagulation proteins, particularly among bleeding patients. It is often used to treat patients with DIC or TTP. FFP is also effective in treating specific clotting factor deficiencies (i.e. factors II, V, VII, IX, X, and XI). FFP is also commonly used to quickly reverse the effects of warfarin therapy (which disables the vitamin K dependent coagulation factors II, VII, IX, and X, as well as the anticoagulant proteins C and S). Note that vitamin K can also be given for this purpose, but it takes two to three days to reverse the effects of warfarin. Therefore, FFP is more a more appropriate therapy for patients who are actively bleeding or who require an invasive procedure.

5. Cryoprecipitate

Cryoprecipitate is a frozen blood product prepared from plasma, and contains factor VIII, fibrinogen, vWF, and factor XIII. It is indicated for hemophilia (when factor VIII/IX concentrates are not available), vWD (however, DDAVP is first line), hypofibrinogenemia (as can be seen after massive blood transfusions), bleeding from excessive anticoagulation (although FFP is a better choice for this), and DIC.

6. vWF

Von Willebrand factor (vWF) is a blood glycoprotein involved in hemostasis. vWF binds to and stabilizes factor VIII, and plays a role in platelet adhesion to wounded tissue. vWF is deficient or defective in von Willebrand disease. It also plays a role in the pathogenesis of thrombotic thrombocytopenic purpura (TTP) and hemolytic uremic syndrome (HUS), in which a deficiency or inhibition of the enzyme responsible for breaking down von Willebrand multimers (ADAMTS13) leads to deposition of fibrin and platelets in small vessels, capillary necrosis, and microangiopathic hemolytic anemia having disastrous systemic consequences.

VII. General Concepts in Surgery

VII.A. Indicators of Morbidity and Mortality

The most significant perioperative risk factor is albumin less than 2.5. Additional major risk factors for surgical morbidity and mortality include high ASA class, poor functional status, need for emergency surgery, advanced age, anemia, and elevated WBC.

The Goldman index assigns points for various risk factors and is a method to estimate cardiac risk from noncardiac procedures. From greatest to least risk, S3 (an extra heartbeat consistent with CHF), recent MI, arrhythmia, numerous PVCs, advanced age, need for emergency surgery, poor functional status, major abdominal or vascular procedure, and clinically-significant valve stenosis are each assigned points. The highest scores imply that patients have a nearly 80% risk of experiencing a major cardiac complication from their surgery.

The Child-Pugh scoring system takes into account the presence of encephalopathy, ascites, hyperbilirubinemia, low albumin, and elevated PT/INR to rate the extent of liver dysfunction. Class A cirrhotics have a 10% risk of mortality from intraabdominal procedures; class B has a 30% risk, and class C has a 75% risk.

1. Hypothermia

Hypothermia is a drop in the core body temperature below 35°C leading to a destabilization of body temperature regulation. Hypothermia presents with chills, dyspnea, shivering, and ataxia. More severe hypothermia has J waves on EKG, slow reflexes, cold diuresis, delirium, cessation of shivering, and eventually, ventricular fibrillation, hypotension, pulmonary edema, and coma. Treatment of hypothermia is to start ACLS, O_2, NG tube, warm hydration, external warming, and core rewarming. Death cannot be established until hypothermia has been corrected.

2. Hyperthermia

Hyperthermia is the result of uncontrolled heat buildup in the body leading to end-organ damage. Hyperthermia evolves after heat exhaustion and presents with myalgia, and muscle cramps. Sudden onset of CNS symptoms and psychosis herald hyperthermia. Orthostatic hypotension is present along with piloerection and tachycardia. With heat exhaustion, the body temperature is less than 41°C. With hyperthermia, the temperature is more than 41°C (106°F). Treatment involves cooling the patient with tepid water and large fans.

3. Radiation Exposure

Radiation exposure of up to 4 Gy leads to pancytopenia, bleeding, and infection. Exposure up to 10 Gy presents with nausea, vomiting, and watery diarrhea, followed by bloody diarrhea, fluid losses, and renal failure. Exposure up to 50 Gy leads to major mental status changes, vasodilation, and some partial recovery within 6 hours but death within 3 days.

4. Blast Trauma

Blast waves lead to death from air embolism, parenchymal hemorrhage, and pulmonary contusion. The most sensitive sign of serious underlying injury is perforation of the tympanic membranes.

Surgical Principles

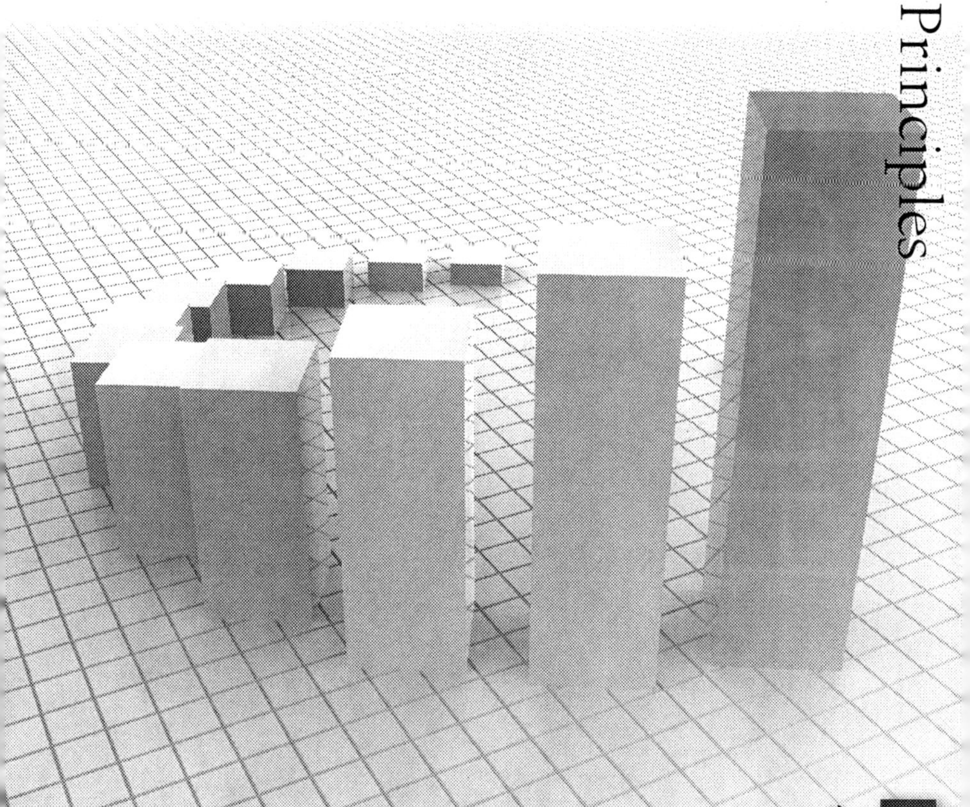

HEAD & NECK

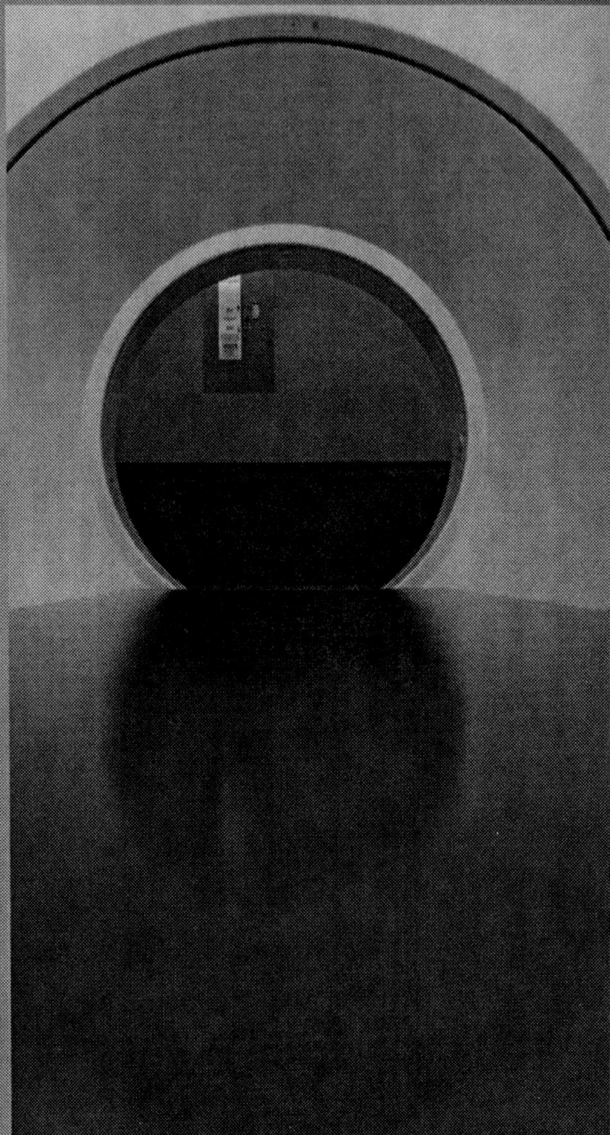

A good surgeon should be acquainted with liberal studies, with medicine and above all with anatomy.

Guy de Chauliac
Inventarium sive chirurgia magna, 1363

SURGISPHERE

HEAD AND NECK SURGERY

Daniel Murariu, M.D.

I. General Concepts

I.A. Introduction

Head and neck surgery encompasses a variety of topics that a general surgeon must be familiar with. Whether it is in the context of completing a difficult thyroidectomy, interfacing with our colleagues as part of a multisystem trauma, or coordinating a complex cancer operation, a familiarity of basic disease states and surgical anatomy is paramount. This short chapter focuses on the essentials – a basic overview of what one needs to be familiar with in the operating room and on the exams.

I.B. Anatomy

1. Nerves of the Head and Neck

Some of the twelve cranial nerves play a major role in general surgery procedures involving the head and neck. A special familiarity with them is necessary to avoid trauma to these structures. Their role is described in the table below.

Table 1. Cranial nerves and their role in surgical procedures.

Nerve	Function	Surgical Relevance
CN I – Olfactory	Smell	Rarely injured.
CN II – Optic	Vision	Rarely injured. Indirectly affected by loss of the ophthalmic artery secondary to giant cell arteritis.
CN III – Oculomotor	Motor to muscles of the eye, except superior oblique and lateral rectus	May cause internuclear ophthalmoplegia, the initial presenting sign of multiple sclerosis. This leads to loss of right or left eye conjugate gaze, impaired adduction, and nystagmus.
CN IV – Trochlear	Motor to superior oblique	Rarely injured.

Nerve	Function	Surgical Relevance
CN V – Trigeminal	Sensory to face, motor to muscles of mastication	Disorders of the superior cerebellar artery or very poor dentition with infection may lead to trigeminal neuralgia, which is severe, debilitating pain that can lead to suicide.
CN VI – Abducens	Motor to lateral rectus	Rarely injured.
CN VII – Facial	Motor to muscles of facial expression. Taste from anterior 2/3s of tongue.	Uncommonly injured. More likely involved with deep malignant tumors of the parotid gland, in which case total parotidectomy with resection of the nerve is necessary. Symptoms may be mitigated by nerve graft.
CN VIII – Vestibulocochlear	Audition and vestibular sense	Rarely damaged but may be affected by tumors or trauma. Manifestation depends on region of disruption and can lead to loss of the vestibular sense or hearing.
CN IX – Glossopharyngeal	Taste from posterior 1/3 of tongue, motor to parotid. Gag reflex.	Damage is rare but can occur with very superior exposures during carotid endarterectomy and other neck procedures, leading to loss of parotid secretions and gag reflex.
CN X – Vagus	Parasympathetic. Motor to pharynx and larynx.	Damage to the vagus nerve specifically can occur as part of a carotid endarterectomy and present with hoarseness (see page 146) Damage to the recurrent laryngeal nerve branch leads to cord paralysis and need for direct laryngoscopy and cord medialization. Bilateral nerve damage requires a permanent tracheostomy to prevent loss of the airway. Damage to the superior laryngeal nerve changes voice timber and loss of high-pitched sounds. This nerve is also sensory to the supraglottic region and may be transected when working with the superior thyroid artery as part of a thyroidectomy.
CN XI – Spinal Accessory	Motor to trapezius.	Damage is rare but can occur with trauma. May lead to inability to shrug one's shoulders.
CN XII - Hypoglossal	Motor to tongue	Unilateral damage leads to deviation of the tongue in the direction of damage upon protrusion.

2. Nerves of the Upper Extremity

a) Overview

The brachial plexus forms the backbone of the network of nerves that supplies the entire upper extremity and emanates from spinal nerves C5, C6, C7, C8, and T1. Although these roots, trunks, divisions, cords, and branches anastomose to various degrees, a simplified model of the function of each of these roots is illustrated in the following table:

TABLE 2. Major function of various nerve roots.

C5	Shoulder abduction, extension, and external rotation; some elbow flexion
C6	Elbow flexion, forearm pronation and supination, some wrist extension
C7	Diffuse loss of function in the extremity without complete paralysis of a specific muscle group, consistently supplies the latissimus dorsi
C8	Finger extensors, finger flexors, wrist flexors, hand intrinsics The ulnar nerve is responsible for innervations to the intrinsic muscles of the hand. Transection of this nerve is not repaired primarily.
T1	Hand intrinsics

b) Long Thoracic Nerve

The long thoracic nerve (C5, C6, C7) supplies the serratus anterior muscle, and is commonly tested in the context of a modified radical mastectomy with axillary dissection. Damage to this nerve during that operation can lead to "winged scapula," which is evident when the patient pushes against a wall with an outstretched arm. The long thoracic nerve descends along the lateral border of the pectoralis minor and medial border of the teres major.

c) Thoracodorsal Nerve

The thoracodorsal nerve (C6, C7, C8) travels with the subscapular artery, crosses the axilla, and innervates the latissimus dorsi. Variations in its course may take the crossing somewhat more inferiorly. Care must be taken to avoid transaction of this nerve during an axillary dissection as part of a mastectomy.

d) Pectoral Nerves

The lateral pectoral nerve (C5, C6, C7) passes through the coracoclavicular fascia to supply the pectoralis major. The medial pectoral nerve (C8, T1) supplies the pectoralis minor and major muscles.

e) Musculocutaneous Nerve

The musculocutaneous nerve (C5, C6, C7) is the chief nerve supply to the coracobrachialis, biceps brachii, and brachialis. This nerve travels along the lateral aspect of the arm between the biceps and brachialis. Direct damage to this nerve is therefore rare given the extensive muscular protection.

f) Median Nerve

The median nerve (C5, C6, C7, C8, T1) is a major nerve from the brachial plexus and travels along the medial aspect of the arm just lateral to the brachial artery. It crosses the brachial artery at its bifurcation within the cubital fossa and travels medially. The median nerve primarily supplies the flexors and pronators of the distal upper extremity. Branches also supply the hand. The median nerve travels deep to the flexor retinaculum and may be affected in carpal tunnel syndrome.

g) Axillary Nerve

The axillary nerve (C5, C6) supplies the teres minor and deltoid muscles. Damage to this nerve may occur with anterior dislocation of the shoulder or fracture of the head of the humerus.

Erb-Duchenne palsy occurs following damage to the superior roots of the brachial plexus (C5, C6), leading to paralysis of the deltoid, biceps, brachialis, coracobrachialis, brachioradialis, supraspinatus, infraspinatus, teres minor, and subscapularis. The upper limb is adducted at shoulder, medially rotated, and extended at the elbow. Erb-Duchenne palsy is the result of excess traction on the neck as can occur during delivery or from falls.

h) Radial Nerve

The radial nerve (C5, C6, C7, C8, T1) supplies the triceps brachii and the extensor compartment of the arm. This nerve initially travels in the posterior compartment of the upper arm, and then crosses through the lateral intermuscular septum to travel in the anterior compartment. In the upper arm, it is located along the radial groove of the humerus and is therefore susceptible to damage in a midshaft fracture. The nerve is also located in close proximity to the lateral epicondyle. The superficial branch of the radial nerve travels deep to the brachioradialis. The radial nerve also supplies muscles of the hand.

Saturday night palsy is due to injury to the radial nerve as a result of a midshaft humerus fracture. It leads to wrist drop. The deep branch of the radial nerve can be injured by deep puncture wounds to the forearm, leading to extension of the thumb and the metacarpophalangeal joints. Superficial damage leaves a coin-shaped area distal to the bases of the 1st and 2nd metacarpals without sensation.

i) Ulnar Nerve

The ulnar nerve (C8, T1) is a mostly unprotected nerve that supplies several flexors and muscles of the hand. It is most likely to be injured at the medial epicondyle of the humerus. The ulnar nerve travels along the posterior and medial aspect of the humerus, then travels with the ulnar artery in the forearm. This nerve passes superior to the flexor retinaculum.

Klumpke palsy is due to lower brachial plexus injury. It occurs when a person grabs something to break a fall. The dorsal and ventral roots of the spinal nerves that form the inferior trunk of the brachial plexus (C8 and T1) may be avulsed. As a result, the short muscles of the hand are affected. It presents as claw hand.

3. Nerves of the Lower Extremity

a) Overview

There are three major plexuses that provide innervation to the pelvis and lower extremities. The lumbar plexus includes a variety of cutaneous and motor nerves to the inguinal region and proximal lower extremity. The sacral plexus predominantly supplies the distal lower extremity, while the coccygeal plexus supplies structures of the perineum and anus.

b) Lumbar Plexus

The chief nerves of the lumbar plexus are the iliohypogastric, ilioinguinal, genitofemoral, lateral femoral cutaneous, obturator, and femoral nerves. The iliohypogastric, ilioinguinal, and genitofemoral nerves are discussed in more detail with hernia surgery on page 276.

The lateral femoral cutaneous nerve provides sensory innervation to the lateral thigh. The obturator nerve (L2, L3, L4) passes through the psoas major, deep to the common iliac artery, and through the obturator canal. It provides sensory innervation to the medial thigh and motor to the adductor muscles. The femoral nerve (L2, L3, L4) travels with the femoral vessels deep the inguinal ligament and provides sensory innervation to the majority of the lower leg and motor to the quadriceps (i.e. the rectus femoris, vastus lateralis, vastus medialis, and vastus intermedius). The major sensory branch is the saphenous nerve, which travels with the great saphenous vein deep to the sartorius.

c) Sacral Plexus

The common fibular, tibial, and sural nerves are major branches of the sciatic nerve, itself a major derivative of the sacral plexus. The superior and inferior gluteal nerves and cutaneous nerves to the thigh also emanate from the sacral plexus. In conjunction with the cutaneous nerves from the lumbar plexus, branches of the sural nerve provide sensory innervation to the entire leg. The sacral plexus includes nerve roots from L4, L5, S1, S2, S3, and S4.

d) Coccygeal Plexus

The coccygeal plexus is formed by roots S4 and the coccygeal nerve. It gives rise to the pudendal nerve, a somatic nerve that regulates the function of the bulbospongiosus and ischiocavernosus muscles, external anal sphincter (via the inferior rectal branch), scrotum (via the superficial perineal nerve), and genitalia (via the dorsal nerve of the penis or clitoris).

4. Major Reflexes

These nerves also play a role in several important reflexes. Testing these reflexes is especially important as part of a trauma workup, as a specific dysfunction may be an indicator of spinal cord injury. The major reflexes are indicated in "Table 3. Major reflexes of the upper and lower extremities.".

Table 3. Major reflexes of the upper and lower extremities.

Biceps Reflex	C5, C6 – Musculocutaneous nerve
Triceps Reflex	C6, C7 – Radial nerve
Patellar Reflex	L3, L4 – Femoral and common peroneal nerves
Ankle Reflex	L5, S1 – Tibial nerve

5. Other Relevant Anatomy

The zones of the neck are discussed on page 146 in conjunction with extracranial vascular surgery. The specific branches of the carotid artery are discussed on page 130 Disorders of the thyroid (page 361) and parathyroid (page 374) are discussed in the Endocrine Surgery chapter.

I.C. Physiology

1. Cerebral Perfusion Pressure

The cerebral perfusion pressure (CPP) is the pressure generated by blood flow to the brain. There are three constituents that modify the CPP, including the mean arterial pressure (MAP), intracranial pressure (ICP), and jugular venous pressure (JVP). Cerebral perfusion pressure is defined as the difference between the MAP and ICP. CPP divided by the cerebral vascular resistance (CVR) yields cerebral blood flow, a quantity that is difficult to measure directly.

$$CPP = MAP - ICP$$

The major constituents that affect ICP include brain volume, cerebral spinal fluid (CSF), and blood. Changes in one or more of these variables can lead to a rise in intracranial pressure, which in turn can reduce cerebral perfusion pressure, decrease, blood flow to the brain, and cause cerebral ischemia with stroke.

Normal MAP ranges between 60 and 150 mmHg and ICP is typically about 10 mmHg. Autoregulation within the brain modulates CPP to between 70 and 90 mmHg. Once the limits of autoregulation are exceeded, a drop in CPP below 70 mmHg leads to cerebral ischemia. In selected, stable patients, the tolerated range for CPP can vary between 50 and 150 mmHg, and a lower limit for children of 60 mmHg may be tolerated.

Urgent correction of potential causes of CPP derangement is required. Rising ICP should be treated with a ventriculostomy drain. Rapid sequence intubation, sedation, mannitol, hypothermia, paralysis, and raising the head of the bed are all means of mitigating a rise in ICP. Pressors may be used to increase MAP to overcome a continuing rise in ICP. Hyperventilation to cause a $PaCO_2$ of 35 mmHg may reduce cerebral vasospasm and improve circulation. Hypotonic saline can also be used to control ICP to some extent.

Severe derangements in intracranial pressure may lead to uncal herniation and death. Early signs include papillary dilation with a sluggish reaction, suggesting compromise of the ipsilateral oculomotor nerve from overstretching.

II. Metabolic and Degenerative

II.A. Delirium

Table 4. Hallmarks of delirium.

Etiology	Alcohol or benzodiazepine withdrawal, anticholinergics drugs, shock, surgery, UTIs.
Presentation	Disturbance of consciousness leading to deficits in attention and arousal, an alteration in cognition and memory, relatively rapid development over a period of hours, and a distinct medical condition or substance-related trigger profound psychomotor agitation.
Differential diagnosis	Delirium is reversible, develops relatively quickly, and the presence of an obvious, immediate precipitating factor, dementia does not.
Treatment	Address underlying cause, supportive therapy, haloperidol, benzodiazepines.

II.B. Multiple Sclerosis

1. Etiology and Pathophysiology

Multiple sclerosis (MS) is a progressive, inflammatory, demyelinating disorder of the CNS that leads to physical disability. Infiltration of lymphocytes and macrophages into nervous tissue cause inflammation and disruption of the nerve. Surgery and other external stressors may be a trigger for onset.

2. Presentation and Diagnosis

The initial presenting sign may be acute blindness, followed by rapid resolution. After a waxing and waning course, neurodegeneration progresses rapidly. Weakness and fatigue are universal. Cognitive changes occur in some, ataxia in others, along with hemiparesis, depression, and psychomotor changes. Bilateral facial weakness and trigeminal neuralgia are strongly indicative of MS. CSF studies reveal oligoclonal banding, normal glucose, normal or high protein, and high WBC count with excess IgG. MRI is used to localize the regions of sclerosis.

3. Treatment

MS is treated with supportive care while minimizing the effects of intercurrent illness and psychomotor stressors. Amantadine or modafinil are beneficial for fatigue mitigation. Disease progression can be slowed with interferon beta-1[a], interferon beta-1b, and glatiramer acetate. Acute exacerbations can be minimized with methylprednisone, and high-dose IV steroids may be beneficial in certain situations.

II.C. Myasthenia Gravis

1. Etiology and Pathophysiology

Myasthenia gravis is a rare autoimmune disorder that leads to weakness and fatigue as a result of antibody-mediated loss of the acetylcholine receptor (AChR) and neuromuscular junction (NMJ). MG is exacerbated by a number of drugs, including penicillamine.

2. Presentation and Diagnosis

MG presents as variable weakness worsened on exertion and improved with rest. Extraocular muscles (EOM) are weak and ptosis may be present in many patients. CXR is used to rule out thymoma, which affects 25% of patients, and thymectomy may forestall symptoms for many years. Electromyography (EMG) is diagnostic, and the edrophonium test can be used when other studies are deemed inconclusive.

3. Treatment

MG has no clear treatment. Inhibitors of AChE have been used with some effect; medications include pyridostigmine and neostigmine. Immunomodulation with prednisone, azathioprine, and cyclosporine A (CsA) has some benefit. Plasmapheresis can remove antibodies emergently and prevent relapse.

II.D. Pseudobulbar Palsy

Pseudobulbar palsy is bilateral dysfunction of cranial nerves IX through XII, leading to a dysfunction in speech, deglutination, and mastication. Failure of deglutination may lead to aspiration. The cause is an upper motor neuron lesion within the pyramidal tract. There are a variety of causes, including head trauma, MS, and bilateral hemisphere infarction.

III. Inflammatory and Infectious

III.A. Sinusitis

Infection of the sinuses and air spaces of the skull presents with malaise, aural fullness, and nasal drainage. More severe symptoms, including fever, headache, and vision changes portend disruption of the sinuses with rupture into the orbits and brain.

Diagnosis proceeds with a CT scan of the head. Immunocompromised and diabetic patients in particular should have an early workup due to their risk of complications from devastating fungal infections such as Mucor. In addition to antibiotics, the treatment for more complicated cases involves drainage of all fluid collections.

III.B. Pharyngitis

Pharyngitis is most commonly secondary to gram positive streptococcus and presents with odynophagia and fever. The back of the oropharynx is erythematous, and a purulent drainage may be evident. The formation of all loculated collections of pus require drainage due to potential complications from Ludwig angina. Signs of complicated pharyngitis include trismus and changes to the voice. Pharyngitis is treated with augmentin or clindamycin, and drainage of all fluid collections. Severe and aggressive infection may require intubation to protect a swollen airway.

III.C. Suppurative Parotitis

Suppurative parotitis is now a rare complication of dehydration in the postsurgical, severely ill patient. Once a highly morbid and frequently fatal illness, early identification and treatment with aggressive rehydration and intravenous antibiotics makes this disease readily amenable to cure. The most common population that now presents with this disorder is the elderly, commonly secondary to use of anticholinergic medications. Other causes include HIV, Sjogren syndrome, and sarcoid. Pain, swelling, and edema are present at Stensen's duct. The most common cause of infection is S. aureus. It sufficient therapy is not started soon, Ludwig's angina can develop leading to significant morbidity and mortality. Surgical interventions include superficial parotidectomy with facial nerve sparing and ligation of the parotid duct.

III.D. Bacterial Meningitis

1. Etiology and Pathophysiology

Bacterial meningitis occurs with infection of the pia and arachnoid membranes by Streptococcus pneumoniae (over half of all cases), Neisseria meningitidis, Listeria monocytogenes, gram-negative rods, Haemophilus influenzae, and group B streptococcus (GBS). Young adults are likely to have meningitis from N. meningitidis; immunocompromised patients with L. monocytogenes; and neonates with GBS perinatally. Infection may occur through the bloodstream, direct invasion, or from otitis or sinusitis.

2. Presentation and Diagnosis

Meningitis presents with headache, neck stiffness, fever, and photophobia. Mental status changes and seizure are present in some patients. Kernig's sign is typically positive with extension of the knee and thigh leading to pain in the back. Blood cultures are positive in about half of all individuals. Lumbar puncture indicates increased neutrophils, increased protein, low glucose, and high opening pressure.

3. Treatment

Treatment of bacterial meningitis is empirical and includes vancomycin plus cefotaxime or ceftriaxone. This is also the standard treatment for Streptococcus pneumoniae. If N. meningitidis is the cause, treatment can proceed with penicillin G or ceftriaxone. L. monocytogenes infection is treated with ampicillin and gentamicin.

III.E. Viral Meningitis

1. Assessment and Management

Table 5. Viral meningitis.

Etiology	Virus
Presentation	Similar to bacterial meningitis.
Diagnosis	LP with high WBCs, normal protein and glucose, normal or high opening pressure.
Treatment	Supportive

III.F. Brain Abscess

Table 6. Brain abscess.

Etiology	Common causes are S. aureus, S. intermedius, Bacteroides, Prevotella, Fusobacterium, Enterobacteriaceae, Pseudomonas, and other infectious agents.
Presentation	Neurologic impingement, headache, fever, seizures, nuchal rigidity, papilledema.
Diagnosis	CT
Treatment	Surgical excision with long-term antibiotic use is the standard of care following precise planning of the surgical approach with the aid of CT.

IV. Vascular

IV.A. Arteriovenous Malformation

Arteriovenous malformations are abnormal, congenital connections between arteries and veins, and may present with headache and epilepsy when involving the brain. Most AVMs are asymptomatic. Coil embolization, surgical resection, or radiation can be used for particularly dangerous AVMs and to forestall a potentially devastating hemorrhagic stroke. For a more detailed discussion on AVMs elsewhere in the body, please see page 187.

Table 7. Symptoms of infarction from major arterial distributions in the head.

Anterior Cerebral Artery	Altered mental status, change in judgement and personality, apraxia, contralateral lower extremity weakness, incontinence.
Middle Cerebral Artery	Contralateral hemiparesis, hemianopsia, hemiplegia, agnosia, and aphasia. Deficits in upper extremities are prominent.
Posterior Cerebral Artery	Change in vision, memory, and mental status. Contralateral hemiplegia (CN III palsy), ataxia, and homonymous hemianopsia with macular sparing (occipital lobe).
Anterior Spinal Artery	Flaccid paralysis, spastic paresis, and loss of pain and temperature. Hyperactive deep tendon reflexes.
Vertebrobasilar Artery	Vestibular derangement, loss of pain and temperature on ipsilateral face and contralateral body, loss of descending motor pathways, and even "locked-in" syndrome from disruption of the pons.

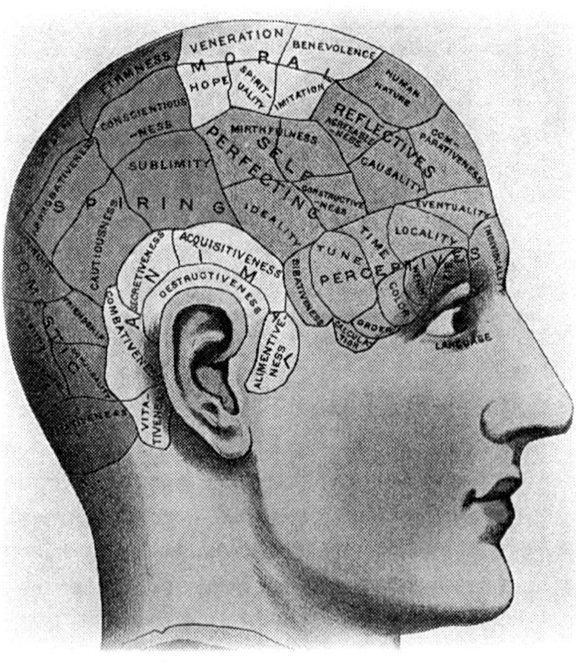

V. Trauma

V.A. Tracheotomy

The need for a long term but temporary airway when prolonged endotracheal intubation is indicated can best be achieved by way of a tracheotomy. Tracheotomies reduce the high resistance found in the oropharynx, improve clearance of pulmonary secretions, and permit continued mechanical ventilation in patients with significant respiratory compromise.

Tracheotomy is indicated in patients with no immediate plans for extubation, and in patients who have failed a trial of extubation. Most practitioners will proceed with a tracheotomy in patients who are intubated for more than 3-7 days. Patients with permanent respiratory failure who will require long term, permanent access can have a tracheostomy created. The difference between a tracheotomy and tracheostomy is that the latter will remain open even if it is decannulated.

Serious complications of tracheotomy creation include the development of a tracheoinnominate fistula, which is more likely when the opening is created too inferior. A tracheoesophageal fistula can form if there is disruption of the posterior wall of the trachea. Finally, there is the potential for damage to the recurrent laryngeal nerves, surrounding vasculature leading to hematoma formation, and aspiration.

A cricothyroidotomy is a form of tracheotomy in which an incision is made through the cricothyroid membrane into the trachea. The thyroid cartilage is first palpated; the cricothyroid membrane is immediately inferior to the thyroid cartilage. Below this membrane is the cricoid cartilage. Following the formation of a tracheotomy, an artificial airway can be inserted once the existing endotracheal tube is removed.

Percutaneous tracheotomy can also be completed by way of serial dilations of the tracheal rings after identification of the lumen via a needle passed through the cricothyroid membrane. Needle cricothyroidotomy is a form of percutaneous tracheotomy that is preferred in children under 12. This airway can be maintained for nearly one hour before intubation or a more long term solution is necessary.

V.B. Head Trauma

1. Etiology and Pathophysiology

Trauma to the head consists of lacerations to the scalp, fractures of the skull, and intracranial damage. The closed space of the calvarium makes it especially susceptible to intracranial injury, as the resulting hematoma and cerebral edema can lead to a significant alteration in cerebral blood flow and potential herniation of the brain.

2. Presentation and Diagnosis

The initial approach to a trauma patient with suspected intracranial injury is to complete the ATLS protocol. The airway, breathing, and circulation should all be secured. Attention should be paid to the patients neurologic examination. A concise but complete head to toe examination should be completed, and the entire examination carefully documented. Should the patient require urgent intubation, the neurologic examination prior to sedation and/or paralysis should be documented. Once the patient is stabilized and is a suitable candidate for imaging, a diagnostic CT of the head and neck should be completed. Plain films of the thoracic, lumbar, and sacral spine should be completed unless there is a specific focus of concern, in which case CT reformats of the entire spine should be completed.

3. Glasgow Coma Scale

The Glasgow coma scale is used for rapid neurologic assessment following acute head injury or stroke. It is closely tied to outcome and is often used to dictate therapy in certain instances. The GCS ranges between 3 and 15, with 3 being the worst. Three responses are gauged ("Table 8. Glasgow coma scale (GCS)." on page 79): eye , verbal, and motor responses. A GCS of 13 or more correlates with mild or nonexistent brain injury. GCS between 9 and 12 is considered a moderate injury, and less than 9 is usually consistent with a severe injury. The motor element is the most important response. A patient is usually intubated for a GCS less or equal to 8.

Table 8. Glasgow coma scale (GCS).

Eye response	No eye opening (1 point), eye response to pain (2), eye response to verbal command (3), and spontaneous eye response (4).
Verbal response	No verbal response gets 1 point, incomprehensive sounds (2), inappropriate words (3), confused (4), and oriented gets 5 points.
Motor response	No response (1), extension to pain (2), flexion to pain (3), withdrawal from pain (4), localizing pain (5), and obeying commands (6).
Interpretation	> 13 mild or nonexistent brain injury; 12-9 moderate injury; 8 or less is severe and requires intubation

4. Treatment

a) Scalp Lacerations

Due to the thin soft tissue overlying the bone, there is little potential for soft tissue to occlude bleeding and promote hemostasis. As a result, scalp lacerations tend to bleed profusely. Hemostasis is the first line of management and consists of applying stitches or staples to close the laceration once it has been thoroughly irrigated and debrided. More extensive injuries that disrupt all of the layers of the scalp may require a split thickness skin graft for closure.

b) Skull Fractures

Severe injuries to the head may lead to skull fractures; these injuries are divided into displaced and non-displaced. Non-displaced fractures can typically be managed conservatively, but a thorough workup for intracranial injury and potential hematoma formation should be completed. Displaced injuries require retrieval of the bony fragments and intraoperative irrigation, debridement, and repair. All open skull fractures should also be managed surgically. Basilar skull fractures can lead to drainage of CSF. Most cases will resolve spontaneously, but continuing drainage 7 days after the injury may require operative repair. Severe basilar skull fractures may lead to disruption of the vestibulocochlear complex and require urgent repair to minimize the risk of damage to this nerve.

c) Intracranial Injury

Intracranial injury is commonly secondary to severe acceleration or deceleration causing diffuse axonal injury from the excessive shearing forces. Intracranial injury can also lead to shearing forces on the bridging veins and intracranial arteries, causing hemorrhage and additional damage. Mild intracranial injury leads to a temporary loss of consciousness, referred to as a concussion. Supportive management and observation are typically all that is required for concussions. More severe injuries may lead to cerebral edema and hemorrhage with an increase in ICP and reduction in CBF. Aggressive surgical management may be necessary in severe cases to avoid neural compromise from hernation and ischemic injury.

Following severe head trauma, spinal cord function may remain intact with brisk deep tendon reflexes in patients who are brain dead. A patient with a closed head injury who has hypernatremia and a urine osmolarity greater than 300 should receive DDAVP for the treatment of diabetes insipidus. The Cushing response involves bradycardia, hypertension, and irregular respirations, and is a sign of a head injury. Hypotension in the setting of head trauma requires urgent fluid resuscitation. Most patients with head injury will receive 24 hours of seizure prophylaxis.

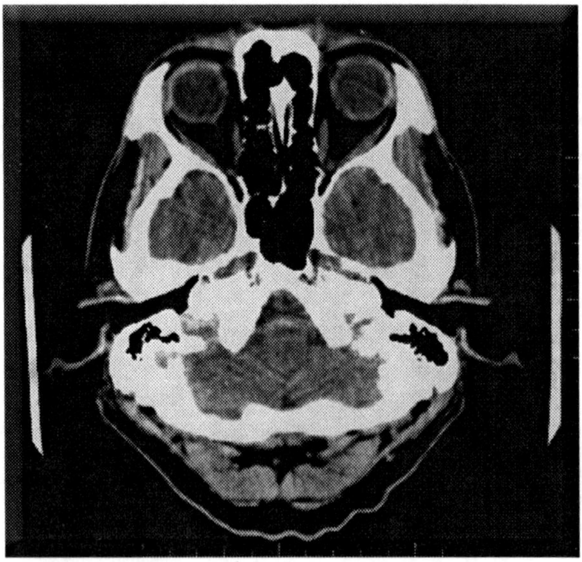

TABLE 9. Common intracranial bleeds and injuries from trauma.

Type	Etiology	Presentation	Findings	Treatment
Epidural hematoma	Temporal bone fracture with middle meningeal artery rupture (branch of maxillary artery)	Lucid interval followed by rapid deterioration	Convex-shaped mass that does not cross suture lines; may lead to midline shift	Surgical evacuation in most cases
Subdural hematoma	Trauma in the elderly leading to rupture of bridging veins	Delayed symptoms followed by rapid deterioration	Concave / crescent-shaped mass that crosses suture lines	Surgical evacuation if large or symptomatic Associated with high mortality due to underlying brain contusion
Subarachnoid hemorrhage	Ruptured Berry aneurysm at circle of Willis bifurcation point (associated with APKD, Ehlers-Danlos, Marfan syndrome, HTN, and traumatic brain injury)	Severe headache, vomiting, neck stiffness, and mental status changes	Diagnosed by CT and/ or lumbar puncture	Coil embolization or surgical clip placement High morbidity and mortality
Diffuse axonal injury	Severe shear forces from trauma leading to disruption of white and gray matter interface	Altered mental status, low GCS scores	Diffuse loss of separation between white and gray matter	Symptomatic

V.C. Spinal Trauma

1. Etiology and Pathophysiology

Patients with trauma to the head and neck are also at risk for specific trauma to the spinal cord. Direct trauma to the vertebral column can also lead to herniation of discs, bony fragments, and direct injury to the spinal cord. Hematoma formation can lead to occlusion, while vascular disruption can lead to ischemia. All patients who are suspected of head, neck, or back trauma should be stabilized in a hard cervical collar (i.e. a Miami J) and backboard. Expeditious clearing of the cervical spine and removal of the backboard should be completed.

2. Presentation

Injuries to the spinal cord are most likely to occur at the cervical level (55%), followed by the thoracic (30%) and lumbar (15%) regions. Spinal shock may occur with injuries above T5, leading to loss of background excitability from loss of lower pathways, decreased reflex function for at least 1 week and perhaps permanently, and loss of vestibulospinal and reticulospinal pathways. This leads to bradycardia, vasodilation, and hypotension. Treat spinal shock with fluids and pressors.

Nonpenetrating injuries of the spinal cord that occurred within 3 hours should be treated with 24 hours of methylprednisolone. Injuries that occurred within 8 hours should be treated with 48 hours of methylprednisolone. Injuries that occurred greater than 8 hour ago should not be treated with steroids. These findings are based off the somewhat controversial NASCIS trials.

3. Clearance of the C-Spine

Clearance of the C-spine in an intubated and sedated patient without neurologic findings can be done with a CT scan through T1, but ligamentous injury cannot be excluded. If suspected, extension/flexion films and physical exam are key. An MRI is also a sensitive test for detecting ligamentous injury.

4. Spinal Cord Compression

Cord compression is commonly the result of tumor, disk herniation, abscess, or hematoma formation – especially in the thoracic levels. Disturbances to the upper central cord lead to loss of sensory and motor function in the distal upper extremities with sparing of the lower extremities.

5. Partial Cord Transection

Brown-Sequard syndrome occurs in the setting of severe trauma in which anatomic or functional hemisection of the spinal cord has occurred. It presents with hemiparesis with limb drift, hyperreflexia, spasticity, Babinski sign, and loss of contralateral pain and temperature. Damage above T1 leads to Horner syndrome, which presents with miosis, ptosis, and anhidrosis. This particular manifestation can occur with metastatic lung cancer.

6. Complete Cord Transection

Complete spinal cord transection above T6 will lead to autonomic dysreflexia in about half of all patients and leads to cardiovascular instability, hypertension leading to hemorrhage and seizures, and vasoconstriction below the level of injury. Unopposed parasympathetic activation leads to diaphoresis, vasodilation, and headache. Autonomic dysreflexia often occurs in response to an uncomfortable stimulus below the level of injury.

VI. Cancer

VI.A. Nasal Cancer

Masses of the nasal spaces usually takes the form of a benign papilloma or potentially malignant squamous cell carcinoma. Both tumors should be excised; the former has a high chance of recurrence and may contain foci of squamous cell cancer. Most tumors are found within the maxillary or ethmoid sinuses and can be defined via CT or MRI for staging and operative planning. Full en bloc resection is necessary for all resectable tumors. Adjuvant radiotherapy is part of the overall management.

VI.B. Salivary Tumors

Tumors of the salivary glands may affect the parotid, submandibular, sublingual, or minor salivary glands. The larger glands are more likely to have benign tumors, while the smaller glands are more likely to present with malignant masses. The most common site for a salivary tumor is the parotid gland. Malignant tumors typically present with an enlarging mass, paresthesia of cranial nerves (i.e. CN VII, IX), and discomfort. All masses should have a fine needle aspiration for pathologic evaluation, along with a CT or MRI for staging and surgical planning.

Pleomorphic adenomas are the most common benign parotid gland tumors. This tumor may be superficial or deep. Superficial tumors are best treated with a facial nerve-sparing superficial parotidectomy. Deep tumors should be treated with careful resection of the parotid gland with sparing of the facial nerve. Papillary cystadenomas (Warthin tumor) may also occur in the tail of the parotid gland and are treated similar to pleomorphic adenomas. While 80% of parotid gland tumors are benign, 20% may be malignant and typically present as a mucoepidermoid or adenoid cystic tumor. Low grade malignant tumors of the parotid gland can be treated a nerve-sparing parotidectomy. However, high-grade, aggressive tumors should elicit a total parotidectomy with modified radical neck dissection and adjuvant radiotherapy. Resection of the facial nerve with nerve interposition can be completed if there is any evidence of perineural invasion, which is especially common with the high-grade cancers.

VI.C. Squamous Cell Cancer

Squamous cell cancer of the head and neck is a complex entity that requires individualized medical and surgical planning. Risk factors for this type of cancer include smoking and alcohol abuse. Continuing abuse even after successful treatment of the original insult is associated with a high risk of recurrent disease. A thorough workup is necessary for appropriate diagnosis and to optimize surgical planning.

Similar to the workup of other cancers affecting the head and neck, all masses of the head and neck should be biopsied by fine needle aspiration. All palpable lymph nodes should also be sampled. Staging CT and MRI is invaluable and also guides operative planning. Triple endoscopy, which includes a direct laryngoscopy, esophagogastroduodenoscopy, and tracheobronchoscopy, should be completed for direct evaluation of all major tubular structures. Most tumors of the head and neck may present with more than one focus (i.e. synchronous cancers) and a thorough workup is necessary so that asymptomatic masses are not inadvertently missed.

Low-grade tumors should be fully resected and are more likely to lead to cure. Radiotherapy is necessary for recurrent disease but does not necessarily need to be utilized following the initial resection unless a change in tumor stage occurs. High-grade tumors should be treated with aggressive en bloc resection followed by adjuvant chemoradiation. Cancer that involves major vascular structures should still be excised whenever it is safe to do so; reconstruction of the carotid vessels may be necessary. Metastatic disease, particularly to the lungs, occurs with high-grade tumors and should be treated with resection and chemotherapy.

Cancers of the lip can be treated by resection of up to 50% of the lip with care taken to preserve the delineation and curvature of the lip. Complex flaps may be necessary if more tissue is resected. Tumors affecting the tongue should be excised with 2 cm margins and a neck dissection unless the tumor is less than 2 mm in size. All affected structures, including the mandible, should also be resected if there is invasive cancer. Tumors of the oropharynx should be treated with radiation therapy if they arelow-grade, or surgical resection and radiotherapy if they are high-grade and invasive. Laryngeal cancers are likely to present sooner due to their effect on the voice. Whenever possible, low-grade tumors should be fully resected or given radiotherapy. High-grade tumors are resected first, and then treated with radiation. Invasive cancers also require a bilateral modified radical neck dissection. Alternative management of complex laryngeal tumors is with neoadjuvant chemoradiation followed by wide local excision of any remaining tumors.

Skin cancers affecting the face are discussed separately in the Surgical Oncology chapter on page 412.

VI.D. Brain Tumors

Tumors of the central nervous system are classified according to their age of onset (juvenile vs. adult) and by source (i.e. cell line). Primary tumors of the brain are less common than tumors that are metastatic to the CNS. The latter is nearly ten times more common.

As a general rule, brain tumors present with headache, altered mental status, increase in intracranial pressure due to an expanse in the brain matter within the fixed volume of the calvarium, nausea, and seizure. Occasionally, specific cranial nerve deficits may be present depending on the origin of the tumor and the mass effects it produces.

The diagnosis is similarly universal for patients suspected of having a brain tumor. A CT scan and MRI of the brain are completed. The CT is an invaluable tool to rapidly identify hemorrhagic foci, while the MRI is an excellent imaging medium for soft tissue changes and for staging. Prior to surgery, cerebral edema should be stabilized with dexamethasone. Seizure prophylaxis with dilantin is used in most patients. Specific tumors of the CNS are discussed below.

TABLE 10. CNS tumors.

Tumor	Pathophysiology	Presentation	Treatment
Astrocytoma	Most common tumor Typically found in cerebellum Infiltrative, enhancing tumor	Low-grade in children Glioblastoma multiforme in older adults Seizures	Radical resection, external beam radiotherapy High grade tumors have a 2-3 year survival
Oligodendroglioma	Primarily affects the frontal lobe "Fried egg" appearance	Seizures	Surgical resection and chemotherapy
Meningioma	Slow growing, benign, typically asymptomatic Psammoma bodies	Asymptomatic	Surgical resection, radiotherapy
Schwannoma	Benign tumors, commonly at vestibulocochlear nerve	Tinnitus, loss of balance, change in hearing	Resection and radiotherapy

Head and Neck Surgery

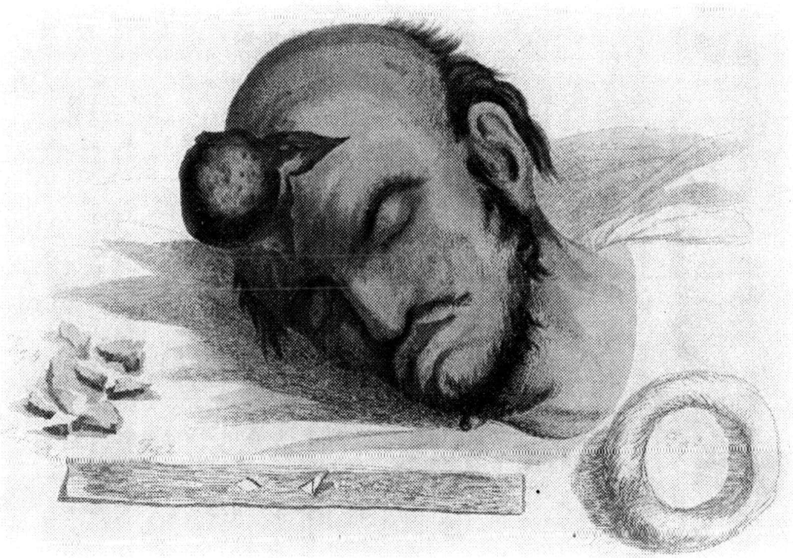

THORACIC

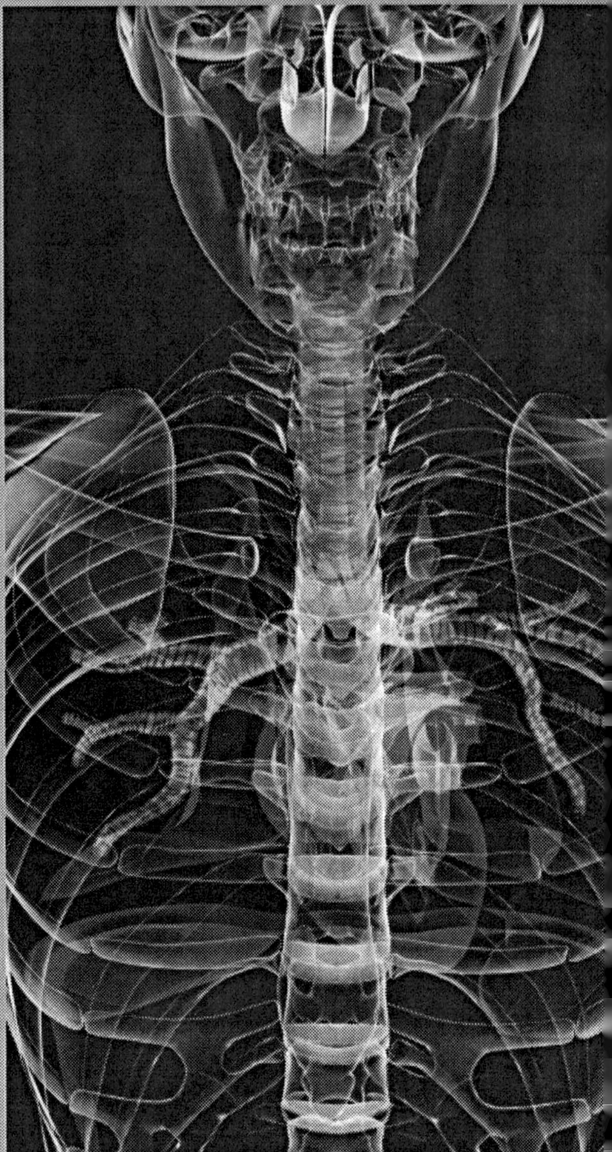

Operative surgery, which was formerly in the hands of a few privileged persons, is becoming more and more the common property of medical men.

Theodor Kocher
Textbook of Operative Surgery, 1903

SURGISPHERE

THORACIC SURGERY

Judson B. Williams, M.D., and Charles E. Murphy, M.D.

I. General Concepts

I.A. Anatomy

1. Lung

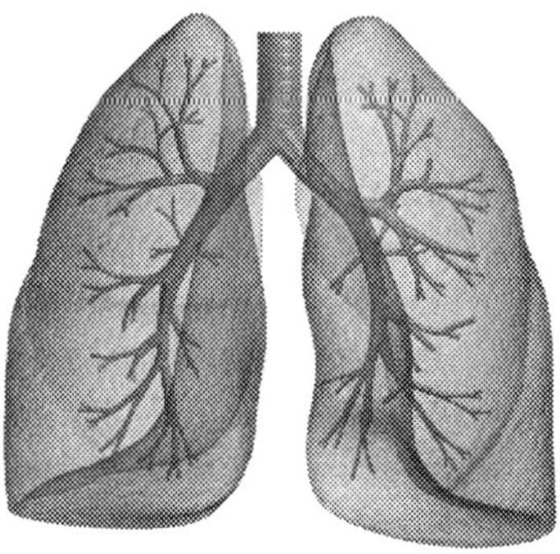

The right lung has three lobes—the upper, middle, and lower. The horizontal fissure separates the upper from the middle lobe, and the oblique fissure separates the lower lobe from the middle lobe.

The left lung has only two lobes—the upper and lower lobes separated by an oblique fissure. The lingula represents a portion of the left upper lobe and is the embryologic correlate of the right middle lobe.

2. Alveoli

Type I cells comprise 90% of the alveolar lining and take part in gas exchange. Type II cells secrete surfactant to decrease the surface tension, maintaining alveolar stability and preventing atelectasis and edema. Type III cells are immune cells that destroy foreign invaders.

3. Esophagus

Unlike the other layers of the alimentary tract, the esophagus has no serosal layer. The layers of the esophagus include the innermost mucosa (which includes the epithelium, the lamina propria, and the muscularis mucosa), the submucosa, the muscularis propria (the inner circular and outer longitudinal muscle layers), and the adventitia. The mucosal layer consists of squamous epithelium for most of its course until it transitions to junctional columnar epithelium at the distal 1-2 cm of the esophagus, known as the Z-line. The submucosal neural plexus is known as Meissner plexus; the muscular propria neural plexus is known as Auerbach plexus. The outer muscular layer consists of striated muscle in the upper esophagus, a mixture of striated and smooth muscle fibers in its midportion, with a transition to smooth muscle in the distal esophagus.

I.B. Physiology

a) Pulmonary Function Testing

Pulmonary function tests (PFTs) measure different aspects of lung volumes and flow rates. These reflect the mechanical properties of lung elasticity, recoil, and compliance. The specific measures include the total lung capacity (TLC), residual volume (RV), forced expiratory volume over 1 second (FEV_1), forced vital capacity (FVC), and midmaximal forced expiratory flow (FEF). The diffusion capacity of carbon monoxide (DL_{CO}) is a measure of the efficiency of gas exchange from alveoli to blood. The DL_{CO} is decreased with interstitial lung disease and emphysema. DL_{CO} levels less than 40% of predicted are associated with increased perioperative risk. Bronchial hyperreactivity is tested with a methacholine challenge test, and is contraindicated in asthmatics. FEV_1 (or other PFT measures) may be expressed as an actual value such as 0.9 liter per second or as a percentage of the predicted values based on height and weight in normal patients. By accounting for body habitus, the percent predicted value is more accurate.

PFTs are required before lung resection and must have a predicted post-op FEV_1 greater than 0.8. An FEV_1 > 2 L is required prior to pneumonectomy, > 1 L for a lobectomy, and 0.6 L for a wedge resection. If the FEV_1 is less than 60% predicted, then a quantitative xenon-133 ventilation-perfusion lung scan may be considered to quantify the contribution of each lung to overall pulmonary function and improve the accuracy of predicted postoperative pulmonary function.

b) Lung Volumes

The total lung capacity (TLC) is the entire volume of air that the lung can retain with maximal inspiration. Residual volume (RV) is the remaining volume after maximum expiration, and is a volume of air that is always present in the lung. The vital capacity (VC) is the difference in volume between the TLC and RV. The functional reserve capacity (FRC) is the volume that remains after a normal exhalation and includes the RV. The inspiratory capacity (IC) is the maximum inspiratory volume that can be taken in with

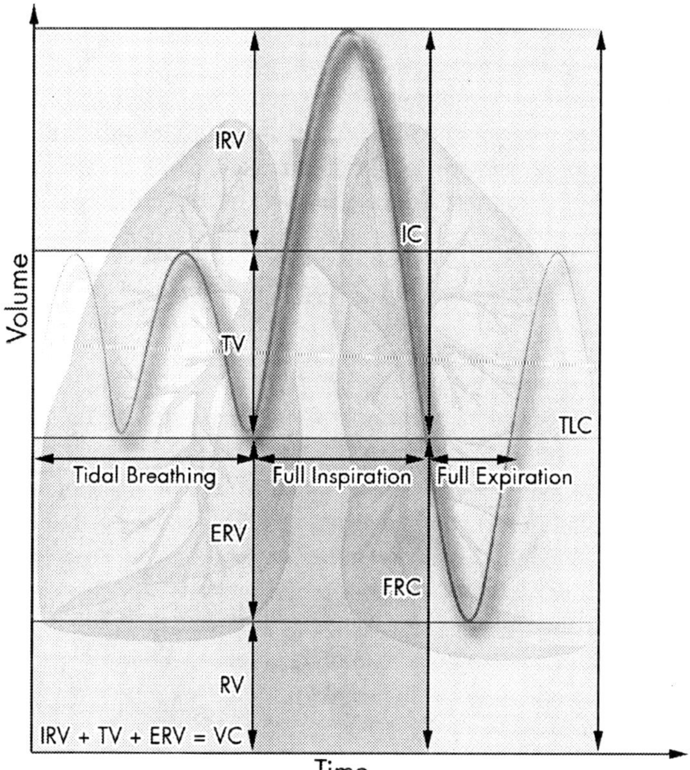

a normal breath. The IC and FRC add up to the TLC as does the VC plus the RV. With a normal breath, the inspiration is known as the tidal volume (VT). The additional volume that is available for inspiration is known as the inspiratory reserve volume (IRV), while the additional volume available for expiration is the expiratory reserve volume. The IRV plus VT plus ERV equal the VC.

Improving oxygenation can be done by "recruiting" additional alveoli to participate in gas exchange. This is done by increasing the positive end-expiratory pressure (PEEP), which in turn increases FRC.

In restrictive disease, the FEV_1/FVC ratio is approximately normal - both FEV_1 and FVC are reduced. In obstructive disease, the FEV_1/FVC ratio is low - FEV_1 is low, and FVC is high.

c) Oxygenation and Delivery

Disorders with gas exchange can lead to impaired oxygen delivery to vital tissues and present with symptoms of hypoxia. Oxygen transport relies on sufficient cardiac output (CO) and hemoglobin (Hgb) of sufficient saturation and quantity. In patients with low CO or Hgb, giving the patient 100% oxygen does little to improve the oxygenation. Calculating oxygenation can be done with the alveolar-arteriolar gradient:

$$PAO_2 = 150 - (PaCO_2 \div 0.8)$$

$$\text{A-a gradient} = PAO_2 - PaO_2$$

Faulty gas exchange can manifest as hypoxia. Causes of hypoxia can be attributed to: (1) ventilation-perfusion (V/Q) mismatch leading to poorly ventilated alveoli or ventilation of poorly perfused alveoli; (2) a right to left cardiac shunt that moves poorly oxygenated blood into the systemic circulation; (3) anemia that leads to decreased oxygen carrying capacity in the blood and poor oxygenation; (4) poor perfusion from MI or shock; (5) increased oxygen demand without a compensatory increase in supply; (6) impairment in oxygen delivery due to cyanide or carbon monoxide poisoning; and (7) low inspired oxygen at higher altitudes.

The most significant contributor to oxygen carrying capacity is hemoglobin. Increasing PO_2 over 100 increases oxygen only slightly via increased dissolved oxygen in the blood. Fe^{3+} improves oxygen delivery. Oxygen delivery is defined as the amount of oxygen made available to the body in one minute. It is equal to the cardiac output times the arterial oxygen content. This is approximately 1 L O_2 per minute.

Oxygen consumption is the amount of oxygen used every minute. Approximately 25% of the arterial oxygen is used every minute (95%+ saturation of blood leaving the heart, about 70% saturation of venous blood returning to the heart). Oxygen extraction decreases with the volume of oxygen, as it becomes harder to remove oxygen from insufficiently populated hemoglobin molecules. SVO_2 increases with an increase in cardiac output. Oxygen extraction increases with sepsis, leading to a greater A-V oxygen gradient.

d) Oxygen-Hemoglobin Dissociation Curve

Table 1. Oxygen-Hemoglobin Dissociation Curve Factors

Variable	Right Shift	Left Shift
Temperature	High	Low
2,3 DPG	High	Low
PCO_2	High	Low
PCO	Low	High
pH	Acidosis	Alkalosis
Hemoglobin	Adult hemoglobin	Fetal hemoglobin

Thoracic Surgery

II. Esophagus

II.A. Congenital and Structural

1. Achalasia

a) Epidemiology

Achalasia literally means "failure to relax." Achalasia is due to increased LES tone and failure of normal peristalsis of the esophagus, leading to severe dysphagia with solid foods and liquids. Achalasia affects males and females equally. The incidence is 6 per 100,000 persons per year.

b) Pathophysiology

Achalasia stems from a loss of conducting neurons in the esophagus. These neurons are responsible for maintaining the normal progression of peristalsis. Loss of these neurons within Auerbach's plexus is due to scarring, and the primary cause of the scarring is presently being explored. Secondary causes of this scarring can be attributed to invasive lymphoma or gastric carcinoma, scleroderma, and Chagas disease (Chagas leads to dilated cardiomyopathy, toxic megacolon, and achalasia). Normal pressures at the LES range from 10-20mmHg with a length of 3-5 cm.

c) Presentation

Dysphagia, regurgitation, and weight loss represent the classic triad of presenting symptoms. Heartburn, regurgitation of food, postprandial choking, and nocturnal coughing are also seen. Diffuse chest pain may be described after the consumption of food. Dysphagia typically progresses over a number of years and patients adapt by eating slowly and with large volumes of liquids to wash food down. Regurgitation of malodorous undigested food and signs of chronic aspiration such as recurrent pneumonias may be seen.

d) Diagnosis

Diagnosis of achalasia is made by barium swallow, which identifies a dilated esophagus and a bird-beak narrowing at the distal aspect. The narrowing at the inferior aspect occurs as a result of failure of the LES to relax. Manometry is the gold standard test to diagnose achalasia. Findings include a normal to high pressure at the LES with no change after swallowing. Esophagogastroduodenoscopy (EGD) is required to rule out gastric carcinoma and lymphoma, two infrequent causes of achalasia (about 1% of patients with gastric carcinoma have achalasia). The typical gastric bubble is commonly missing on plain films of the abdomen.

e) Treatment

Nonsurgical treatments for achalasia include: the use of nitroglycerin, nitrates, or calcium-channel blockers to relieve symptoms, and injection of botulinum toxin into the LES to block acetylcholine-induced muscle contraction. Botulinum toxin injections are successful in about ⅔s of patients, but must be repeated over time.

Surgical treatment includes pneumatic dilation at the LES that tears the muscle fibers (and thereby decreases LES pressure), and permits the semi-normal transport of food and liquid to the stomach. Balloon dilation of the LES can cause perforation in about 1-2% of patients. A post-procedure esophagogram is mandatory to rule out a perforation. Surgical esophagomyotomy is considered superior to balloon dilation.

The operation of choice is the modified laparosopic Heller myotomy. Ten to thirty percent of patients will suffer reflux postoperatively. Most surgeons choose to perform an antireflux procedure (usually a partial fundoplication) to decrease the frequency of this complication. Esophagectomy is considered in patients who have failed multiple myotomies, have an undilatable stricture, or a tortuous esophagus.

2. Diffuse Esophageal Spasm

a) Epidemiology

Diffuse esophageal spasm (DES) presents in a similar fashion to achalasia and is often found in patients with multiple complaints. DES is five times less common than achalasia and is seen most commonly in women.

b) Pathophysiology and Presentation

DES is a generalized spasm of the esophagus secondary to failure of activity of the inhibitory neurons within Auerbach's plexus. Spontaneous contractions of the esophagus occur that do not resemble peristalsis. The diffuse contractions in DES lead to dysphagia and chest pain. Acid reflux is usually not seen but regurgitation of saliva and esophageal contents is common.

c) Diagnosis

Diagnosis of DES is made by barium swallow and manometry. Barium swallow reveals a corkscrew-like pattern due to the uncoordinated activity of various parts of the esophagus. Large waves are seen after swallowing. Manometry confirms the uncoordinated activity of the esophagus and detects high amplitude contractions that may extend into the upper ⅓ of the esophagus. The LES is typically at normal or slightly low pressure.

d) Treatment

Fewer treatments are available for DES than for achalasia. Nonsurgical management is the mainstay of treatment with calcium-channel blockers, nitroglycerin, and anticholinergics sometimes giving relief. A randomized, double-blinded crossover trial demonstrated the effectiveness of diltiazem in relieving chest pain. Elimination of trigger foods and treatment of any gastric reflux are essential. Bougie dilation and botulinum toxin injections are also used.

3. Nutcracker Esophagus

a) Epidemiology

Nutcracker esophagus is the most common esophageal hypermotility disorder and is the most painful. It occurs is patients of all ages with equal gender distribution.

b) Pathophysiology and Presentation

Nutcracker esophagus is due to high-amplitude contractions that arise from increased activity of the neurons within the esophageal plexuses. It presents similarly to DES, with dysphagia, diffuse chest pain, and large waves of contraction.

c) Diagnosis and Treatment

Nutcracker esophagus is diagnosed by manometry, which indicates high-amplitude peristaltic contractions. Barium swallow distinguishes between nutcracker esophagus and DES, as the latter has a corkscrew appearance. Treatment is similar to that of DES with the use of nitroglycerin, calcium-channel blockers, and anticholinergics for temporary relief of acute spasms.

4. Esophageal Rings and Webs

a) Etiology and Pathophysiology

Schatzki rings and Plummer-Vinson syndrome are two of the most common anatomic esophageal obstructions. Schatzki rings are narrow mucosal rings located in the lower esophagus just proximal to the LES with concomitant dysphagia. Schatzki rings affect both males and females, and appear to target individuals with pre-existing symptoms of intermittent dysphagia. Nearly 10% of are asymptomatic.

Esophageal webs are thin membranous structures that occlude the lumen. They may be congenital or acquired. Plummer-Vinson syndrome is characterized by hypopharyngeal webs in conjunction with iron-deficiency anemia. It is most common in middle-aged women. Plummer-Vinson syndrome presents with complaints of dysphagia immediately after swallowing food.

b) Diagnosis and Treatment

Both Plummer-Vinson syndrome and Schatzki rings are diagnosed with barium swallow. The preferred method of treating a Schatzki ring is balloon dilation. Plummer-Vinson syndrome often requires more involved surgical management. Complications of Plummer-Vinson syndrome include an elevated risk of squamous cell carcinoma.

5. Zenker Diverticulum

a) Etiology and Pathophysiology

Zenker diverticulum is the presence of a mucosal pouch extending outside of the esophagus due to a defect in the muscular layer. These diverticuli are located between the lower inferior constrictor and cricopharyngeus muscles. They occur at the junction between the posterior hypopharynx and the esophagus, just above the upper esophageal sphincter.

b) Presentation and Diagnosis

Zenker diverticulum presents with halitosis, regurgitation of foul-smelling food, and esophageal obstruction leading to dysphagia. Noisy eating with progressive dysphagia is a hallmark. Diagnosis is by barium swallow that identifies the outpouching as a contrast-filled region. Endoscopy and intubation should not be done due to the risk of perforation.

c) Treatment

Surgical treatment options include: (1) diverticulectomy, (2) cricopharyngeal myotomy with diverticulectomy or diverticulopexy, or (3) cricopharyngeal myotomy. Most experts recommend performance of a cricopharyngeal myotomy during definitive surgery. Long-term good or excellent results are found in 90% of patients with a recurrence rate of only 3-4%. Intraluminal techniques using rigid or flexible endoscopes to divide the wall between the diverticulum and esophagus with a variety of coagulation and cutting devices or staplers have also been reported with good outcomes. The presence of a large diverticulum is a relative contraindication to these procedures, because of poor emptying of the resultant pharyngeal cavity.

II.B. Inflammatory and Infectious

1. Gastroesophageal Reflux Disease

a) Epidemiology

According to a journal article in "Gastroenterology", gastroesophageal reflux disease (GERD) affects nearly 20% of the population on a weekly basis, and nearly 40% of people on a monthly basis. GERD increases the risk of developing Barrett's esophagus and subsequently, esophageal adenocarcinoma.

b) Pathophysiology

Gastroesophageal reflux disease is predominantly due to incompetence of the lower esophageal sphincter (LES), leading to reflux of stomach contents into the esophagus. Other causes include the presence of a hiatal hernia, delayed emptying of the stomach, and decreased motility of the esophagus.

c) LES Incompetence

Failure of the LES to properly function may be attributed to one or more causes. The high level of progesterone in pregnancy contributes a great deal to the symptoms of heartburn and substernal burning in these patients. Consumption of acidic foods and fatty foods, in addition to chocolate, peppermint, alcohol, and coffee can exacerbate LES dysfunction and potentiate the symptoms of GERD. Smoking has also been linked to a decrease in LES tone. Finally, a variety of medications that have effects on muscle tone, such as calcium-channel blockers, β-blockers, anticholinergics, nitrates, and theophylline have been implicated as having a negative effect on maintaining the tone of the LES.

d) Presentation

The signs and symptoms of GERD include heartburn, dysphagia, increased salivation, cough, and asthma-like symptoms. The hydrochloric acid secreted by the stomach travels up the esophagus due to LES incompetence, and leads to a burning feeling in the epigastric or substernal region, known as heartburn. This pain may occasionally present as chest pain, and GERD should be in the differential diagnosis of angina and chest pain. Dysphagia in GERD is often a result of the formation of anatomic defects in the esophagus, such as webs and strictures. Increased salivation in GERD leads to a water brash. Cough in GERD is often dry and non-productive. GERD may also exacerbate underlying asthma or may present as symptoms of asthma in certain individuals.

e) Diagnosis

Diagnosis of GERD is made by a careful consideration of the history and confirmed through the use of a 24-hour pH probe, barium swallow, esophagoscopy, and biopsy. The latter tests are more commonly used in longstanding cases of GERD to rule out histologic changes that may lead to the formation of adenocarcinoma and to detect any underlying anatomical defects. Endoscopy with biopsy is recommended to evaluate patients with GERD symptoms who fail empiric treatment with twice-daily PPI. Manometry is recommended in this group of patients who have normal endoscopy. Patients who then have normal manometry should undergo pH probe monitoring.

f) Treatment

GERD is treated by inducing lifestyle changes in the patient in conjunction with the use of medications. In patients highly compliant with lifestyle changes, the use of medications may not be necessary. Lifestyle modifications include obese patients losing weight, promoting the consumption of smaller meals to avoid overburdening the stomach and thereby minimizing reflux, discontinuing foods which precipitate reflux, and cessation of smoking. Eating several hours before bedtime to allow food to travel to the small intestine and elevating the head of the bed can be recommended in patients with symptoms of nighttime reflux. A Nissen fundoplication should be performed in patients who are intolerant of PPIs or who have persistent symptoms despite good medical therapy. Significant retching following this repair requires a gastrograffin swallow study to ensure that the wrap is not too tight. Fundoplication has an 80% success rate.

g) Medications

The first line of medications that is often tried by patients is oral antacids, such as Mylanta and Tums. In GERD that is refractory to lifestyle changes and over-the-counter medications, H_2 blockers and/or proton pump inhibitors are commonly used. H_2 blockers tend to be curative in about half of all patients, while proton pump inhibitors are even more successful. In patients with an identified anatomical defect, or those who are refractory to medical management, Nissen fundoplication can be used to position the stomach around the lower esophageal sphincter to allow the normal contractions of the stomach and to keep the LES closed.

h) Complications

GERD is commonly thought of as a relatively benign complaint, but serious complications can develop over a long period of time, if GERD is not appropriately managed. GERD can lead to esophageal damage, which can lead to bleeding and friability. These inflammatory changes are known as esophagitis. In about 10% of patients, peptic strictures can form that further heighten the symptoms of dysphagia. Columnar cell metaplasia of the lower ⅔s of the esophagus can also occur in a condition known as Barrett esophagus. This transformation from the normal squamous cell epithelium predisposes individuals to developing adenocarcinoma of the esophagus. Finally, continuing smoking in the face of GERD, in conjunction with damage to the upper ⅓ of the esophagus, can lead to the development of squamous cell carcinoma.

2. Scleroderma

a) Etiology and Pathophysiology

Scleroderma is the autoimmune disorder that causes significant fibrosis throughout the body with numerous systemic effects. Induction of collagen production and a general increase in the extracellular matrix (ECM) proteins leads to diffuse fibrosis that affects numerous organs.

b) Presentation

Scleroderma occasionally presents with the CREST syndrome, including calcinosis, Raynaud phenomenon, esophageal dysmotility, sclerodactyly, and telangiectasis. The esophageal dysmotility that may occur with scleroderma and the CREST syndrome is similar to achalasia in that fibrotic changes of the esophagus lead to dysphagia and defects in peristalsis. Unlike achalasia, the LES is incompetent.

Esophageal dysmotility in scleroderma presents with progressive dysphagia from solids to liquids and GERD from LES incompetence. Skin changes are among the initial changes detected and lead to a wrinkling and aged appearance in an otherwise younger person. Fibrosis of arteries can lead to malignant HTN. Pulmonary HTN occurs due to fibrosis of pulmonary vessels, which can lead to right heart failure. Telangiectasiae are noted throughout the body. Other causes for esophageal dysmotility include SLE, polymyositis, and dermatomyositis.

c) Diagnosis and Treatment

Esophageal dysmotility in scleroderma is diagnosed with a barium swallow, which demonstrates decreased peristalsis in the lower ⅔ of the esophagus and decreased smooth muscle contraction on manometry and motility studies. Treatment consists of minimizing the symptoms of GERD, but there is no known treatment for the esophageal dysmotility. Diagnosis is confirmed by the presence of an SCL-70 antibody to topoisomerase, antibodies to centromeres and various components of the nuclei, a normocytic normochromic anemia, elevations in ESR and CRP, and restrictive lung disease (diminished VC on PFT).

II.C. Trauma

1. Esophageal Perforation

a) Etiology and Pathophysiology

Perforation or rupture of the esophagus is commonly due to trauma to the esophagus, whether through medical procedures or severe vomiting. Iatrogenic causes are the most frequent (60%), followed by traumatic (20%) and idiopathic (15%). Common iatrogenic causes include endoscopy, esophageal dilation, the use of Blakemore tubes, intubation of the esophagus instead of the trachea, and the use of nasogastric (NG) tubes. Leakage of air and ingested contents may occur into the mediastinum, causing mediastinitis and rampant infection. Treatment involves primary repair with drainage of the mediastinum and NGT decompression. A Nissen repair is performed for abdominal esophagus perforations. Early detection and surgical repair within the first 24 hours results in approximately 80% survival but survival decreases to less than 50% when repair is delayed beyond 24 hours.

b) Boerhaave Syndrome

Esophageal rupture following emesis is known as Boerhaave syndrome. Boerhaave syndrome is a full-thickness tear of the esophagus, usually located in the left posterolateral portion of the distal ⅓ of the esophagus. Presentation of Boerhaave syndrome is typically with severe chest pain following retching. Mortality approaches 90% with a delay in diagnosis over 36 hours.

c) Mallory-Weiss Tear

Mallory-Weiss tears of the esophagus are usually not associated with perforation. Mallory-Weiss tears of the esophagus most commonly occur at the squamocolumnar junction near the LES. This is a partial-thickness tear that is commonly on the right posterolateral portion of the distal ⅓ esophagus.

Patients usually present with transient upper GI bleeding following forceful vomiting or retching. Active bleeding can usually be managed by endoscopic methods including hemoclipping, band ligation, electric coagulation, or local epinephrine injection. Surgery, in which the bleeding vessel is oversewn, is rarely required.

d) Presentation

Boerhaave syndrome generally presents with the sudden onset of severe pain that radiates to the chest, back, and abdomen following an episode of retching or vomiting. Dyspnea, tachypnea, and cyanosis often occur. Mediastinal and subcutaneous emphysema are often present in Boerhaave syndrome due to the leakage of air from the esophagus into those areas. Mediastinal emphysema presents with a crunching sound over the precordium known as Hamman's crunch. Chest or abdominal pain after vomiting requires a gastrograffin swallow study in appropriate patients to diagnose this type of tear.

e) Diagnosis

The diagnosis of esophageal perforation is suspected in the appropriate clinical setting, and frequently with a patient who appears profoundly ill. A chest X-ray (CXR) may demonstrate mediastinal or subcutaneous emphysema and usually a pleural effusion and pneumothorax. An esophagogram with water-soluble contrast (Gastrograffin) is the diagnostic test of choice and will show extravasation of contrast outside the esophagus. Barium is not used due to the risk of chemical mediastinitis. Endoscopy and other studies may also be done. Emergent surgical repair is required for all episodes of Boerhaave syndrome.

f) Treatment

Esophageal perforation requires stabilization and resuscitation in an ICU setting. Stable patients who have had perforation for less than 24 hours are candidates for surgical intervention. A free perforation of the cervical esophagus can be treated with primary repair via a left cervical incision, internal drainage, and external drainage. An upper GI series should be repeated within one week.

Free perforation of the thoracic esophagus if less than 24 hour old can be approached via a right thoracotomy if located superiorly, or left thoracotomy if located inferiorly. A two layer closure with intercostal muscle flap, internal drainage, and chest tube placement are required. An esophagogram is completed within 1 week, and a soft diet is started at 3 weeks.

Patients with free perforation of the esophagus longer than 24-48 hours tend to have a significant amount of mediastinitis and an inflammatory reaction unfavorable for primary repair. The majority of these patients will require a cervical esophagostomy, esophagectomy, internal and external drainage, and a feeding G-J tube. A gastric pull-through and potential esophagogastric anastomosis can be completed several months later in selected patients.

Contained perforations of the esophagus are unusual and are managed conservatively. Nil per os, TPN, and potential drainage are necessary. Selected patients can have a primary repair completed if detected early. A contrast study should be completed within one week to evaluate the esophagus.

II.D. Cancer

1. Barrett Esophagus

a) Pathophysiology

Barrett esophagus is the transformation of squamous cell epithelium to mucus-producing columnar cell epithelium. This transformation is due to an attempt by the body to protect the lower esophagus from continuing damage due to acid reflux from an incompetent LES. Barrett esophagus occurs due to chronic reflux and over a period of time of continuing symptoms. These metaplastic changes are most common in patients with GERD, affecting some 20% of these patients. Barrett metaplasia is a strong positive predictor of adenocarcinoma, carrying a relative risk of 30 times that of normal. The risk of developing esophageal cancer is estimated at 0.5% per year. The presence of Barrett metaplasia plus dysplasia is known as Orringer syndrome.

b) Diagnosis and Treatment

Diagnosis of Barrett esophagus is made by examining biopsy specimens for columnar cell epithelium superior to the LES. Biopsies should be performed in all 4 quadrants of each 2 cm length of Barrett esophagus. Initial treatment is to limit the symptoms of GERD with medication. Proton pump inhibitors are favored in this population. There is no convincing data that aggressive medical therapy reduces the incidence of cancer. Anti-reflux surgery is indicated if the reflux is refractory to medical management. Randomized studies have not shown a reduction in cancer prevalence with surgical versus medical therapy. The initial surveillance endoscopy should be performed within one year of the endoscopy which established the diagnosis. If no dysplastic changes are present on two consecutive endoscopies, then EGD should be repeated every 3 years. If low-grade dysplasia is present, EGD should be repeated every 6 months.

Finally, in patients with the finding of high-grade dysplasia, repeat endoscopy with biopsies should occur in 3 months. High-grade dysplasia is a strong predictor of adenocarcinoma. The patient should also be counseled regarding the treatment options for high-grade dysplasia. No management strategy has demonstrated a survival benefit. Treatment options include: (1) esophagectomy (3% operative mortality in high-volume centers); (2) endoscopic ablation therapies (including laser and photodynamic ablation); (3) endoscopic mucosal resection; and (4) intensive surveillance therapy with invasive treatments reserved for biopsy-proven cancer. Therapy in this setting remains controversial. The risk of adenocarcinoma is worsened with concomitant Barrett esophagus with metaplasia extending about six inches, dysplastic changes, and a history of smoking.

2. Leiomyoma

Leiomyomas are often asymptomatic, but sometimes present with retrosternal pain or dysphagia. Leiomyomas present as smooth filling defects on barium swallow. Indications for enucleation include size over 5 cm or the presence of symptoms. Resection is completed via a right thoracotomy if the filling defect is in the middle esophagus, or via a left thoracotomy if in the lower esophagus. Biopsy should not be done.

3. Esophageal Cancer

a) Epidemiology and Etiology

The most common type of esophageal carcinoma is adenocarcinoma (60-85%), which is typically associated with Barrett's esophagus and occurs more frequently in Caucasian males. Squamous cell carcinoma is more common in African American males over the age of 40 and with a history of smoking. Adenocarcinoma is more likely to occur in the distal ⅓ of the esophagus, while squamous cell carcinoma is more likely in the proximal ⅓ of the esophagus. Adenocarcinoma and squamous cell carcinoma have approximately equal incidence in the middle ⅓ of the esophagus.

b) Pathophysiology

Squamous cell carcinoma has a number of risk factors, including a history of alcohol consumption, a long-standing history of smoking, esophageal motility disorders such as achalasia, anatomic defects such as Plummer-Vinson syndrome, and consumption of carcinogens such as foods rich in nitrates and certain spices. The risk factor with the largest positive predictive value for squamous cell carcinoma is smoking.

c) Presentation

With squamous cell carcinoma and adenocarcinoma, the esophageal cancer spreads inward circumferentially to cause progressive dysphagia. Initially, the dysphagia occurs with solid foods, but it progresses with time to affect the transport of liquids in the esophagus. The decrease in food consumption, in addition to the effects of the cancer, leads to weight loss, poor nutritional status, and substernal or back pain. Hypercalcemia is sometimes present in patients with squamous cell carcinoma, which may be related to the production of a parathyroid hormone-related protein.

d) Diagnosis

Diagnosis of esophageal cancer is often initially made through barium swallow, which demonstrates an intraluminal mass with jagged edges. Upper endoscopy allows direct visualization and biopsy of the mass. Endoscopic ultrasound establishes the depth of penetration of the tumor through the wall of the esophagus and detects the presence of enlarged periesophageal nodes. Bronchoscopy may be necessary to rule out invasion of the tracheobronchial tree in cancers involving the upper and middle thirds of the esophagus. PET scans are indicated to look for the presence of distant metastases.

e) Treatment

Surgery has historically been the definitive treatment of early stage esophageal cancer. Options include a transhiatal esophagectomy (THE) versus a transthoracic esophagectomy (TTE). Advantages of THE include avoiding a chest incision and creating the anastomosis in the neck. This avoids a potentially devastating intrathoracic leak. The operation has been criticized for not being as good a cancer operation as the TTE, but studies indicate no difference in survival between the two procedures. Modern series put the 5-year survival rate at 15-20%. Perioperative mortality rates are lower in high-volume centers and are in the 5% range. Recent data demonstrate improved survival with neoadjuvant chemoradiation.

Contraindications to surgery include: (1) metastases to N2 nodes or solid organs; (2) invasion of adjacent structures; and (3) severe comorbid conditions. Cisplatin based chemotherapy and radiation therapy has demonstrated a survival benefit versus radiation alone. Current studies are looking at the additional benefit of induction chemotherapy versus traditional chemotherapy, but no definite conclusions can yet be made. The benefit of post-chemoradiation surgery is controversial. Two trials demonstrated equivalent 2 year survival and quality of life; however, there were more local failures in the chemoradiation cohort (40-50%).

The goal of palliation is to treat dysphagia. Dysphagia is improved in 50% of patients treated with radiation alone. This result is improved by the addition of concurrent chemotherapy, which gives ⅔ of patients good palliation until death. Other options include laser therapy with the Nd:YAG laser with good relief of dysphagia in 70% of patients. The development of a tracheoesophegeal fistula is associated with a dismal prognosis. These patients are usually treated with stents.

III. Diaphragm and Mediastinum

III.A. Congenital and Structural

1. Pneumomediastinum

a) Pathophysiology

Pneumomediastinum, sometimes referred to as mediastinal emphysema, is the result of air in the mediastinum. It is commonly due to rupture of the esophagus, alveolar rupture (with dissection of air retrograde along the airways rather than into the pleural space), or damage to the tracheobronchial tree.

b) Diagnosis

This diagnosis is established by air in the mediastinum on either plain films or CT scans of the chest. Hamman's sign is present in 50% of the cases. The presence of pneumomediastinum should prompt a targeted work-up to look for the source. A patient with recent vomiting should undergo a gastrograffin swallow to rule out a leak. A blunt trauma patient would undergo bronchoscopy to rule out a tracheobronchial injury.

c) Treatment

The underlying cause of the pneumomediastinum should be corrected.

III.B. Inflammatory and Infectious

1. Mediastinitis

a) Assessment

Inflammation of the mediastinum may be due to: (1) rupture of the esophagus; (2) anthrax infection leading to hemorrhage (nearly 100% fatal); (3) infection by TB or Histoplasma; (4) extension of infection from the neck (peritonsillar abscess); and as a (5) complication of cardiac surgery. Mediastinitis presents with symptoms including fever, chills, chest pain, and shortness of breath. Significant leukocytosis is usually present. CT scans of the chest may demonstrate fluid collections or air within the mediastinum. Needle aspiration of fluid collections may be helpful in some cases.

b) Management

Mediastinitis requires prompt medical and often surgical attention. The underlying etiology is rapidly treated with antibiotics and surgical drainage as necessary.

III.C. Cancer

1. Lymphomas

a) Hodgkin Disease

(1) *Etiology and Pathophysiology*

Hodgkin lymphoma (HL) is a distinct malignant lymphoma with a clonal B-cell population proliferating as Reed-Sternberg (RS) cells. These cells propagate the effects of HL while numerous inflammatory cells lead to local insult and injury. HL accounts for less than 1% of all cancers and has a good

5 year survival rate, if caught early. It is more common in Caucasian males. It has been postulated that infection by EBV is a predecessor to HL.

(2) *Presentation and Diagnosis*

HL presents with supradiaphragmatic lymphadenopathy (typically seen in the neck and axilla), numerous constitutional symptoms, chest pain, intermittent fever, and pruritus. Hepatosplenomegaly is typically evident on physical exam. On laboratory workup, ESR and LDH are elevated. CBC typically indicates an anemia of chronic disease. CT scans are used to identify the extent of disease, and flow cytometry is the key for diagnosis. The most common site for a single positive lymph node is the axilla. Stage 2B disease indicates presence of supraclavicular and mediastinal lymph nodes without abdominal disease in a symptomatic patient. Staging requires a laparotomy except in Stage I disease; however, this procedure is becoming less common with the advent of sensitive MRI and CT scans.

Table 2. Hodgkin Lymphoma Staging

Stage	Features
Stage I	Single lymph node or single extralymphatic site involvement
Stage II	Two or more lymph nodes on the same side of the diaphragm or one lymph node region and one contiguous extralymphatic site
Stage III	Involvement of lymph nodes on either side of the diaphragm (including spleen), or limited contiguous extralymphatic organ involvement
Stage IV	Disseminated disease in extralymphatic organs

(3) *Treatment*

HL is treated with radiation and chemotherapy. The MOPP or ABVD regimen is often used; MOPP stands for the trade names of mechlorethamine, vincristine, procarbazine, and prednisone and ABVD stands for adriamycin, bleomycin, vinblastine, and dicarbazine. Other regimens are also used for HL therapy. One side effect of bleomycin is pulmonary fibrosis. Adriamycin leads to DNA template disruption and the formation of free radicals. Vinblastine leads to inhibition of mitosis via tubulin binding and subsequent disruption of spindle formation. Bone marrow transplant is sometimes necessary. PET scans are used to assess the success of therapy and look for recurrence.

b) Hodgkin Disease

(1) *Etiology and Pathophysiology*

Non-Hodgkin lymphoma (NHL) is a lymphoid tumor with several distinct presentations. It may be due to malignant expansion of B cells, T cells, natural killer (NK) cells, or macrophages, but the majority are due to B cell expansion. NHL leads to over 25,000 deaths a year with over 50,000 new cases annually. Patients tend to be middle-aged adults at the time of diagnosis. Causes of NHL include: (1) a chromosomal translocation that predisposes the patient to the development of lymphoma; (2) a history of infection by EBV, human T-cell leukemia virus (HTLV), HCV, or herpesvirus 8 (HHV 8); (3) exposure to certain environmental toxins or chemotherapeutic agent; (4) various congenital causes (severe combined immunodeficiency disease [SCID]); (5) a state of chronic inflammation; or (6) H. pylori infection.

(2) *Presentation and Diagnosis*

NHL usually presents as a painless peripheral adenopathy. Other presentations include pancytopenia caused by bone marrow extension, multiple constitutional symptoms, or extranodal manifestations. Bowel obstruction may occur. Significant growth of the lymphoma may lead to cranial nerve impingement. Hepatosplenomegaly is common, and more advanced disease may also present with testicular enlargement, skin lesions, or a mediastinal mass. Workup includes a CBC to detect the extent of the pancytopenia and lymphocytosis, an LDH (which is tied to prognosis), and various enzyme function tests to screen for involvement of other organ systems. Imaging studies help to identify the extent of the tumor. Stage IV disease is confirmed by bone marrow biopsy. Laparotomy is not indicated for staging for NHL; CT scanning is sufficient.

(3) *Treatment*

Early stage NHL is treated with radiation therapy, but chemotherapy is sometimes used in high-risk patients. More advanced stages have both radiotherapy and chemotherapy with the CHOP regimen (trade names for cyclophosphamide, hydroxydaunomycin, vincristine, and prednisone) or CVP (cyclophosphamide, vincristine, and prednisone). Monoclonal antibodies such as rituximab have been used with success. More aggressive tumors are treated with high dose chemotherapy, radiotherapy, followed by BMT.

IV. Pleural Cavity

IV.A. Congenital and Structural

1. Thoracic Outlet Syndrome

Thoracic outlet syndrome may occur in neurologic, venous, or arterial forms. Anatomically, the subclavian artery, subclavian vein, or brachial plexus is compressed where it passes between the scalene muscles and over the first rib. The neurologic form is the most common, typically presenting as compression of the ulnar nerve leading to symptoms in the C8-T1 distribution. Symptoms are worsened with abduction of the arm. Nerve conduction studies are required for definitive diagnosis. Physical therapy for 2-12 months is usually effective. Venous thoracic outlet syndrome with vein thrombosis is initially treated with thrombolysis, anticoagulation, and then excision of the first rib. Effort thrombosis is also known as Paget-Schroetter disease. If suspected by history, the Adson or scalene test for thoracic outlet syndrome may be employed at bedside: the patient extends the neck maximally, turns head towards the affected side, and holds a deep breath, while the ipsilateral radial pulse is palpated/auscultated. The test is positive if pulse amplitude decreases. Thoracic outlet syndrome is discussed in more detail on page page 154.

IV.B. Metabolic and Degenerative

1. Atelectasis

a) Assessment

Collapse of a portion of the lung is one of the most common causes of early postoperative fever due to activation of alveolar macrophages and secretion of IL-1. Poor inspiratory effort in this period, lack of sufficient coughing and lung expansion, and failure to use devices that aid in inspiration and expiration have all been implicated in the development of lung collapse. Atelectasis presents with fever, tachycardia, dyspnea, tachypnea, and hypoxemia. Deviations of the trachea or elevations of the diaphragm may be present on CXR, while more significant atelectasis may have mediastinal shifts.

b) Management

Treatment of atelectasis involves incentive spirometry, inducing cough, and deep breathing in an attempt to re-expand the affected lung regions. Treating any concomitant pulmonary disorders is also necessary, along with removing any obstructions or foreign bodies via bronchoscopy. Early ambulation following surgery reduces the risk. Fever is induced by alveolar macrophages. Aspiration leading to atelectasis may be treated with nasotracheal suctioning and bronchoscopy. Positive end-expiratory pressure ventilation may be used to treat associated hypoxia..

2. Chronic Obstructive Pulmonary Disease

a) Etiology and Pathophysiology

Chronic obstructive pulmonary disease (COPD) includes emphysema and chronic bronchitis. A long-standing expiratory obstruction is present with decreases in FEV_1. COPD is an irreversible airway obstruction and presents with significant anatomical and functional changes. Chronic bronchitis presents with a chronic productive cough for at least three months within a two year period. Emphysema presents with airway enlargement distal to the terminal bronchioles. COPD is more common in men and carries a greater mortality in Caucasians. The most common cause of COPD is smoking, followed by air pollution, infection, allergy, and alpha-1-antitrypsin deficiency. Up to 90% of patients with COPD are smokers. Alpha-1-antitrypsin deficiency is an autosomal recessive disorder that is more common in patients of Mediterranean descent. Liver abnormalities are commonly present in this disorder. The underlying pathophysiology of COPD is increased airway resistance in bronchitis, and decreased lung recoil in emphysema. Patients with chronic bronchitis are typically known as blue bloaters and present with right heart failure, polycythemia, and high PCO_2 with low O_2 on ABG. Patients with emphysema are typically known as pink puffers with a barrel chest, anorexic appearance, and a low PCO_2 with normal PO_2 on ABG. Congenital lobar emphysema is accompanied by compression of normal alveoli.

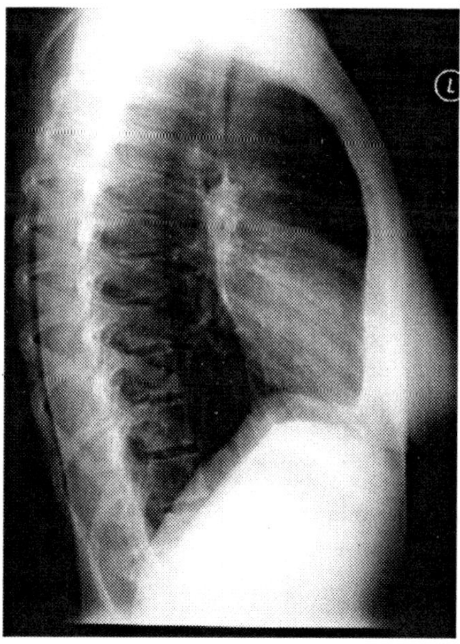

b) Presentation and Diagnosis

The diagnosis of COPD is established by physical exam, CXR, and PFTs. Chronic bronchitis presents with ronchi and wheezes upon auscultation; emphysema presents with distant breath sounds. The CXR shows increased pulmonary markings with chronic bronchitis. Emphysematous changes on CXR include lung hyperinflation, flattening of the diaphragms, small heart size, and increased retrosternal space. PFTs indicate an increased TLC and RV, but a reduction in FEV_1, FVC, and FEF. DL_{CO} is decreased in emphysema. As COPD is irreversible, there is typically little change in FEV_1: FVC after administration of bronchodilators. Obtaining PFTs is the diagnostic method of choice for COPD.

c) Treatment

COPD is primarily treated with oxygenation via home oxygen support. The goal is to maintain PaO_2 over 60 and hemoglobin saturated over 90%. Vaccinations against influenza and Streptococcus pneumoniae are mandatory. Antibiotic treatment is given empirically against Haemophilus influenzae and Streptococcus pneumoniae to reduce hospitalization and acute symptoms. Inhaled beta agonists are used along with ipratropium bromide, and steroids are used during exacerbations. Surgical options are limited, but include lung volume reduction to improve FEV_1. Lung volume reduction appears to benefit COPD patients with primarily upper lobe disease with decreased exercise tolerance. Lung transplantation is an option for selected patients. Regardless of what treatment is used, smoking cessation is mandatory to slow the progression.

d) Prognosis

Survival in COPD is best predicted by FEV_1, with a rapid decline indicative of increased morbidity and mortality. Dyspnea often occurs with exercise (DOE) when FEV_1 drops below 50% predicted. FEV_1 below 25% often portends dyspnea at rest.

3. Acute Respiratory Distress Syndrome

a) Etiology and Pathophysiology

Adult respiratory distress syndrome (ARDS) is a severe diffuse alveolar injury that leads to pulmonary infiltrates, hypoxemia, and failure of normal lung function. Increased permeability of the alveoli leads to fluid infiltration into the alveoli and subsequent damage to the sensitive epithelial cells. Damage occurs primarily to the vascular endothelium or alveolar epithelium, depending on the nature of the infiltrate. Vascular congestion occurs with alveolar collapse, inflammatory cell infiltration, and edema. Pulmonary edema occurs with destruction of type II pneumocytes. Longstanding damage leads to hypoxemia, pulmonary HTN, and in more severe cases, fibrosis with permanent and progressive pulmonary damage. Limited acute injury typically resolves.

b) Presentation and Diagnosis

ARDS presents with acute onset of dyspnea and hypoxemia following an identifiable cause (i.e. drug overdose, sepsis, acute pancreatitis, aspiration). Physical findings include tachypnea, tachycardia, dyspnea, oxygen supplementation, signs of hypoxia, and signs of the underlying etiology. ARDS often occurs with sepsis and shock. Criteria for diagnosis include acute onset, bilateral pulmonary infiltrates on CXR, hypoxemia (i.e. PaO_2 / FiO_2 less than 200), and absence of cardiogenic pulmonary edema (PAWP < 18 mmHg).

c) Treatment

Treatment of ARDS is primarily supportive with treatment of the underlying etiology. Respiratory support may be necessary. Maintaining an FiO_2 as low as possible is helpful. Permissive hypercapnia is a strategy often employed to achieve minimal ventilator settings. Utilizing a low tidal volume strategy of 6 ml/kg provides a survival benefit.

IV.C. Inflammatory and Infectious

1. Pneumocystis Carinii

P. carinii infection is a serious concern in HIV patients with a CD4 T-cell count below 200 / mm^3. Prophylaxis should be started in these and otherwise symptomatic patients with bactrim. Aerosolized pentamidine can also be given, although this has been associated with spontaneous pneumothorax and extrapulmonary pneumocystosis. Dapsone has also been shown to be an effective therapy.

2. Lung Abscess

a) Assessment

A lung abscess is an infectious cavity within the lung parenchyma. A lung abscess may occur distal to a blocked bronchus. Infectious sources are commonly anaerobic and associated with aspiration, alcohol abuse, foreign body, advanced age or debilitated state, immunosuppression, IV drug use, or esophageal disease. Staphylococcus, Streptococcus, Klebsiella, HIB, Actinomyces, Aspergillus, and Nocardia are all potential pathogens. Lung abscess presents with fever, productive cough, night sweats, and weight loss with foul smelling sputum. Blood culture and sputum culture are collected, and bronchoscopy should be performed. Plain films and CT are also done to precisely identify the location and extent of infection. When due to aspiration, the right lung is more commonly involved due to the less acute angle of the right mainstem bronchus.

b) Management

Medical management is with antimicrobials tailored to the causative organism. Bronchoscopy may assist in drainage or removal of obstructing matter. Surgical intervention is needed for persistent cavities, failure to clear sepsis, thick cavity wall, hemoptysis, or to exclude cancer.

3. Pleural Effusion

a) Etiology and Pathophysiology

Pleural effusions are fluid collections within the pleural cavity, classified as either transudative or exudative. Common causes of a transudative effusion are increased hydrostatic pressure or decreased oncotic pressure (as in CHF), cirrhosis, fluid overload, PE, lobar collapse, and nephrotic syndrome. Transudative effusions are likely to be due to systemic causes and tend to be bilateral in nature. Exudative effusions contain cells and are due to local processes such as cancer, infection, trauma, post-coronary bypass grafting, or pancreatitis. Exudative effusions tend to be unilateral. Pleural fluid has a turnover of 1-2 liters per day.

b) Presentation and Diagnosis

Pleural effusions are diagnosed by thoracentesis and the LDH and protein titers are measured. An LDH > 200, a ratio of effusion LDH to serum LDH > 0.6, or a protein effusion to serum ratio > 0.5 are indicative of an exudative effusion. A parapneumonic effusion is considered if the leukocyte count is greater than 10,000 with a high PMN number; these are always exudative effusions due to the high cellular content. Blood in the effusion brings the differential to trauma, infection, aortic dissection, and malignancy. Low glucose in the effusion leads to the consideration of tuberculosis, empyema, rheumatoid arthritis, and malignancy. Finally, elevated amylase titers require ruling out pancreatitis, renal failure, esophageal rupture, and tumors.

c) Treatment

Transudative and exudative effusions should be treated by treating the underlying cause(s). Tube thoracostomy or thoracoscopic drainage with or without chemical pleurodesis may be needed for recurrent symptomatic effusions. Thoracotomy or thoracoscopy with mechanical pleurodesis or pleurectomy is used in cases refractory to all other measures.

IV.D. Vascular

1. Pulmonary Embolism

a) Etiology

Pulmonary embolism (PE) is a challenging diagnosis that must be made to avoid potentially catastrophic outcomes. Untreated PE has a 30% mortality rate in the inpatient setting. PE is commonly due to deep vein thrombosis (DVT) from venous stasis, intimal injury, and hypercoagulability, which comprise Virchow's triad. Most DVTs arise from the iliofemoral circulation. As thrombi become larger and veins become larger in the thigh and pelvis, propensity for dislodging increases. Specific risk factors for PE include use of oral contraceptives, cancer, thrombophilias (including factor V Leiden, antithrombin III (AT III) deficiency), protein C (PrC) deficiency, protein S (PrS) deficiency, and antiphospholipid antibody (APA).

b) Pathophysiology

Respiratory effects of PE include hypoxemia, hyperventilation, and alveolar necrosis. Pulmonary infarction often occurs with untreated PE decreases lung integrity through surfactant loss in the affected region. Arterial hypoxemia is a common finding due to ventilation-perfusion (V/Q) mismatch, shunts, decreased cardiac output from increased pulmonary circulation pressure, and a patent foramen ovale (PFO). Infarction of the lung is rare due to collateral circulation from the bronchial arteries. Increased pulmonary vascular resistance leads to increased RV afterload with subsequent right heart strain. Sudden increases in load can lead to sudden cardiac death from excessive RV load. Large emboli may become lodged at the bifurcation of the pulmonary artery or major branches thereof, leading to a saddle embolus that leads to acute heart failure.

c) Presentation

The most common signs and symptoms of PE include tachypnea, rales, tachycardia, S4 gallop, and accentuated P2 heart sound. A sudden decrease in $ETCO_2$ during surgical procedures likely indicates a pulmonary embolism. A large PE presents with circulatory collapse and death, and is a common cause of death in hospitalized postoperative patients, especially in the elderly. Smaller PEs can present with pulmonary infarction with pleuritic chest pain and hemoptysis. SOB, DOE, pallor, hypotension, and numerous atypical symptoms such as seizures, syncope, abdominal pain, wheezing, CNS changes, and atrial fibrillation complicate the picture. Signs of a PE on EKG include ST-T wave changes, right-axis deviation, S waves in lead 1, Q waves in lead 3, and inverted T waves in lead 3 (S1-Q3-T3).

d) Diagnosis

PE diagnosis involves a host of exams and imaging studies with variable sensitivity and specificity. The diagnostic testing begins after a thorough history and physical exam are completed. ABG may indicate hypoxemia, hypocapnia, and alkalosis with a decreased A-a gradient. D-dimer is a nonspecific test that indicates fibrin breakdown; it should not be used alone for diagnosis but raises the clinical suspicion if positive. In a low risk patient (outpatient with pleuritic chest pain and no risk factors), a normal D-dimer effectively removes PE from the differential diagnosis. D-dimer is rarely indicated in the postoperative period. CXR is normal in the acute phase, but later may show dilation of proximal pulmonary vessels, atelectasis, pleural effusions, and/or decreased pulmonary vascular markings peripherally (Westermark sign). A Hampton's hump is a wedge-shaped subpleural consolidation that is often discussed but rarely seen on CXR. V/Q scanning provides a meaningful diagnosis in many cases; segmental perfusion defects with normal ventilation are highly indicative of PE but many patients fall in the intermediate probability category. Additional testing is warranted, and includes ultrasound to detect a DVT. CT with contrast may be used to identify a significant pulmonary embolus (smaller ones are not detected), and is the most common modality employed when suspicion for PE is high. Pulmonary angiography is considered the gold standard but is an invasive study.

e) Treatment

Any patient with a high or medium clinical suspicion with a high-probability V/Q scan, or those with confirmed results by CT should be treated for PE. Anticoagulation therapy beginning with heparin followed by warfarin is used. Treatment is typically continued for at least 3 months with a goal INR of 2-3. The first occurrence of a DVT is typically treated with six months of anticoagulation, the second occurrence with one year of therapy, and a third occurrence requires lifetime warfarin therapy. Low-molecular-weight heparins (LMWH) are being used with increasing frequency and do not usually require routine laboratory evaluation; the level of anticoagulation is measured with anti-Xa assay or estimated by LMWH level. LMWH is the treatment of choice in pregnant patients. Thrombolytic therapy may be used in hemodynamically unstable patients and must be given shortly after the event to achieve maximal effectiveness. An inferior vena cava filter is placed in patients with contraindications to anticoagulation, fragile patients who cannot tolerate another PE, those with risk of recurrence, and patients who experience a significant PE while being anticoagulated.

Table 3. Indications for IVC filter.

Indications for IVC Filter
DVT or PE in the presence of anticoagulation therapy
DVT or PE with contraindications to anticoagulation therapy (i.e. trauma, head bleeds, GI bleeding)
Persistent DVT or PE with maximum anticoagulation therapy
s/p Pulmonary embolectomy

IV.E. Trauma

1. Overview

Thoracic injuries and complications of chest trauma account for roughly 45% of all trauma-related deaths. Physical examination of the chest in any trauma patient is critical to identify life-threatening conditions amenable to immediate intervention, including cardiac tamponade, tension pneumothorax, massive hemothorax, flail chest, and open pneumothorax. CXR should be obtained following physical examination.

2. Rib Fractures

Fracture of 1-2 ribs without pleural or lung involvement may generally be treated on an outpatient basis. Poor pain control can lead to complications such as pneumonia or atelectasis due to inability to inspire deeply and cough. Elderly patients have twice the risk compared to younger patients. In the event of multiple rib fractures, an epidural catheter should be considered for pain management and an abdominal CT should be obtained due to the risk of intra-abdominal injury (spleen, liver) from a fractured rib. Flail chest is paradoxical movement of the chest wall due to two or more fractures in three or more consecutive ribs.

3. Spontaneous Pneumothorax

a) Etiology and Pathophysiology

Spontaneous pneumothorax is a potentially devastating disorder that leads to air in the pleural cavity from a sudden rupture of a pleural bleb. It is most likely to occur in tall and thin people, or in those who smoke. Other causes include COPD, cystic fibrosis, pneumonia, cancer, and illicit drug abuse.

b) Presentation and Diagnosis

Spontaneous pneumothorax presents with pleuritic chest pain, SOB, and exam findings of decreased breath sounds. Hyperresonance due to increased conduction through the air is present on the affected side. Diagnosis includes upright expiratory CXR, where a collapsed lung may be found. ST changes may be present on EKG. Volume-control mode on ventilation will increase airway pressures in the event of a pneumothorax.

c) Treatment

Initial treatment includes oxygen and observation. A significant pneumothorax or an increasing space mandates placement of a catheter into the pleural space (tube thoracostomy). Most first-time spontaneous pneumothoraces can be treated successfully with a chest tube. Recurrent pneumothoraces should be treated with definitive therapy (bleb resection and pleurodesis) secondary to the risk of further recurrences.

4. Tension Pneumothorax

a) Etiology and Pathophysiology

Tension pneumothorax occurs with air under pressure within the pleural space. Blunt or penetrating thoracic trauma and mechanical ventilation are situations in which tension pneumothoraces occur. Pneumothorax can also be an iatrogenic complication of central line placement.

b) Presentation and Diagnosis

Tension pneumothorax presents similarly to spontaneous pneumothorax, with the addition of tracheal deviation away from the side of the pneumothorax, hypotension, and tachycardia. Diagnosis is made by clinical presentation, not by CXR. Beware of tension pneumothorax following central line placement. A tension pneumothorax exerts its physiologic compromise through vena cava compression, leading to decreased venous return. This leads to hypoxia, hypercapnia, hypotension, and sudden death. A sign of tension pneumothorax while on a mechanical ventilator includes increasing inspiratory pressures using volume-controlled ventilation and decreased tidal volumes with pressure-control modes.

c) Treatment

Tension pneumothorax requires emergency management and is treated with needle decompression followed by tube thoracostomy. An 18 gauge needle is inserted into the second intercostal space at the mid-clavicular line. Trauma patients with a pneumothorax should be intubated first (preserve the airway first).

5. Penetrating Parasternal Injuries

a) Assessment

A parasternal stab wound may present with hypotension and shortness of breath. Diagnosis is made by CXR and EKG. Wounds that are anterior and below the fifth intercostal space also require a FAST or DPL to rule out abdominal injuries. An echocardiogram should be obtained.

b) Management

Treatment includes chest tube placement. If immediate chest tube output is greater than 1.5L or over 250 cc/hr over 4 hours, a thoracotomy is required. Other indications for thoracotomy include pericardial tamponade and hypovolemic shock. A median sternotomy may be chosen in the appropriate setting. "Trap door" incisions can be made to the left subclavian or the incision can be extended along the anterior border of the sternocleidomastoid muscle to allow exposure of the carotid artery.

6. Blunt Parasternal Injuries

Deceleration injuries following a fall or motor vehicle accident may lead to shear injuries causing damage to important vascular structures in the chest. This primarily occurs in the proximal descending aorta just distal to the ligamentum arteriosum and the left subclavian artery. The majority of these injuries result in death prior to arrival in the ER. The modern approach to these injuries involves stent grafting of the aorta.

IV.F. Cancer

1. Lung Cancer

a) Epidemiology

The leading cause of cancer-related death is due to lung cancer, and is the number one killer in both men and women. Over 160,000 people die annually in the United States, surpassing the combined total number of deaths from breast, prostate, and colorectal cancer. Lung cancer has very high morbidity and mortality with only a fraction of patients surviving after five years. By the time tumors are found, metastasis has already occurred in most people with rapid spread through lymphatics and blood to the liver, adrenal glands, bones, and brain.

The vast majority of lung cancer can be traced back to a longstanding history of smoking, and this invariably worsens the prognosis of lung cancer. About 95% of all lung cancers are either small cell lung cancer (SCLC) or non-small cell lung cancer (NSCLC). Unusual varieties include carcinoid, lymphoma, metastatic cancers to the lung, and others. Of the NSCLCs, adenocarcinoma (adenoCA) and squamous cell carcinoma (SCC) are the most common. Overall, adenocarcinoma makes up 45% of all lung cancers, followed by squamous cell cancer at 30%, small cell cancer at 20%, and large cell cancer at 10%.

b) Etiology

Without question, the most significant positive predictor of lung cancer risk is a history of smoking. The number of cigarettes smoked, the number of years of smoking, and the age that smoking started are specific positive predictors of risk. Other causes make up about 15% of all lung cancers, and include secondhand smoke, air pollution, chronic lung disease (including TB and COPD), exposure to heavy metals or asbestos, and a prior history of lung cancer. One affected oncogene is K-ras, which is transformed through point mutation.

c) Presentation

Lung cancer presents without symptoms in up to a quarter of patients at the time of diagnosis. The remainder develops a new, progressive cough (occasionally blood-tinged), pleuritic chest pain, SOB, wheezing, hoarseness, recurrent URIs, and systemic effects based on metastasis. Paraneoplastic syndromes can also occur with production of gastrin, ACTH, ADH, calcitonin, ANF, and PTHrP. Squamous cell and small cell cancers tend to occur centrally, while adenocarcinomas tend to occur peripherally.

d) Diagnosis

Lung cancer is diagnosed beginning with a careful smoking history and complete physical exam. CXR is typically the first test ordered, sometimes indicating the presence of a nodule or adenopathy, though in early cases (those potentially amenable to curative resection) the CXR may show no evidence of lung mass.

CT and MRI are more sensitive and can detect smaller nodules, and are also useful for staging; a CT of the chest and abdomen is typically completed, along with the head as indicated. Biopsy, sputum cytology, and bronchoscopy are other methods of obtaining cells and tissue for additional analysis. Collection of fluid via thoracentesis, or open procedures such as thoracotomy may be necessary to collect an adequate tissue sample. Regional spread to lymph nodes is evaluated by mediastinoscopy.

Approximately half of all lung cancers are metastatic at the time of diagnosis. PFTs with $FEV_1 > 0.8$ is required prior to lung surgery. An $FEV_1 > 2$ L is required prior to pneumonectomy, > 1 L for a lobectomy, and 0.6L for a wedge resection. $PCO_2 > 60$ and poor DL_{CO} ratios are prohibitive risks for lung resection due to the elevated chance for permanent mechanical ventilation postoperatively.

e) Small Cell Lung Cancer

SCLC accounts for 20% of lung cancers with 80% centrally located. SCLC tends to be more aggressive and rapidly growing than NSCLC. Histology often indicates dark nuclei with little cytoplasm, an oat-like appearance. SCLC produces gastrin, ACTH, ADH, ANF, and calcitonin, which can lead to a number of paraneoplastic effects. Treatment of SCLC involves radiotherapy and chemotherapy. Surgical resection is typically not possible because of extensive disease at presentation. SCLC has a 5 year survival of approximately 5%.

f) Non-Small Cell Lung Cancer

NSCLC includes adenocarcinoma, bronchoalveolar carcinoma, squamous cell carcinoma, and large cell carcinoma or the lung. NSCLC features cells with pleomorphic nuclei and large amounts of cytoplasm. Adenocarcinoma of the lung is the most frequent NSCLC, accounting for 45% of lung cancers, with 75% occurring peripherally.

Adenocarcinoma tends to metastasize earlier than squamous cell carcinoma and more often to the CNS. Bronchoalveolar carcinoma is a subtype of adenocarcinoma and is associated with the best prognosis of all the types because it is more differentiated and spreads along alveolar walls.

Squamous cell carcinoma (SCCA) accounts for 30% of lung cancers and ⅔ are located centrally. Squamous cell carcinoma may produce PTHrP. Surgical resection is the treatment of choice in early stage disease. Five year survival is better for NSCLC than for SCLC.

Large cell undifferentiated carcinoma accounts for 10% of lung tumors. These tend to occur peripherally and metastasize relatively early.

g) Prognosis

Palliative care is often the final outcome of therapy for lung cancer. This is due to the high rate of recurrence, in which many lung cancers are present again within 2 years. Pain management with hospice care involves the use of high dose opioids and NSAIDs as indicated. Oxygen administration is often the key to patient comfort.

The primary method of avoiding the lethal pitfall of lung cancer is avoidance – smoking cessation is the first and most important step to reducing the risk of lung cancer. Survival with stage I NSCLC is 70% at 5 years; stage II offers a 30% 5-year survival, stage III a 20% 5-year survival, and stage IV offers only a 9 month survival period. SCLC that is treated with chemotherapy has a 10% 5 year survival; advanced SCLC has a 6 month survival period.

h) Screening

Some institutions offer CT scans as a screening test in high risk patients; early data appears to indicate that CT scans can detect lung cancer earlier, and in some patients, this may lead to earlier treatments and potential surgical resection before significant metastasis occurs. Whether this translates into less morbidity and mortality over a 5 year period remains to be determined.

i) Associated Syndromes

Lung cancer is associated with numerous syndromes. Superior vena cava syndrome occurs due to compression of the SVC with swelling of the upper extremity, head, and neck. Cough, headache, epistaxis, and syncope are commonly associated symptoms.

SVC syndrome is most likely due to lung cancer (90%). It is treated with radiotherapy. Horner syndrome presents with paralysis of the sympathetic nerve due to damage to the ganglion; it presents with ptosis, enophthalmos, miosis, and anhidrosis.

Pancoast tumor presents with damage to the 8th cervical nerve, 1st and 2nd thoracic nerve, and damage to the ribs that leads to pain that radiates to the ipsilateral arm. Pancoast tumor can lead to Horner syndrome, vessel or nerve compression, and injury to underlying structures.

SIADH presents with hyposmolality and hyponatremia. Eaton-Lambert syndrome occurs with an autoimmune reaction to nerve terminals leading to decreased release of acetylcholine (ACh). Trousseau syndrome is a hypercoagulable state that leads to venous thrombosis.

j) Staging

TABLE 4. Lung Cancer Staging

Lung Cancer Staging	
Stage I	N0 with no direct invasion and greater than 2cm from the carina
Stage II	N+ with ipsilateral hilar nodes, no metastasis
Stage III	Invasion of chest well, diaphragm, pericardium, or the presence of positive mediastinal lymph nodes
Stage IV	Metastatic disease

k) Key Points

The most important determination to make is the histological presence or absence of tumor cells in any radiographically enlarged (>1 cm) mediastinal lymph nodes. This is done with mediastinoscopy. If mediastinal nodes are positive for tumor, pulmonary resection is only performed as part of a combined program of chemotherapy and radiation. If mediastinal lymph nodes are devoid of tumor, resection and intrathoracic mediastinal lymph node dissection are performed with adjuvant chemotherapy considered for any stage II disease.

2. Mediastinal Masses

Mediastinal masses present due to compression of mediastinal structures or are found incidentally.

The most common masses by mediastinal compartment are as follows:

- Anterosuperior Mediastinum (thymus gland, lymph nodes, fat): Thymoma, thyroid enlargement, T-cell lymphoma, teratoma
- Middle Mediastinum (heart, pericardium, great vessels, phrenic and vagus nerves, trachea/bronchi, lymph nodes): Cysts, vascular lesions, enlarged lymph nodes
- Posterior Mediastinum (esophagus, azygos/hemiazygos veins, thoracic duct, sympathetic chain, lymph nodes): Neurogenic tumors

Mediastinal masses are most commonly located in the anterosuperior mediastinum (54%), followed by the posterior (26%) and middle mediastinum (20%). In adults, mediastinal masses represent malignancy about 40% of the time.

VASCULAR

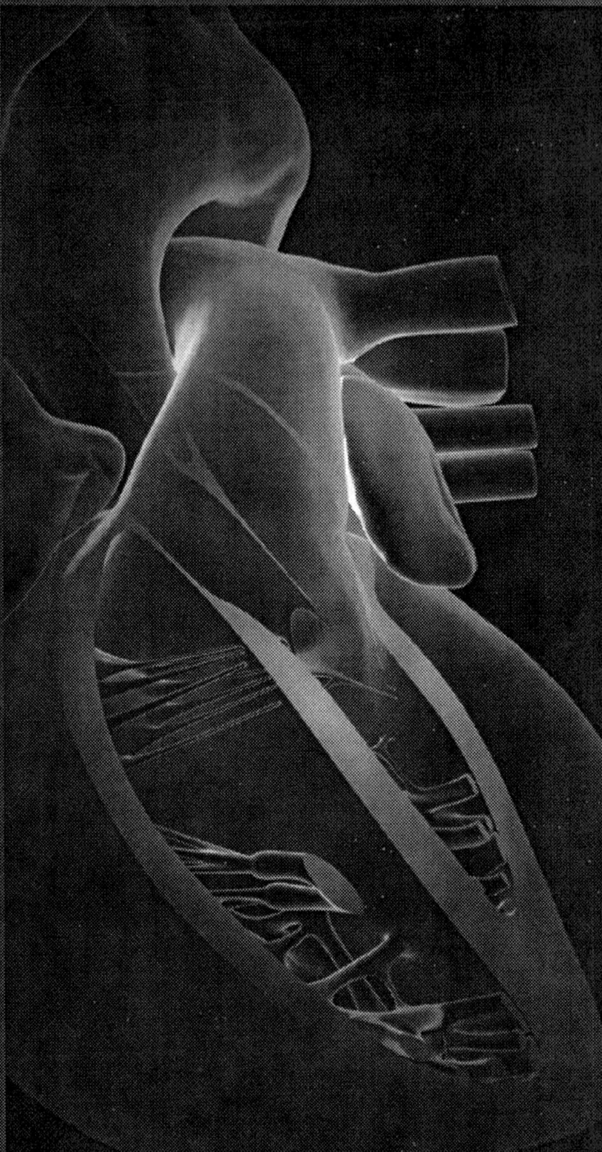

I still have an almost religious sense when I work on the heart. It is something God makes, and we have yet to duplicate.

Michael E. Debakey
Father of Cardiovascular Surgery (1908-2008)

SURGISPHERE

VASCULAR SURGERY

Luigi Pascarella, M.D. and Cynthia K. Shortell, M.D.

I. General Concepts

I.A. Introduction

Vascular surgery is a unique discipline of surgery in that both a gross and fine approach are required, often intimately woven together in an intricate interplay throughout the same procedure. An intimate knowledge of anatomy with familiarity of numerous, but rare, anatomic variations is required.

Vascular surgery involves nearly every part of the body, and a rich three-dimensional grasp of anatomy is basic training for the adept operator. The surgical approach requires careful dissection through multiple tissue planes to establish the optimal exposure, an understanding of the relationship of a vessel to proximal ligaments, tendons, muscles, and fascial planes, and a grasp of fundamental physical relationships to ensure the success of an operation. The small AV fistulas in the wrist depend on the appropriate selection and placement of an artery and vein with an inner lumen measured in millimeters. The more intricate revascularization procedures rely upon properly weaving a graft through specific tissue planes to ensure that the conduit is not later obstructed by something as simple as flexing a knee.

A critical understanding of the anatomical and physical science, sound technical skills, and a vision for what the end result should look like form the cornerstones of modern vascular surgery. This chapter is intended to serve as a relevant overview of major disease processes in vascular surgery and to help establish a fundamental understanding of this branch of surgery.

I.B. Aortic Arch

The aorta arises from the left ventricle, gives off the right and left coronary arteries, and travels 5 cm to the sternum, where it becomes the arch of the aorta. At the apex, it gives rise to the brachiocephalic, left common carotid, and left subclavian arteries before continuing as the descending aorta. The

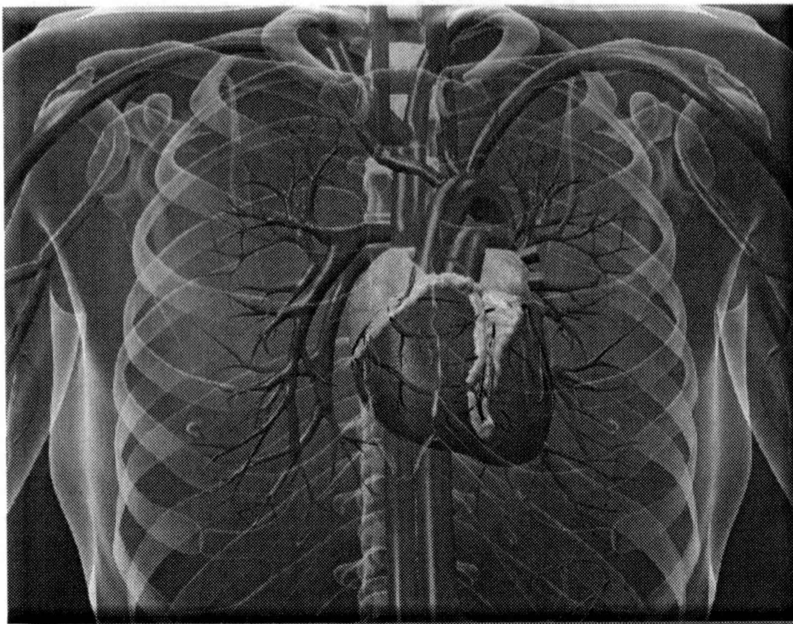

brachiocephalic artery, occasionally referred to as the innominate artery, branches into the right subclavian and right common carotid arteries. At the distal portion of the arch is the ligamentum arteriosum, which shunts blood from the pulmonary artery to the aorta during ontogeny.

Crossing anterior to the arch is the left vagus nerve, which sends the left recurrent laryngeal nerve around the arch and back up to the neck. The right recurrent laryngeal nerve hooks around the right subclavian artery as it comes off the brachiocephalic trunk.

A variety of congenital alterations to the aortic arch exist. The true bovine arch begins as a singular, large common brachiocephalic trunk coming off the apex, rather than having three separate vessels. This common trunk then separates into the right and left subclavian arteries, and a bicarotid trunk. This bicarotid trunk then bifurcates into the right and left common carotid arteries. A true bovine arch is rarer than the "so-called" bovine arch. This variation has the left common carotid artery branch from the brachiocephalic trunk instead of the aortic arch. Up to 20% of patients may have this variation.

Identification of these variations is crucial in carotid artery surgery as it may affect the placement of a shunt and potentially lead to intraoperative ischemia. For example, if a patient has the more common ("so-called") bovine arch variant in which both common carotid arteries come from the brachiocephalic artery, the use of a balloon to reduce flow during a left carotid endarterectomy may compromise distal flow to the right common carotid artery by impeding the flow of blood in the brachiocephalic trunk. Cerebral hypoperfusion may occur if there is insufficient collateralization within the circle of Willis. This variation may be suspected if shunt placement does not alter blood pressure in the left arm.

I.C. Anterior Cervical Triangle

1. Overview

The anterior cervical triangle is bound by the sternocleidomastoid muscle laterally, the inferior border of the mandible superiorly, and the anterior midline of the neck medially. The anterior cervical triangle may be subdivided into four smaller triangles: the submandibular, submental, carotid and muscular.

2. Submandibular Triangle

The submandibular triangle is delimited by the inferior border of the mandible, and the anterior and posterior bellies of the digastric muscle. The submandibular gland is the largest structure within this triangle. Other structures within this triangle are the anterior and posterior facial veins, facial artery, submental branch of the facial artery, the superficial and deep layers of the submaxillary fascia, and hypoglossal nerve. The facial artery is a branch of the external carotid artery and enters the submandibular triangle under the posterior belly of the digastric, the stylohyoid muscle, and the submandibular gland. It then becomes superficial and lies under the platysma when it encounters the mandible.

3. Submental Triangle

The submental triangle is bound by the anterior belly of the digastric muscle laterally, the hyoid bone medially, the mylohyoid muscle posteriorly, the midline medially, and the skin and superficial fascia anteriorly. Lymph nodes draining from the chin, lower lip, floor of the mouth, and tip of the tongue are found in this triangle.

4. Carotid Triangle

The carotid triangle is bound by the sternocleidomastoid muscle posteriorly, the anterior belly of the omohyoid anteriorly, and the posterior belly of the digastric superiorly. The hyoglossus muscle, inferior and middle constrictors of the pharynx, and thyrohyoid are noted medially. The common carotid artery, its bifurcation as the external and internal branches, vagus nerve, spinal accessory muscle, hypoglossal nerve, ansa hypoglossi, and cervical sympathetic nerves are within the carotid triangle. The jugular lymph nodes drain in the supraclavicular lymph nodes.

5. Muscular Triangle

The muscular triangle is bound by the anterior belly of the omohyoid superiorly, sternocleidomastoid muscle inferiorly, midline of the neck medially, prevertebral fascia and muscle posteriorly, and the deep layer of the deep cervical fascia, sternohyoid muscle, and cricothyroid muscle anteriorly. The thyroid and parathyroid glands, trachea, esophagus, and sympathetic trunk are found within the muscular triangle.

I.D. Carotid Anatomy

1. Common Carotid Artery

The left common carotid artery arises as a direct branch of the aortic arch, while the right common carotid artery is a branch of the brachiocephalic artery as it gives rise to the right subclavian. The left common carotid artery is closely associated with the recurrent laryngeal nerve and thoracic duct, and eventually travels with the vagus and phrenic nerves as it goes more superior. The right common carotid artery has a similar relationship with these two nerves in the neck.

Within the neck, the common carotid artery is enclosed by the carotid sheath, an extension of the deep cervical fascia. The sheath also includes the

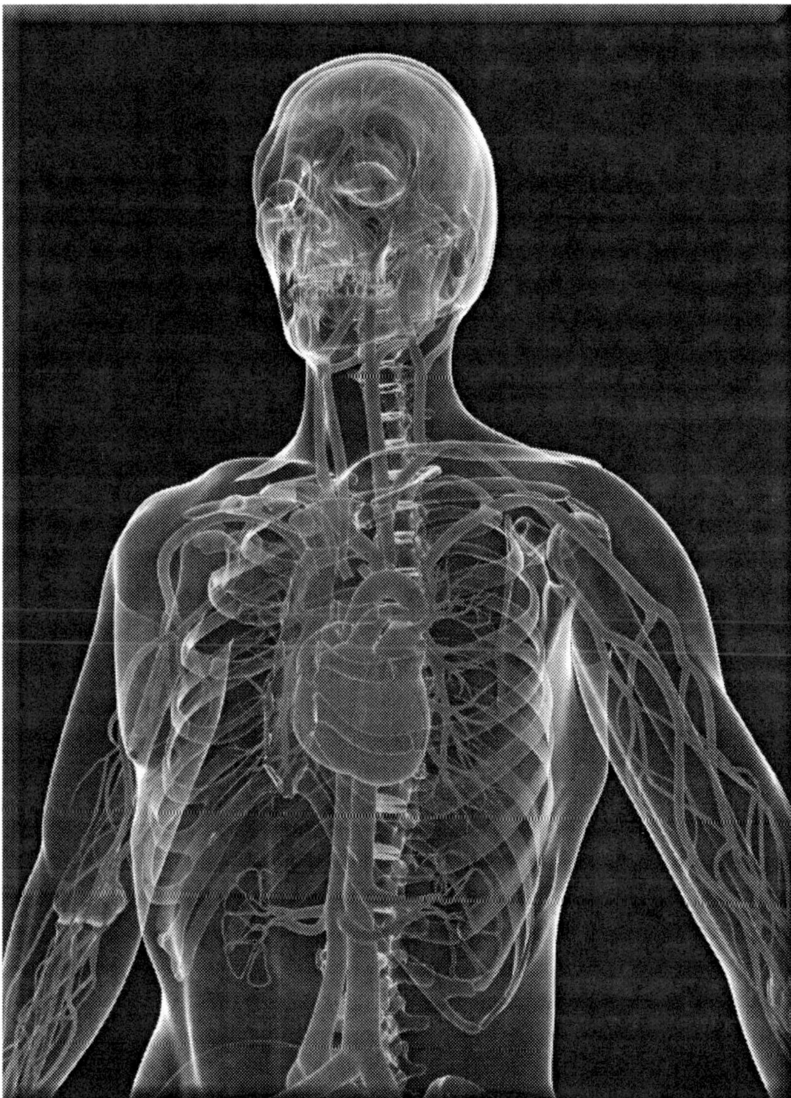

internal jugular vein and vagus nerve. Care must be taken with dissection, as the descending branch of the hypoglossal nerve is occasionally incorporated into the carotid sheath. The common carotid artery divides into the external and internal carotid arteries at the upper border of the thyroid cartilage, near the level of the fourth cervical vertebra. The common carotid artery rarely has other branches, but may occasionally include the thyroid arteries (superior and inferior), pharyngeal artery, and vertebral artery.

2. External Carotid Artery

The external carotid artery bifurcates to form the maxillary artery and superficial temporal artery within the parotid gland. It is anterior and medial to the internal carotid artery. Careful dissection is required as it is crossed by the hypoglossal nerve near its superior extent. The glossopharyngeal nerve is located posterior to this artery. The external carotid artery gives off the superior thyroid artery, facial artery, occipital artery, posterior auricular artery, and the two terminal branches discussed above.

3. Internal Carotid Artery

The Bouthillier classification is used primarily by neurosurgeons to divide the internal carotid artery into seven distinct segments. The internal carotid artery at its take off contains the carotid bulb. The carotid nerve plexus is intimately associated with the internal carotid and emanates from the superior cervical ganglion. The internal carotid artery is the chief supply to the circle of Willis anastomosis that supplies blood to the brain.

4. Carotid Bifurcation

The carotid bifurcation is an important neurovascular structure. Within the bifurcation near the internal carotid artery, the carotid bulb contains mechanoreceptors and baroreceptors. Stimulation leads to bradycardia and vasodilatation via a parasympathetic reaction. The carotid sinus contains chemoreceptors which serve as detectors for CO_2 and acidosis. Stimulation here leads to a sympathetic response.

I.E. Vertebral Arteries

The vertebral artery is the first branch of the subclavian artery and provides extensive collateral blood flow to the brain via the circle of Willis. The vertebral artery travels posterior to the transverse process of C6, then enters the transverse foramina until it reaches C1. It then travels posterior to the arch of the atlas and penetrates the skull through the foramen magnum. Anterior to the vertebral arteries at their takeoff are the internal jugular veins and inferior thyroid artery. The inferior cervical sympathetic ganglion is in close proximity to the artery when it is located proximal to the transverse processes. A portion of the vertebral artery may be uncovered within the suboccipital triangle, bound by the superior oblique, inferior oblique, and rectus capitis posterior major muscle. The suboccipital nerve is in close proximity to the vertebral artery at this point. The left vertebral artery tends to be somewhat larger and have higher flows compared to the right.

I.F. Thoracic Outlet

The thoracic outlet is bound by the first ribs, clavicles, manubrium, and the first thoracic vertebra. It defines the transition between the root of the neck and the superior mediastinum. Hypertrophy of the anterior and middle scalene muscles, narrowing of the space between the clavicle and first rib, or the presence of a cervical rib may lead to compression of the brachial plexus, subclavian artery, or subclavian vein, resulting in clinically-significant thoracic outlet obstruction. There are other rarer causes of obstruction, including the presence of fibrous bands, exostosis of the first rib, bifid clavicle, abnormalities of the omohyoid muscle, and enlargement of the C7 transverse process. Trauma to the upper extremity or chest can cause fractures of the clavicle or dislocation of the head of the humerus and present with disruption of the structures within the thoracic outlet.

The brachial plexus and subclavian artery travel through the scalene triangle, while the subclavian vein passes through the costoclavicular space. The boundaries of the scalene triangle include the anterior scalene muscle (anterior border), middle scalene muscle (posterior border), and first rib (inferior border). The costoclavicular space is bound by the clavicle (superior border), first rib (inferior border), costoclavicular ligament (anterior border), and middle scalene muscle (posterior border).

I.G. Vascular Supply to the Upper Extremity

1. Subclavian Artery

The blood supply to the upper extremity begins as the subclavian artery, a direct branch off the aorta to the left extremity and a branch of the brachiocephalic trunk for the right extremity. The first part of the subclavian artery travels to the medial border of the anterior scalene muscle, and is located anterior to the vagus and phrenic nerves. The artery is posterior to the sternohyoid and sternocleidomastoid muscles, and gives rise to the vertebral artery, internal thoracic artery, and thyrocervical artery. The second part of the subclavian artery travels posterior to the anterior scalene muscle and gives rise to the costocervical trunk. At this location proximal to the clavicle, the subclavian vein is located inferior and anterior to the subclavian artery. The third part of the subclavian artery commences at the lateral border of the anterior scalene muscle and becomes the axillary artery at the lateral border of the first rib; this part gives rise to the dorsal scapular artery.

2. Axillary Artery

The axillary artery is divided into three parts based on its relationship to the pectoralis minor muscle. The first part of the axillary artery is proximal, the second part posterior, and the third part lateral to the pectoralis minor. The second part of the axillary artery is intimately associated with the brachial plexus cords. The internal mammary artery arises from the first part, while the circumflex arteries to the head of the humerus arise from the third part. Due to an anastomosis between the suprascapular artery and dorsal scapular artery, the axillary artery may be clamped proximal to the subscapular artery. The axillary artery supplies the upper arm and becomes the brachial artery at the border of the teres major.

3. Brachial Artery

The brachial artery divides into the radial and ulnar arteries at the cubital fossa. The brachial artery travels with the median nerve for much of its course. Several important collateral vessels are given off from the brachial artery, including the deep brachial, and superior and inferior ulnar collateral arteries. The deep brachial artery has branches that anastomose with recurrent branches emanating from the radial artery along with the inferior ulnar collateral artery. Due to its close proximity to the humerus, a fracture of this bone can compromise the brachial artery.

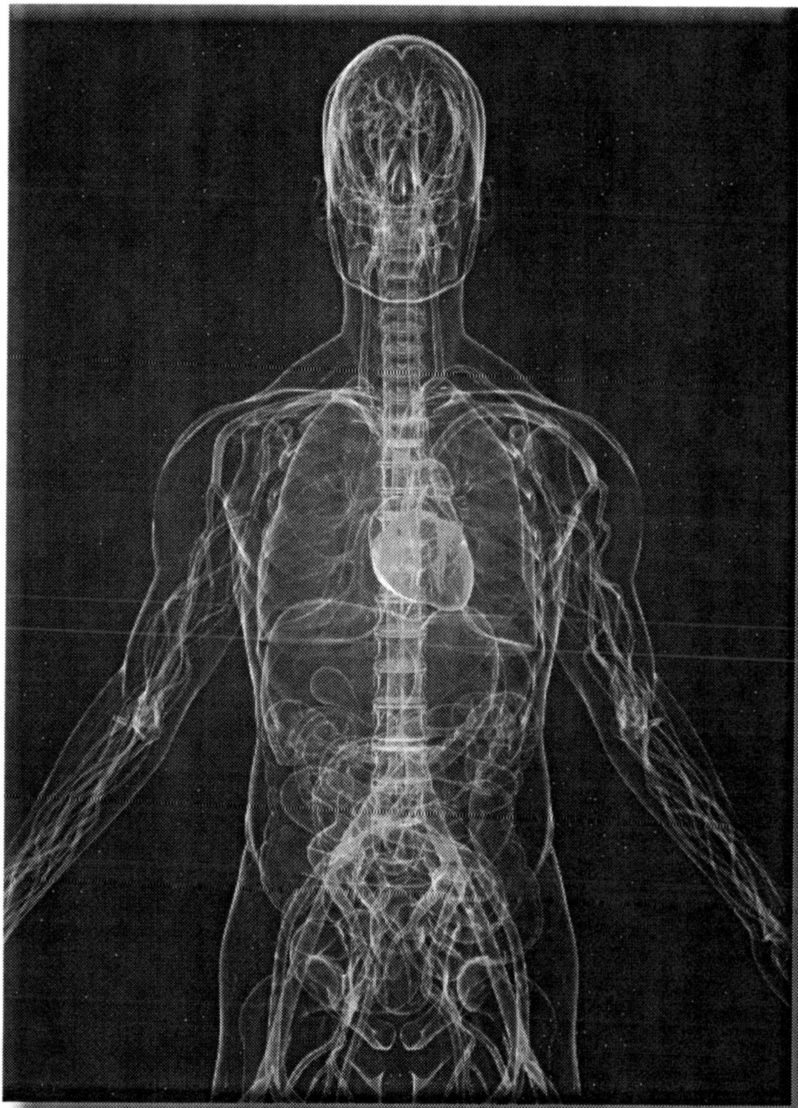

Vascular Surgery

4. Radial Artery

The radial artery is located in the anterior and lateral compartment of the forearm. It ends as the deep palmar arch after passing between the dorsal interosseus muscle and through the anatomic snuff box. The Allen test is done prior to using the radial artery for access as part of an arteriovenous fistula or insertion of an arterial line. This test is done by elevating the hand and making a fist, occluding the radial and ulnar arteries, opening the hand and confirming pallor, then releasing the ulnar artery pressure to verify satisfactory collateral flow to the hand. The ulnar artery is typically the dominant artery to the hand; if the Allen test is abnormal, it implies that the radial artery is the dominant supply and should not be used to avoid vascular compromise to the hand.

5. Ulnar Artery

The ulnar artery travels along the medial forearm and terminates as the superficial and deep palmar arch near the pisiform bone. The artery is proximal to the median nerve at its take off.

6. Venous Drainage

The veins of the upper extremity are divided into a superficial and deep distribution. The superficial distribution starts as the dorsal plexus of the hand and eventually gives rise to two major veins, the cephalic and basilic. The cephalic vein is lateral, while the basilic is medial. The major vein in the deep distribution is the brachial vein, which travels with the brachial artery. The brachial vein eventually joins the basilic at the lateral border of the teres minor; together they join the cephalic vein to form the axillary vein.

I.H. Vascular Supply to the Abdomen and Pelvis

1. Abdominal Aorta

The abdominal aorta gives rise to the major visceral arteries and eventually supplies blood to the lower extremity via the terminal common iliac artery branches. It begins at the diaphragm at T12 to give off the celiac trunk at T12, superior mesenteric and suprarenal arteries at L1, renal and gonadal arteries at L2, inferior mesenteric artery at L3, and the common iliac bifurcation at L4. Various lumbar arteries also arise between L1 and L4.

One collateral around the aorta is the internal thoracic artery, which becomes the superior epigastric artery after it gives off the musculophrenic artery at the diaphragm. The superior epigastric anastomosis with the inferior epigastric artery, a branch of the external iliac artery. There are also collaterals between the inferior mesenteric artery and internal pudendal artery, and occasionally collaterals between the lumbar arteries and internal iliac artery.

2. Celiac Artery

The celiac artery supplies the stomach, liver, duodenum, pancreas, and spleen. Its branches include the left gastric artery, splenic artery, and common hepatic artery. The splenic artery gives rise to six short gastric arteries, left gastroepiploic artery, and continues on to supply the spleen. The common hepatic artery gives rise to the gastroduodenal artery, and then becomes the proper hepatic artery. The gastroduodenal artery becomes the anterior superior and posterior superior pancreaticoduodenal arteries and the right gastroepiploic artery. The proper hepatic artery gives off the cystic artery before dividing into the right and left hepatic arteries.

In a quarter of all individuals, the left hepatic artery arises as a branch off the left gastric artery. In one in ten people, either a branch of or the entire common hepatic artery arises directly from the SMA. A small percentage of patients may have the hepatic artery arise directly from the aorta. The right hepatic artery may be replaced and arise entirely from the SMA; alternatively, an accessory right hepatic artery may arise from the SMA or aorta and complement flow from the natural right hepatic artery arising from the proper hepatic trunk.

3. Superior Mesenteric Artery

The superior mesenteric artery gives rise to the anterior inferior and posterior inferior pancreaticoduodenal arteries, the jejunal and ileal branches, the ileocolic artery, and the right and middle colic arteries. The ileocolic artery also supplies the cecum.

4. Inferior Mesenteric Artery

The inferior mesenteric artery gives rise to the left colic artery, sigmoid arteries, and superior rectal artery. Loss of this artery may occur as part of a graft

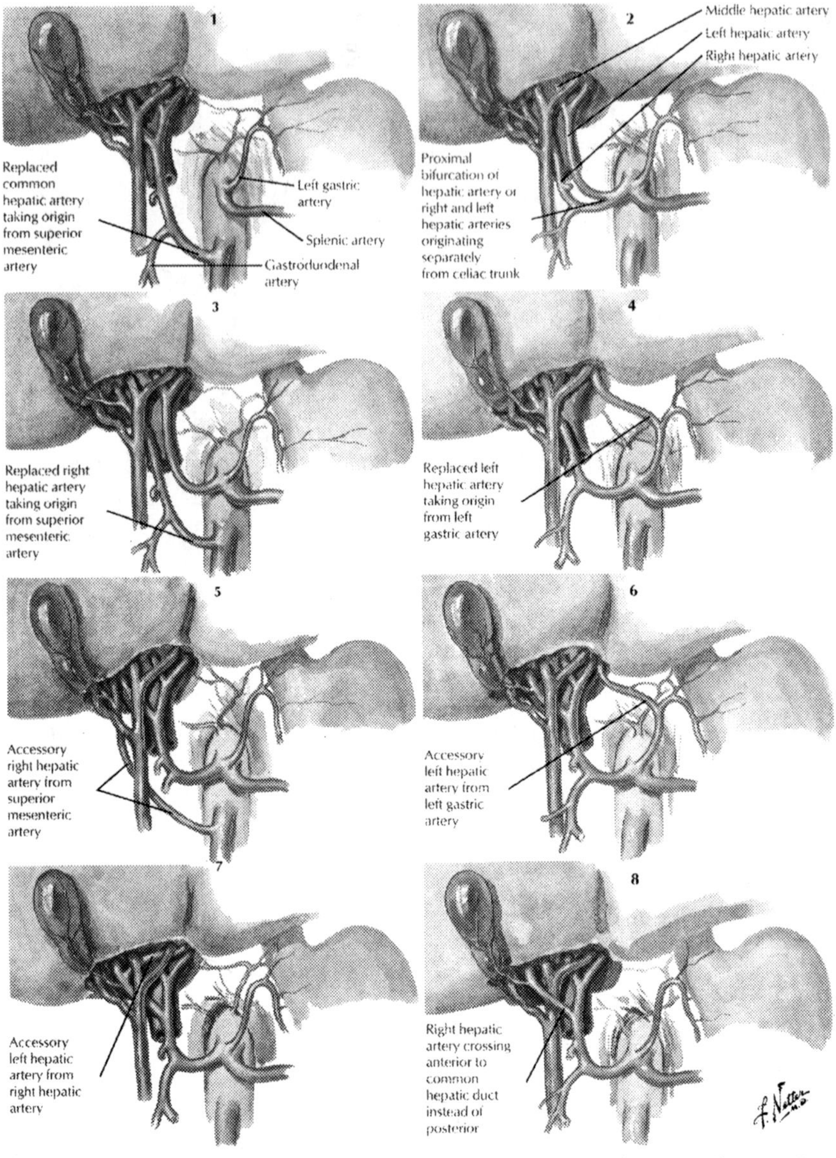

placement to treat an abdominal aortic aneurysm; sufficient collateral flow must be confirmed to avoid a potential compromise of the sigmoid colon.

1.1. Vascular Supply to the Lower Extremity

1. Iliac Artery

The common iliac artery arises at L4 at the bifurcation of the aorta, and travels about 4 cm to the pelvic brim, where it divides into the internal and external iliac arteries. The internal iliac artery, frequently referred to as the hypogastric artery, gives rise to a plethora of branches that supply the pelvis, gonads, rectum, and anus. During open and endovascular repair of abdominal aortic aneurysms, preservation of one hypogastric artery is sufficient to preserve pelvic perfusion due to extensive collateralization. This includes anastomosis between the superior and middle rectal arteries, lumbar and iliolumbar arteries, and the medial and lateral sacral arteries.

The external iliac artery gives rise to the inferior epigastric artery (discussed above), deep circumflex artery, and continues as the femoral artery at the inguinal ligament.

2. Femoral Arteries

The common femoral artery gives rise to the deep femoral artery superiorly within the thigh and continues as the femoral artery. The deep femoral artery forms a cruciate anastomosis around the femoral bone and provides collateral flow via anastomosis with recurrent branches below the popliteal fossa.

3. Popliteal Artery

The popliteal artery is the continuation of the femoral artery after it passes through the adductor canal and hiatus (also known as Hunter's canal). After forming a collateral supply around the knee, the popliteal artery bifurcates into the anterior tibial artery and the tibial-peroneal trunk. This trunk then immediately divides into the peroneal artery and posterior tibial artery. Congenital deformity of the muscle or tendon insertions into the popliteal fossa can lead to compression of this artery, causing popliteal artery entrapment syndrome (see page 187).

4. Tibial Artery and Lower Branches

The anterior tibial artery supplies the anterior compartment of the leg and dorsum of the foot as the dorsalis pedis. A number of recurrent branches are given off, which help provide a small collateral flow with branches of the deep femoral artery. The dorsalis pedis artery is anterior to the ankle and lateral to the extensor hallucis longus tendon. It may be naturally absent in up to 2% of patients.

The posterior tibial artery supplies the posterior compartment of the leg and travels posterior and inferior to the medial malleolus. The peroneal artery supplies the lateral compartment and anastomosis with the anterior tibial artery.

5. Venous Drainage

The venous drainage of the lower extremity is much more extensive than that of the upper extremity, and also more susceptible to venous disorders due to its dependent position. Like the upper extremity, the venous system of the leg is divided into a superficial and deep system.

The superficial veins of the leg start with the dorsal venous arches on the feet, which form the great and small saphenous veins. Various perforator branches and a posterior arch vein join the saphenous veins in the distal lower extremity. As they travel superiorly, the veins of Giaccomini and the anterolateral veins of the thigh join the great saphenous vein. A major confluence is present in the groin, where the circumflex iliac vein, inferior epigastric vein, external pudendal vein, and great saphenous vein come together at the saphenofemoral junction to form the femoral vein. The great saphenous vein is more anterior and medial, while the small saphenous is posterior and somewhat lateral.

The deep veins of the leg include the soleal sinusoids, which join the peroneal, and anterior and posterior tibial veins to form the popliteal vein. The popliteal vein joins the deep femoral vein to form the common femoral vein. After receiving inflow from the superficial system, the common femoral vein continues as the external iliac vein, then the common iliac vein after joining with the internal iliac vein, and finally the inferior vena cava.

I.J. Pharmacology

Table 1. Anticoagulants, antiplatelet agents, vasodilators, and other vasoactive agents.

Please refer to page 142 for this table.

I.K. Diagnostic Evaluation

1. Ankle-Brachial Index

The ankle-brachial index (ABI) is calculated as the ratio of systolic blood pressure at the dorsalis pedis or posterior tibial artery to the highest brachial artery pressure, measured bilaterally. The highest brachial pressure measurement is an accurate reflection of core arterial pressure because bilateral upper extremity occlusive disease is extremely rare. If present, however, the ABI is not an accurate assessment of lower extremity perfusion. ABI measurements are highly sensitive and specific for hemodynamically-significant stenosis, but can be unreliable in patients with extensive calicification of vessels (as may occur in diabetics). Normal values range from 1.0 to 1.2; higher numbers indicate calcification. Claudication is usually seen in patients with ABIs ranging from 0.5 to 0.9. Rest pain and/or tissue loss are often present with values less than 0.4.

An exercise walking test can be completed to determine the severity of disease. During progressive ambulation, patients have a drop in their ABI during exercise, with a return to baseline following completion of strenuous activity. The extent of this drop and the rate of return to baseline are indicators for the extent of stenosis. Patients with iliac artery disease may have normal ABIs at rest and may require an exercise claudication test for diagnosis.

2. Duplex Ultrasound

B-mode ultrasound permits evaluation and measurement of flow vectors and measurement of vessel diameters. It is an extremely accurate test for a variety of vascular diseases in experienced hands. However, its overall performance is operator-dependent and can overestimate disease burden in inexperienced hands, especially for carotid artery stenosis. Duplex ultrasound

Text continued on page 144

Drug / Class	Mechanism of Action
ANTICOAGULANTS	
Warfarin	• Inhibits vitamin K based carboxylation (epoxide reductase and gamma-glutamyl carboxylase) of factors II, VII, IX, and X, protein C, S, and Z • Slower acting but longer half-life compared to heparin; typically effects manifest after 2-3 days • Monitor PT/INR
Heparin	• Binds to antithrombin III to inactivate thrombin and factor Xa • Rapid onset but half-life of 1 hour • Monitor PTT
LMWH	• Inhibition of factor Xa • Monitor anti-factor Xa levels
Direct Xa inhibitors	• Inhibit factor Xa directly • Agents include rivaroxaban and apixaban
Direct thrombin inhibitors	• Inhibits factor II (thrombin) directly • Agents include hirudin (Bivalirudin), and agatroban
ANTIPLATELET AGENTS	
Aspirin	Irreversible COX-1 inhibition and change in function of COX-2 enzyme that blocks TxA2 formation by platelets
Clopidogrel (Plavix)	Inhibits ADP receptor on platelets to block GP IIb/IIIa activation
Cilostazol (Pletal)	Selective phosphodiesterase inhibitor that causes vasodilation and inhibits platelets
Abciximab (ReoPro)	Direct inhibitor of GP IIb/IIIa
Dipyridamole (Persantine)	Inhibits platelet phosphodiesterase and induces PGI2; adenosine reuptake inhibitor

Contraindications	Notes
• Pregnancy due to fetal bleeding; existing bleeding risk • Interacts with statins, macrolides, metronidazole, and hypo/hyperthyroidism • Related to osteoporosis in men	• Target INR 2.0-3.0 for most cases; 2.5-3.5 for mechanical heart valves • Early deficiency of protein C can cause warfarin skin necrosis and therefore requires a heparin bridge • Purple toe syndrome from cholesterol deposits in feet • Reverse with FFP and vitamin K
• Heparin-induced thrombocytopenia due to autoantibody formation against platelets • Can lead to osteoporosis and hyperkalemia	• Requires antithrombin III to function; give FFP if suspected unavailability • Naturally stored in basophils and mast cells • Reverse with protamine sulfate
Less risk for osteoporosis and HIT	• Renal clearance • Reacts less well to protamine • More effective for cancer-induced thrombosis than warfarin (CLOT study)
	Used when rapid anticoagulation is desired but heparin cannot be used
No readily available monitoring test	Used when rapid anticoagulation is desired but heparin cannot be used
• Gastric ulcers, tinnitus, and children (Reye's syndrome) • Selective COX-2 inhibitors do not block COX-1 and increase the risk of MI	• TxA_2 leads to vasoconstriction and releases platelet granules • Wide variety of indications and usage
• Safer than aspirin in patients with gastric ulcers, unless aspirin is used with a PPI • May lead to neutropenia and TTP	GP IIb/IIIa receptor induces fibrinogen release; blockade inhibits platelet aggregation and cross-linking
Similar drugs related to increased death in patients with CHF	Used for intermittent claudication due to PVD
	Used with percutaneous coronary interventions and stent placement
Avoid in patients with highly stenosed arteries due to risk of steal syndrome from vasodilation of healthy arteries	• PGI2 inhibits TxA_2 • Used in pulmonary HTN, prevents AVF failure, reduces reperfusion injury, impairs platelet aggregation, and causes some vasodilation

Drug / Class	Mechanism of Action
THROMBOLYTICS	
tPA	Synthetic agent that catalyzes plasminogen conversion to plasmin
VASODILATORS	
Nitric oxide	• Produced by L-arginine and leads to an increase in cGMP • Suppresses free radical formation

uses flow velocities to calculate the extent of stenosis, and ultrasound to locate the stenosis and determine vessel characteristics.

3. CT Angiography

Computed tomographic angiography (CTA) is a superior imaging study that highlights vascular anatomy in three-dimensions. The resulting high-quality images are invaluable for surgical planning. CTA more accurately projects the extent of stenosis compared to ultrasound and MRA, and can mitigate the need for diagnostic arteriography. It is a highly sensitive and specific test for vascular trauma. Extravasation of contrast (a "blush") is indicative of vascular compromise with need for close observation, coil embolization by interventional radiology, or even surgery. CTA plays an important role in the evaluation of aortic stent grafts and the identification of an endoleak.

The major contraindication to CTA is the high contrast dye load that cannot be tolerated in patients with renal disease. There is also the risk of anaphylaxis, which can be avoided through premedication with steroids in susceptible patients.

4. MRA

Magnetic resonance angiography (MRA) images blood flow patterns and has a high sensitivity for clinically-significant stenosis. However, positive

Contraindications	Notes
• Hemorrhagic stroke • May lead to reperfusion injury in penumbra with free radical formation, edema, and compromise of a limb necessitating fasciotomy	• Must be given within 3 hours if IV, or 6 hours if catheter-directed • Reversed with aminocaproic acid • Streptokinase is produced by beta-hemolytic streptococcus
Hypotension or use of other nitrates	• Vasodilator and inhibitor of platelet aggregation • Produced by endothelial cells, macrophages, neutrophils, and smooth muscle cells • Pulmonary hypertension

findings are not necessarily specific for vascular disease. The combination of ultrasound and MRA can reveal a satisfactory picture of clinically-significant vascular disease; this modality is preferred in renal patients who will not tolerate a contrast dye load. However, the use of gadolinium dye in patients with renal disease may lead to systemic nephrogenic fibrosis.

5. Arteriography

Arteriography offers real-time imaging of a vessel through catheter-directed injection of a radio-opaque contrast agent. Combined with fluoroscopy, arteriography can precisely identify a compromised vessel. When used following the completion of a vascular intervention, arteriograms can confirm distal patency and flow.

I.L. Graft Patency

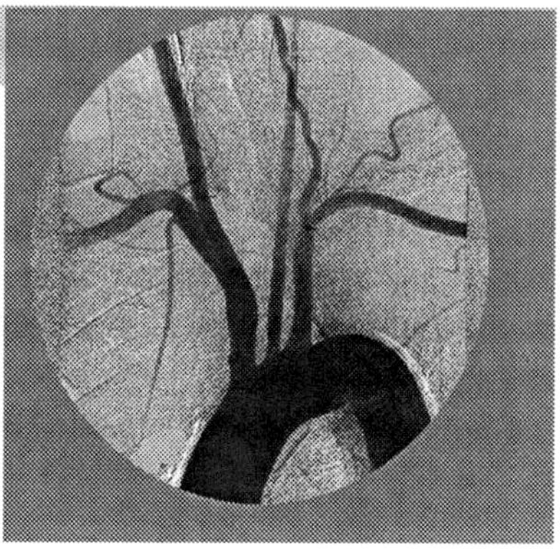

Primary patency is defined as continuing arterial flow and ceases with the need for an intervention or thrombosis of a graft. Primary-assisted patency is continuing arterial flow following an endovascular intervention due to stenosis or other impending compromise of a graft. Secondary patency is thrombosis or other loss of a graft requiring an intervention to reestablish flow. Unsurprisingly, long-term outcome for a graft is best when no intervention is necessary.

II. Extracranial Cerebrovascular Disease

II.A. Carotid Artery Disease

1. Etiology

Carotid artery disease has a number of distinct causes, including atherosclerosis, fibromuscular dysplasia, anatomic malformations, and inflammatory arteritides. Atherosclerosis most commonly affects the carotid bifurcation and is a major risk factor for stroke. Anatomic malformations include coils, kinks, and aneurysms. Radiation therapy has also been identified as cause of accelerated carotid artery atherosclerosis.

2. Pathophysiology and Presentation

Stroke is the third most common cause of death in the United States with an incidence of over 160 events per 100,000 people annually. Stroke has an initial mortality between 20 and 30%; of the patients who survive the initial event, half will die from a new stroke within 5 years.

A neurologic deficit is the initial clinical presentation of patients with symptomatic occlusive disease of the extracranial carotid artery. Aphasia, combined motor and sensory deficits, as well as visual disturbances, are associated with the anterior cerebral circulation. Vertigo, dizziness, ataxia, and drop attacks are associated with disturbances of the posterior cerebral circulation, especially to the vertebral artery.

These neurologic deficits can be due to thrombosis of an atherosclerotic plaque that produces a critical reduction in blood flow, cerebral embolism from an ulcerated carotid plaque, and occasionally from a cerebral low flow state. Neurologic deficits may take the form of a TIA, crescendo TIA, stroke, and amaurosis fugax. A TIA is a transient focal neurologic deficit that may last from several seconds to several hours, but subsides within 24 hours.

A crescendo TIA is a focal neurologic deficit with a rapid succession of focal deficits followed by complete recovery. Crescendo TIAs carry a high risk of progression to a permanent deficit and must be promptly diagnosed and treated. A focal neurologic deficit that persists over 24 hours is a stroke. A stroke that continues to worsen is defined as a stroke in evolution and requires immediate treatment.

Amaurosis fugax is a transient mono-ocular blindness usually described as a shade coming down over an eye. It is caused by an ophthalmic artery embolism. Hollenhorst plaques are cholesterol plaques that can be identified with a fundoscopic examination.

3. Diagnosis

A careful neurologic evaluation should precede any testing in patients with extracranial carotid artery and vertebral artery disease. Imaging of the carotid artery allows the classification of carotid artery lesions as follows:

- Mild (< 50% stenosis)
- Moderate (50-69% stenosis)
- Severe (70-99% stenosis)
- Occlusion (100% stenosis)

Noninvasive testing by way of carotid artery duplex ultrasound, CTA, and MRA can identify patients with carotid artery disease. Preoperative angiogram has lost its utility with the advent of high-quality CTA imaging. The correlation between preoperative angiogram and inspection of the plaque at time of surgery was analyzed in the 540 patients that were enrolled in the NASCET study. The sensitivity and specificity for detecting ulcerated plaques was 45.9% and 74.1%, while the positive predictive value for identification of an ulcer was 71.8% (see detailed discussion on page 148).

4. Treatment

a) Overview

Treatment of carotid artery lesions is beneficial for both symptomatic and asymptomatic patients. The Asymptomatic Carotid Atherosclerosis Study (ACAS) evaluated the efficacy of CEA in patients with asymptomatic high-grade stenosis. The Asymptomatic Carotid Surgery Trial (ACST) is the largest multicenter study to evaluate the benefit of CEA in asymptomatic patients with high-grade stenosis. The North American Symptomatic Carotid Endarterectomy Trial (NASCET) and the European Carotid Surgery Trial (ECST) have demonstrated the efficacy of carotid endarterectomy (CEA) in symptomatic patients. The Stenting and Angioplasty with Protection in Patients at High Risk for Endarterectomy (SAPPHIRE) study found that carotid stenting in patients who were otherwise poor candidates for CEA due to medical comorbidities is effective.

b) ACAS and ACST

ACAS randomized 1,662 patients with 60-99% stenosis as assessed by ultrasound and arteriography to the CEA or ASA (325 mg/day) group. The initial endpoint was TIA or cerebral infarction in the distribution of the study artery, or any TIA, stroke or death in the perioperative period. The median follow up was 2.7 years.

ACST was carried over from 1993 to 2003. It randomly assigned 3,120 patients with 60% or greater asymptomatic carotid artery stenosis to immediate CEA or deferred CEA groups. Median follow up was 3.4%. The study showed a perioperative stroke risk of 3.1 % at 30 days and a net five-year stroke risk of 6.4 % in the immediate CEA arm vs. 11.8% in the deferred arm.

Early CEA was also favored for fatal and disabling strokes in both men and women. However, in women the absolute risk reduction at 5 years was 4.1 vs. 8.2 in men. The benefit was significantly better in patients younger than 75 years of age, but remained obscure in patients over the age of 75 (but see NASCET findings below). The most significant finding of the ACST trial was that benefit from CEA was demonstrated in contralateral CVA.

c) NASCET

NASCET is a prospective, randomized, multicenter trial initiated in the mid-80s to investigate the efficacy of CEA in symptomatic patients. It enrolled 659 patients that had a hemispheric TIA, amaurosis fugax, or a non-disabling stroke within 120 days with a stenosis of 70-99% in the ispilateral carotid artery. The study was prematurely terminated by the NIH because of clear evidence of benefit from surgery. At the time of termination, median follow up was 18 months. NASCET measured the residual lumen diameter at the most stenotic portion of the vessel and compared it with the lumen diameter of the internal carotid artery distal to the stenosis.

A lower cumulative risk of any ipsilateral stroke (9% vs. 26%; $p<0.001$) and a lower risk of major and fatal ipsilateral stroke (2.5% vs. 13.1%; $p<0.001$) were noted in the CEA arm. CEA is highly beneficial in symptomatic patients with ispilateral carotid stenosis of 70 to 99%.

In a subsequent report, NASCET demonstrated that CEA had a moderate degree of benefit in symptomatic patients with stenosis between 50 and 69% in the ipsilateral carotid artery, but the statistical significance was more marginal. The 5 year rate of any ipsilateral stroke for endarterectomy vs. medical treatment was 15.7% vs. 22.2% ($p=0.045$). No benefit of CEA vs. medical therapy was shown in symptomatic patients with stenosis less than 50%.

CEA was also beneficial at a 7 year follow-up. A further analysis of the NASCET data found that older patients (>75 years of age) benefited more from the CEA than younger patients. This has been confirmed by several reports in the literature.

d) ECST

The European Carotid Surgery Trial (ECST) is a multicenter, randomized, controlled trial that enrolled over 3,000 patients over a 10 year period to evaluate the risks and benefits of carotid endarterectomy as a surgical treatment for patients with symptomatic carotid stenosis. A control arm avoided surgery unless there was symptomatic recurrence, while the treatment arm underwent a planned carotid endarterectomy.

The ECST study measured the lumen at the most stenotic segment of the vessel and compared it to the estimated probable original diameter at the site of maximum stenosis. This method required assumption of true lumen diameter and led to an increase in inter-observer variability.

Overall, the ECST confirmed the results of the NASCET and demonstrated a benefit with CEA in symptomatic patients with ipsilateral carotid lesions. In the ECST, the risk varied with age and gender with benefit being less pronounced in women and over a narrower range of carotid stenosis in younger patients. As in NASCET, the ECST demonstrated long term (10 years) benefit of CEA in symptomatic patients.

No value of emergent CEA has been found in patients with acute stroke. In both NASCET and ECST, the incidence of stroke was significantly lower in the surgical group (relative risk reduction 0.53 with 95% CI). A subgroup analysis suggested that CEA was less effective in women. In all of these trials, low dose ASA therapy (81-325 mg daily) is recommended prior to surgery and for at least three months after surgery.

e) SAPPHIRE

The Stenting and Angioplasty with Protection of Patients with High Risk for Endarterectomy (SAPPHIRE) trial is a multicenter, prospective study that has enrolled over 2,000 patients who have contraindications to carotid endarterectomy. These patients underwent angioplasty and stent placement and were followed for a 30 day period to determine the incidence of adverse events.

The SAPPHIRE trial indicates that carotid artery stent (CAS) placement in lieu of carotid endarterectomy is suitable for patients who are not candidates for CEA due to medical or surgical comorbidities but would have otherwise benefited from a CEA.

5. Complications

Following CEA or CAS, approximately 3% of asymptomatic patients and 6% of previously symptomatic patients may have a stroke or die. The risk of hemorrhage may occur in about 2-3% of patients and may lead to obstruction of the airway through tracheal compression. This may require opening of the incision and drainage of the hematoma at the bedside if the airway is in danger. There is about a 1% chance of damage to the hypoglossal nerve, leading to deviation of the tongue toward the affected side. A dangerous but rare complication is cerebral hyperperfusion and may present with a spectrum of symptoms ranging from headache to fatal intracranial hemorrhage. MRI is the imaging test of choice; treatment involves correction of high blood pressure with some indications that beta-blockers may be protective.

Recurrence of carotid artery stenosis after CEA occurs in up to 20% of cases. Early restenosis within 1-2 years is commonly due to intimal hyperplasia. A late manifestation of stenosis 2 years following surgery may be secondary to recurrent and progressive atherosclerosis. Abu Rhama and colleagues suggest that patch closure can reduce the risk of fibroplasia so that only 7% of patients are affected. This was also confirmed by the ACAS study.

Predictors of medical complications include history of MI, angina and HTN. Based off subgroup analysis completed in the NASCET trial, the risk of perioperative stroke and death at 30 days and stroke severity at 90 days is correlated to 5 major variables predictive of increased surgical risk:

- Hemispheric vs. retinal TIA as the qualifying event
- Left-sided procedure
- Contralateral carotid occlusion
- Ipsilateral lesion at CT Scan
- Irregularity and/or ulceration of the plaque

II.B. Carotid Artery Aneurysm

1. Etiology and Pathophysiology

Extracranial carotid artery aneurysms are rare, affecting only 1 out of 200 patients with carotid artery disease, and comprising less than 2% of all aneurysmal disease. The most important predisposing risk factors are atherosclerosis and trauma. Other major causes are cystic medial necrosis from syphilis, fibromuscular dysplasia, polyarteritis nodosa, and Marfan syndrome. Atherosclerotic disease can lead to weakening of the arterial wall from the inflammatory response. Both blunt and penetrating trauma can lead to a disruption of the arterial wall and cause false aneurysms (see page 180).

2. Presentation and Diagnosis

Carotid aneurysm disease may be entirely asymptomatic, or lead to thromboembolic phenomenon causing TIA and stroke. Rupture can occur into the esophagus, trachea, or soft tissues of the neck and lead to exsanguination, cerebral ischemia, and loss of the airway. An uncomfortable, pulsatile mass in the neck is the most common finding on exam.

3. Treatment

Management for extracranial carotid aneurysmal disease is by way of surgery in all satisfactory candidates. Simple ligation of the common carotid artery is fraught with up to a 50% rate of death from cerebral hypoperfusion and thromboembolism to the brain; however, this may be the only option in some patients with extensive life-threatening disease of the supraclinoid carotid artery in which surgical exposure is nearly impossible. Mitigation of this risk is possible with full anticoagulation and gradual carotid artery occlusion over a period of time; this approach has reduced the risk of stroke to 25% and mortality to about 10%.

By far the most optimal treatment for carotid aneurysm disease is reconstruction of the artery with an end-to-end anastomosis or PTFE interposition graft to ensure patency of the carotid artery. Patch repair is possible after excision of a small saccular aneurysm with a small neck. It is important to place the distal clamp first and to heparinize the patient to avoid embolism to the brain. Shunt placement is the preferred option to help minimize this complication.

II.C. Giant Cell Arteritis

1. Assessment

Giant cell arteritis is a chronic inflammatory process affecting the tunica intima and media of large- and medium-sized vessels especially common in elderly women. This disorder is also known as temporal arteritis and reflects the predisposition of this disorder to the temporal artery and other arteries of the head. However, giant cell arteritis may present anywhere in the body and symptoms including myalgia, arthritis, and inflammation of the joints throughout the proximal and distal extremities can occur. In this form, the disorder is typically referred to as polymyalgia rheumatica. The axillary artery is commonly affected.

When present with the temporal artery or other branches of the external carotid artery, the primary presentation involves fever, headache, jaw claudication, and sudden blindness. Tenderness over the temporal artery is present; involvement of the ophthalmic artery presents with amaurosis fugax and can lead to permanent blindness.

Regardless of the distribution, a diagnostic biopsy of an affected artery is necessary for confirmation. A conglomeration of giant cells (large, multinucleated macrophages) is evident on histology. A halo sign is seen on diagnostic imaging.

2. Management

Treatment is by way of corticosteroids and is started immediately upon a clinical diagnosis. The goal is to avoid occlusion of the ophthalmic artery and subsequent blindness. Low dose aspirin is particularly effective in the prevention of blindness and stroke.

III. Upper Extremity Vascular Disease

III.A. Subclavian Steal Syndrome

1. Etiology

Subclavian steal is retrograde flow of blood from the vertebral artery into the subclavian artery. It occurs secondary to stenosis of the subclavian artery proximal to the vertebral artery take off. As a result, any instance where increased blood flow is required to the extremity, the source is from the vertebral artery. The most common cause of the stenosis is atherosclerosis, but it is also present in Takayasu disease and congenital malformations of the subclavian artery or aortic arch.

2. Presentation

Subclavian steal syndrome, symptomatic in only 10% of patients with underlying structural disease, presents with neuronal ischemia leading to lightheadedness and syncope. Onset of symptoms is with increased use of the extremity and may also lead to arm ischemia depending on the extent of stenosis; a baseline low blood pressure is typically present in the affected limb. Nearly one in four patients over the age of 70 develop this syndrome, particularly of the left subclavian artery.

3. Diagnosis

The workup for subclavian stenosis begins after a sufficient history and physical examination heightens the suspicion for this disease. Ultrasound demonstrates retrograde flow, while CT angiography demarcates the anatomy and may identify the area of stenosis.

4. Treatment

Treatment for subclavian steal syndrome is with endovascular subclavian artery stenting, the preferred surgical treatment. Balloon angioplasty, extra-anatomic carotid to subclavian bypass, extra-anatomic axillary-axillary bypass, and transposition of the subclavian artery are other available options if an endovascular stent placement is not possible.

The optimal treatment for subclavian steal syndrome is carotid to subclavian artery bypass with conduit. If there are significant contraindications to surgery, a variety of alternative procedures exist including endovascular subclavian artery stenting and balloon angioplasty. If carotid to subclavian bypass is not possible due to anatomic restrictions, an alternative is extra-anatomic axillary-axillary bypass or transposition of the subclavian artery.

III.B. Thoracic Outlet Obstruction

Thoracic outlet obstruction is secondary to compression of neurovascular structures at the thoracic outlet, commonly due to structures within the scalene triangle or costoclavicular space.

1. Neurogenic

Neurogenic thoracic outlet obstruction typically presents with compression of the entire brachial plexus cords. Weakness of the extremity, headache, and back pain are common, reproducible symptoms. Involvement of the sympathetic plexus can lead to changes in the color and temperature of the hand. The brachial plexus passes through the scalene triangle (see page 133).

2. Venous

Venous thoracic outlet obstruction is secondary to compression of the subclavian vein within the costoclavicular space (see page 133). The subclavian vein passes through this quadrangle. Compression by any of these bounding structures can lead to venous manifestation of disease. Proximal structures include the phrenic nerve and thoracic duct (on the left). The lateral thoracic nerve traverses the middle scalene muscle.

3. Arterial

The most common cause of an arterial manifestation of thoracic outlet obstruction is from a cervical rib leading to compression, stenosis, and thromboembolism of the second part of the subclavian artery. This compression commonly occurs within the scalene triangle. The subclavian artery and brachial plexus pass through this triangle, while the vein passes through the costoclavicular space.

4. Diagnosis and Treatment

Diagnosis of thoracic outlet obstruction is made clinically after exclusion of other causes by CT and MRI. Angiography or venography can be completed if either an arterial or venous manifestation is suspected. Ultrasound is used to identify collateral vessels and to optimize surgical planning.

Definitive treatment includes physical therapy, anticoagulation for arterial or venous disease, and surgical correction of the anatomic defect. Venous manifestation is repaired by correcting any abnormalities within the subclavian vein, thrombectomy, and open decompression. Arterial or neurologic manifestation is treated by release of one or more components of the scalene triangle. Great care must be taken to protect the vital nerves that travel in this region.

III.C. Raynaud Phenomenon

1. Assessment

Raynaud disease is arterial vasospasm of small and medium vessels in the distal extremity leading to pallor and cyanosis. The major trigger is cold exposure. Following resolution of the vasoocclusion, reactive hyperemia occurs with resumption of arterial flow. Primary manifestations of disease may be symptomatic but typically do not lead to clinically-significant deterioration or irreversible physical findings.

Secondary Raynaud phenomenon is associated with hypercoagulable states and connective tissue disease, and can lead to poorly healing wounds, gangrene, and auto-amputation. Diagnosis is confirmed by digital video capillaroscopy and laser Doppler evaluation.

2. Management

The mainstay of therapy is minimization of triggers that lead to the symptoms. Nifedipine can be used for symptomatic management. Serious disease can be forestalled with a sympathetic nerve block or sympathectomy. Surgery may be needed for severe secondary manifestations, such as gangrene.

III.D. Takayasu Arteritis

1. Assessment

Takayasu arteritis, first described in 1908, is a large vessel inflammatory disease that primarily affects young Asian women. Granulomatous disease of the major vessels leads to arterial stenosis and aneurysm formation. There is marked fibrosis and thickening of the arterial wall. It presents with loss of peripheral pulses, particularly in the carotid artery and upper extremity. Reactive changes in the eye from the stenosis leads to loss of vision from angiogenesis in the retina. Recently, some cases of atypical aortic coarctation have been found to have similar lesions and are now considered as variants of Takayasu arteritis. Two phases of the disease have been described. In the early phase systemic flu-like symptoms predominate but subside with no further complication. Months or years later, vascular occlusion takes place.

Four different types of Takayasu arteritis have been identified:

1. Involvement of the aortic arch and its branches
2. Involvement of the descending and abdominal aorta only
3. Combination of types 1 and 2
4. Features of types 1, 2 and 3 plus involvement of the pulmonary artery.

2. Management

Takayasu arteritis is treated with prednisone. Advanced cases may require arterioplasty, stent placement, and bypass.

III.E. Buerger Disease

Buerger disease, also known as thromboangiitis obliterans, is inflammation and subsequent thrombosis of small arteries in the distal extremities. The largest risk factor is smoking. Buerger disease presents with ulceration and gangrene of the hands and feet from thrombosis, leading to amputation. An arteriogram illustrates 'corkscrew' vessels, stenosis, and occlusion. A biopsy is contraindicated due to the risk of no healing. Smoking cessation is required, but there is no definitive cure. Angioplasty, stent placement, and bypass of affected vessels can sometimes forestall amputation.

IV. Lower Extremity Vascular Disease

IV.A. Limb Ischemia

1. Epidemiology and Etiology

Intermittent claudication is the most common symptom in patients with compromised blood flow to the lower extremities. It is defined as a reproducible myalgia induced by exercise and relieved by rest. The most important pathogenic factor is atherosclerosis of the lower extremity vasculature. Reversible risk factors include diabetes, hyperlipidemia, smoking, and hypertension.

The prevalence of peripheral arterial disease increases with age. The Inter-Society Consensus (TASC) II guidelines published in 2007 estimate that peripheral arterial disease affects over 27 million individuals and leads to 88,000 hospitalizations annually throughout North America and Europe.

2. Pathophysiology and Presentation

The area affected by claudication is related to the level of arterial blood flow impairment:

- Claudication of the buttocks and hips is due to aorto-iliac disease and defined as Leriche syndrome. Leriche syndrome presents with buttock claudication and impotence. The distal aorta and both internal and external iliac arteries may be compromised.
- Claudication of the thigh is secondary to low aorto-iliac disease or common femoral disease.
- Claudication of the upper third of the calf is due to compromise of the superficial femoral artery.
- Claudication of the lower third of the calf is due to compromise of the popliteal artery.
- Claudication of the foot is secondary to compromise of the tibial or peroneal artery.

Clinically significant disease presents with claudication and is accompanied with paresthesias, muscular atrophy, and loss of hair. Advanced disease may lead to tissue loss, hyposphigmia, and even complete loss of the distal pulses.

3. Diagnosis and Classification

Following a thorough history and physical examination, a Doppler evaluation should be completed of the major vessels in the lower extremity. A biphasic signal indicates direct flow to the artery, while a monophasic signal implies indirect flow via a collateral.

Noninvasive arterial examination should follow with calculation of segmental limb pressures, volume plethysmography, and duplex ultrasound. These values will provide a physiologic assessment of the lower extremity. CT angiography is an invaluable tool to provide anatomic imaging and to permit surgical planning. CTA has an outstanding sensitivity and specificity for a clinically significant stenosis with over 50% narrowing. If the contrast load cannot be tolerated, an MRA can be completed with a similar resolving power as CTA.

Peripheral arterial disease can be classified by the Fontaine scale:

- Stage 1: Asymptomatic
- Stage 2A: Mild claudication when walking > 200 m
- Stage 2B: Moderate to severe claudication with walking < 200 m
- Stage 3: Pain at rest
- Stage 4: Ulceration or gangrene

Critical limb ischemia is defined as Fontaine class III or IV, an ABI < 0.4, or an ankle systolic pressure < 50 mmHg.

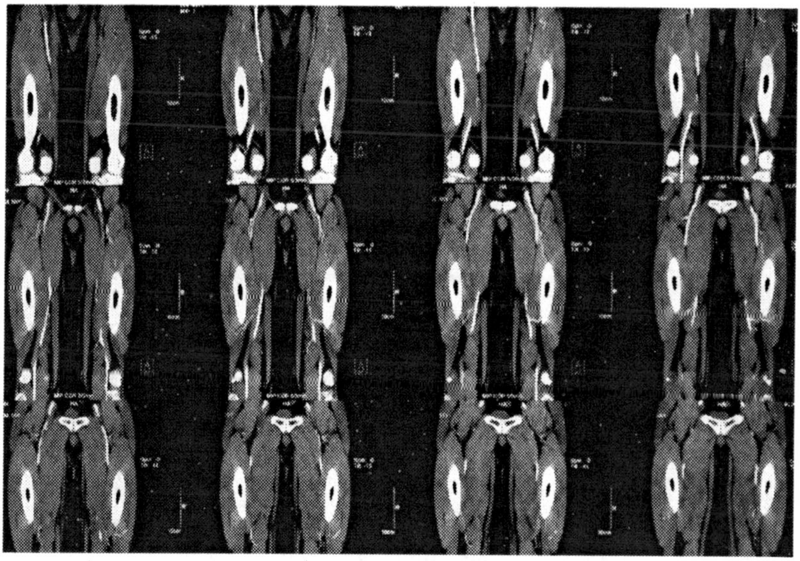

4. Treatment

The preferred treatment in patients with peripheral arterial disease is mitigation of clinical risk factors, smoking cessation, and an aggressive exercise regimen. Treatment with antiplatelet agents such as cilostazol and pentoxyfiline are used in concert with lifestyle changes. Continuing symptoms of lifestyle-limiting disease or critical limb ischemia requires surgical revascularization. Frank wet gangrene of the affected limb can only be treated with amputation. Based on the gangrene level, relevant comorbidities, and rehabilitation potential, toe, transmetatarsal, below the knee (BKA), or above the knee amputations (AKA) may be recommended.

The primary treatment option is bypass of the affected region delineated by CTA. Autologous graft via a saphenous vein or synthetic conduit via Dacron or PTFE can be used as the conduit. Both inflow and outflow disease must be addressed in order to have successful distal revascularization; achieving this goal may even require an extra-anatomic bypass such as a femoral-femoral bypass with PTFE or an axillary-femoral bypass. Regular postoperative surveillance with ultrasound and ABIs is necessary for early detection of graft failure.

The ACC/AHA guidelines note that the expected patency rates with different types of bypass for aorto-iliac disease are as follows:

- Aorto-bifemoral, aortoiliac or aorto-femoral: 85-90% at 5 years
- Femoral-femoral 70% at 5 years
- Axillary-femoral 50-80% at 3 years

The patency rates for inguinal disease are:

- Femoral-popliteal vein graft above or below the knee: 65% at 5 years
- Femoral-popliteal with synthetic PFTE graft: 50% at 5 years above the knee and 33% at 5 years below the knee
- Femoral-tibial with vein: 75-80 % at 5 years
- Femoral-tibial with synthetic PTFE graft: 25% at 3 years

Patients who are poor surgical candidates from related co-morbidities or from anatomic limitations may be candidates for percutaneous interventions such as angioplasty and stent placement. A focal lesion is amenable to this approach. Surgical management vs. endovascular management was compared in the BASIL trial, which was a randomized trial with 450 patients with severe limb ischemia and infrainguinal disease. Over 20% of the patients in the percutaneous intervention arm had an immediate technical failure. Patients in the surgery group had a higher rate of morbidity compared to the percutaneous group (57% vs. 41%), but overall mortality was the same. Surgery was superior to percutaneous intervention with regard to the rate of recurrent disease and amputation risk.

The conclusion of the study was that percutaneous interventions are satisfactory in patients with high-risk disease with a limited life expectancy. Treatment with a percutaneous intervention requires post-procedure therapy with aspirin and Plavix, a conclusion drawn from the extensive cardiac literature on similar interventions.

5. Complications

Predictors of poor outcome following vascular reconstruction for lower extremity occlusive disease include severe peripheral disease with poor outflow circulation, advanced age, uncontrolled diabetes mellitus, renal insufficiency, female gender, and systemic hypertension. The most important complications include thrombosis, infection, and pseudoaneurysm formation.

Early failure of a vein graft is likely due to technical error and presents as thrombosis. Mid- and late-graft failure are due to neointimal hyperplasia and atherosclerosis, respectively. Antiplatelet agents are used for all patients, but those with an especially high risk of graft occlusion or limb loss should be fully anticoagulated with heparin and warfarin.

V. Splanchnic Vascular Disease

V.A. Mesenteric Ischemia

1. Pathophysiology and Presentation

Mesenteric ischemia is the compromise of gastrointestinal blood flow. Atrial fibrillation leading to thromboembolic phenomenon, low flow states contributing to hemostasis, mesenteric thrombi, and hypercoagulable states contribute to mesenteric ischemia. Acute mesenteric ischemia presents with severe abdominal pain out of proportion to exam, typically secondary to acute thromboembolism and impending bowel infarction. Late signs include metabolic lactic acidosis, BRBPR, and necrotic bowel. Mortality is nearly 75%.

Chronic mesenteric ischemia presents with severe abdominal pain that worsens with ingestion, leading to anorexia from decreased oral intake. Patients with a history of CAD may have chronic mesenteric ischemia.

2. Diagnosis

There are four distinct types of acute mesenteric ischemia, including acute mesenteric arterial embolism, acute mesenteric arterial thrombosis, nonocclusive mesenteric ischemia, and mesenteric venous thrombosis. Insufficient blood flow to the bowel is the common pathway and eventually leads to hemorrhagic infarction, sepsis from disruption of the mucosa, and death. Early findings include bowel wall thickening along a specific vascular pathway, free fluid in the pelvis, pneumatosis intestinalis, and eventually, signs of free perforation and frank necrosis. The SMA near the middle colic artery is most commonly affected.

Diagnosis of mesenteric ischemia is confirmed by CTA demonstrating a sharp cut-off of contrast along a particular arterial pathway. Ultrasound can be done as a highly sensitive test, but is relevant only in thromboembolic disease. MRA is superior to CTA in its sensitivity and specificity.

3. Treatment

Treatment of acute mesenteric ischemia depends on the particular cause of the disease. Papaverine can be infused via angiography in an attempt to dilate the affected vessels. Catheter-directed thrombolysis is effective when a thromboembolic cause is suspected. Angioplasty is possible, but fraught with difficulty due to the anatomy of the SMA. Stent placement is possible in selected patients.

Surgical interventions by Fogarty thrombectomy is possible if there is little compromised bowel and the occluded area can be identified. Revascularization with an anterograde aortomesenteric bypass is possible with proximal SMA occlusion; an acceptable alternative is transaortic endarterectomy. Mesenteric vein thrombosis should be treated with heparinization and medical support, as thrombectomy is rarely possible due to the longstanding and extensive nature of the clot.

Selected cases of chronic mesenteric ischemia can be treated with surgical reconstruction or angioplasty with stenting of the affected portion of SMA. In many cases, diagnosis is missed for a prolonged period and patients require nutritional support prior to surgical intervention because of poor oral intake.

V.B. Renal Artery Stenosis

1. Pathophysiology and Presentation

Renal artery stenosis leads to a decrease in flow to the kidney, which is sensed at the macular densa and leads to activation of the renin angiotensin-aldosterone pathway. The net effect is sodium reabsorption, fluid salvage, and elevated blood pressure. Renal artery stenosis causes hypertension in up to 10% of patients with high blood pressure and should be suspected in patients refractory to maximum medical management. Stenosis can lead to chronic renal insufficiency and progress to end stage renal disease. Atherosclerosis and fibromuscular dysplasia are two common causes of disease; the former primarily affects older males, while the latter affects younger females.

2. Diagnosis

Renal ultrasound demonstrates asymmetric flow between the two kidneys, unless bilateral disease is present. CTA and MRA are satisfactory anatomical imaging studies, but may not be options in patients with renal dysfunction from longstanding disease. Fibromuscular dysplasia is presents with bilateral disease and a 'string-of-beads' sign on radiographic imaging (see below).

3. Treatment

The ideal treatment for renal artery stenosis is surgical or percutaneous correction of the stenotic defect. Angioplasty and stent placement are satisfactory percutaneous interventions and highly effective for atheromatous disease. The success of percutaneous interventions makes them the favored approach in most patients. Refractory disease or technical limitations with an endovascular intervention requires a revascularization procedure with surgical bypass. Any variation of aortorenal, hepatorenal, ileorenal, or splenorenal bypass can be completed using autologous or synthetic conduit.

Reimplantation of the kidneys can also be accomplished. The treatment of choice for fibromuscular dysplasia is angioplasty; stent placement is contraindicated in this disorder.

V.C. Fibromuscular Dysplasia

1. Assessment

Fibromuscular dysplasia is stenosis of the renal, iliac or carotid arteries leading to flow-limiting ischemic disease, hypertension, stroke, and aneurysm formation. It is most common in young women and leads to eccentric arterial stenosis with interspersed dilation, leading to a 'string of beads' sign on angiography. The right renal artery is more likely to be affected than the left, and is the most common cause of arterial stenosis in young females.

Fibromuscular dysplasia was first described in the carotid artery in 1964 and has been recognized as a cause of cerebrovascular symptoms, especially in women. In 25% of cases fibromuscular dysplasia is associated with atherosclerotic lesions, while 65% of cases are bilateral. Four histologic types have been recognized:

- **Medial fibroplasia** is the most common form and is a consequence of smooth muscle cell fibrosis within the tunica media. Focal stenosis and multiple lesions with intervening small aneurysms are found.
- **Intimal fibroplasia** results from accumulation of mesenchymal cells in the intimal subendothelium, resulting in long tubular stenosis in young patients and focal stenosis in older patients.
- **Medial hyperplasia** is a rare variant and results from the accumulation of smooth muscle cells in the media.
- **Perimedial dysplasia** is characterized by accumulation of elastic tissue between the media and the adventitia. It usually affects the renal arteries and is correlated with aneurysm development.

2. Management

Treatment involves ACE-inhibitors for unilateral disease but is contraindicated in bilateral disease due to the risk of renal failure. Angioplasty and stent placement are used for refractory disease, while bypass of the affected vessel can be done in more extreme cases.

VI. Systemic Vascular Disease

VI.A. Atherosclerosis

Plaque formation occurs in a three step process starting with deposit of lipid within the vessel wall. This stimulates recruitment of macrophages that attempt to resorb this lipid, leading to the formation of foam cells. Intimal hyperplasia sets in with smooth muscle cell proliferation. This is followed by sudden plaque rupture and thromboembolism. Significant atheroma formation leads to peripheral arterial occlusive disease. Stenosis of over 50% causes significant arterial flow disruption, while symptoms are present with over 75% stenosis. However, friable plaques and anatomic location play a major role in the risk assessment of stenotic disease; for example, symptomatic patients with carotid stenosis over 50% will undergo a carotid endarterectomy.

A related idiopathic condition leading to accelerated atherosclerosis is Mönckeberg medial arteriosclerosis, leading to osteoporosis, peripheral arterial occlusive disease, and MI through calcium deposition within the tunica media.

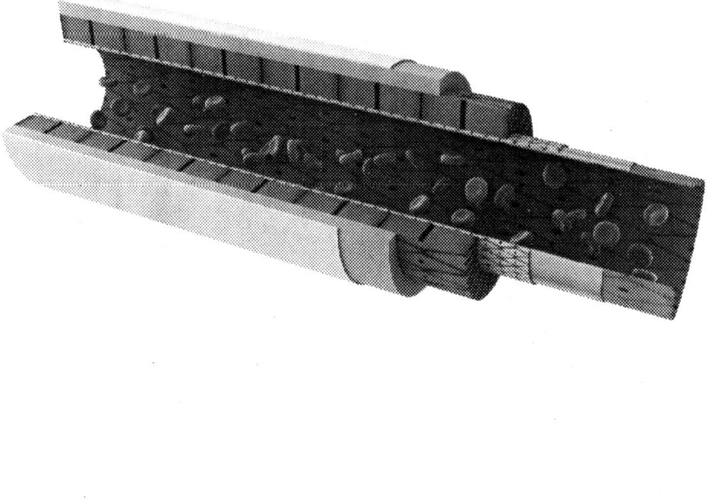

VI.B. Wegener Granulomatosis

Table 5. Wegener Granulomatosis

Etiology	Formation of necrotizing granulomas in the respiratory tract and renal parenchyma.
Presentation	Inflammation of the respiratory tract, vasculitis of smaller vessels, and focal glomerulonephritis. Triad of sinusitis, pulmonary infiltrates, and nephritis.
Diagnosis	Elevated C-ANCA and confirmation by biopsy from kidney or lung.
Treatment	Steroid-induced immunosuppression. Cyclophosphamide and methotrexate for serious disease. TMP-SMX to avoid relapse.

VI.C. Churg-Strauss Disease

Table 6. Churg-Strauss Disease

Etiology	Systemic vasculitis of medium sized arteries.
Presentation	Vasculitis, bronchospasm, and maculopapular rashes.
Diagnosis	Hypereosinophilia
Treatment	Corticosteroids, azathioprine, and cyclophosphamide.

VI.D. Henoch-Schonein Purpura

Table 7. Henoch-Schönlein Purpura (HSP)

Etiology	Aggregation of IgA and deposition within vessel walls and renal mesangium due to allergic reaction from foreign object or viral infection. Primarily affects young children.
Presentation	Erythematous macular rash on the lower extremities followed by purpura, edema, and arthralgia. Eosinophilia is often present along with IgA.
Diagnosis	Skin biopsy. The distinguishing feature of HSP is the presence of arthralgias.
Treatment	Corticosteroids if disease progresses.

VI.E. Thrombotic Thrombocytopenic Purpura

Table 8. Thrombotic Thrombocytopenic Purpura (TTP)

Etiology	Vascular injury from inflammatory or toxic damage.
Presentation	Widespread capillary thrombosis to kidney and brain. Evolves over a week with fever and purpura. Hematuria and hematochezia with hemorrhage in mucosal membranes and retina. Pancreatitis and arthralgia also evolve. HUS may be preceded by a viral or bacterial prodrome and presents with abdominal pain, nausea and vomiting, diarrhea, GI bleeding, ARF, uremia, HTN, CNS changes, and high fever. A microangiopathic hemolytic anemia with hematuria and proteinuria occur in both TTP and HUS.
Diagnosis	Biopsy is typically required to detect the focal necrotizing arteritis.
Treatment	Plasmapheresis, FFP, and corticosteroids. Splenectomy. HUS requires blood transfusions in most patients. Dialysis is necessary in about half of all patients due to the severe ARF. Fluid and electrolyte management is required, and correction of HTN is necessary. Anticoagulation, thrombolysis, plasmapheresis, and prostacyclin infusion are used in some cases. Mesenteric infarction leading to ischemia of the colon in HUS may necessitate bowel resection.

VI.F. Polyarteritis Nodosa

1. Assessment

Polyarteritis nodosa (PAN) is a necrotizing, inflammatory vasculitis of medium and small arteries leading to hemorrhage and thrombosis. Involvement of the musculoskeletal, renal, and gastrointestinal systems is especially common; this presents as myalgia, anorexia, diastolic hypertension, renal insufficiency, and livedo reticularis. Causes include a variety of viral infections, rheumatoid arthritis, and leukemia. Diagnosis is confirmed by angiography, which may indicate aneurysmal disease in the affected organs. ANCA is elevated and PMNs are found on arterial biopsy, which is required for a definitive diagnosis.

2. Management

Treatment for PAN is via immunosuppression to forestall further damage. Antivirals are given whenever a viral prodrome is suspected as the underlying etiology. Surgery is primarily reserved for complications associated with advanced disease.

VII. Arterial Aneurysms

VII.A. Visceral Artery Aneurysmal Disease

1. Thoracoabdominal Aortic Aneurysm

a) Etiology and Pathophysiology

Aneurysms are defined as dilation over 50% of the normal diameter of the vessel. The normal width of the thoracoabdominal aorta is about 2.3-2.8 cm. The normal width of the infrarenal aorta is closer to 2 cm. As a result, aneurysm of the thoracoabdominal aorta begins at about 3.5 cm, and 3.0 cm for the infrarenal aorta.

Laplace's law describes the physical relationship between wall tension as it directly relates to pressure and radius. It is thought that increased tension leads to increased pressure to a certain extent, before the connective tissue framework dissolves and the radius of the afflicted vessel increases. Disruption of the elastin network can lead to partial rupture and formation of a dissection. Free rupture can occur, but is more likely with an already dilated vessel with a weakened vessel wall. Aneurysm formation is more likely as the aorta travels inferiorly due to a decrease in elastin content.

Thoracoabdominal aortic aneurysms affect the descending aorta as it enters the abdominal cavity. These aneurysms have many of the same complications associated with abdominal aortic disease, but treatment options and indications for repair are different.

Thoracoabdominal aortic aneurysms are separated into various categories.

- **Crawford type I**: Aneurysm beginning distal to the left subclavian artery and terminating proximal to the renal vessels.

- **Crawford type II:** Aneurysm beginning immediately distal to the left subclavian artery and terminating at the aortic bifurcation.
- **Crawford type III:** Aneurysm beginning more than 7 cm distal to the left subclavian artery and terminating at the aortic bifurcation.
- **Crawford type IV:** Aneurysm below diaphragm and extending to the aortic bifurcation.

b) Presentation and Diagnosis

Thoracoabdominal aneurysms are asymptomatic and are an incidental finding on diagnostic imaging completed for other reasons. Early signs of an expanding aneurysm include chest or back pain and may lead to compression of the esophagus or inferior vena cava with thromboembolism. The presence of pain, hypotension, and a pulsatile mass on exam are worrisome for a rupturing aneurysm and require immediate operative management; imaging studies are contraindicated in this instance.

Diagnostic imaging includes ultrasound, aortography, CT, and MRI. Ultrasound is satisfactory for infrarenal disease, but is inadequate in the thoracoabdominal aorta. Aortography defines the anatomy of the aorta and

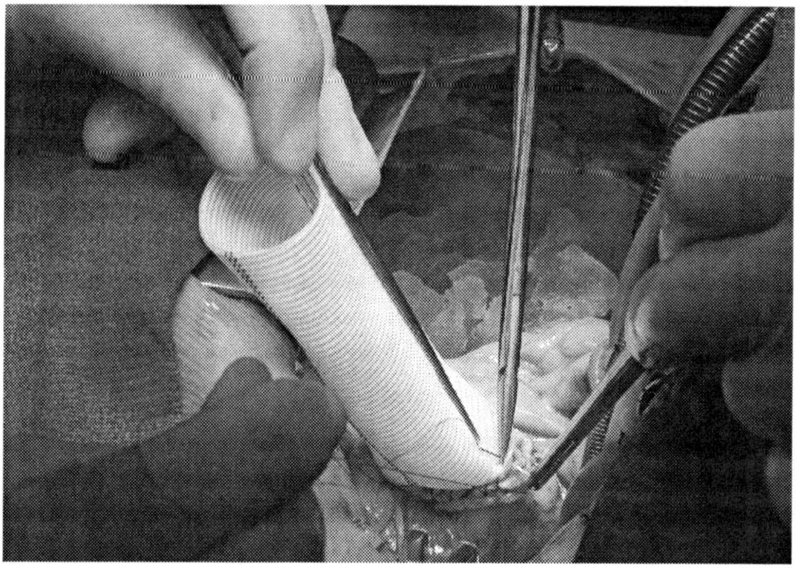

branches but gives no information about the size of an aneurysm as the outer diameter of the aorta is not measured. CT is the preferred test in patients who can tolerate the contrast load and permits three-dimensional reconstruction of the aorta and optimal operative planning.

c) Treatment

Repair is indicated for thoracic segments wider than 5.5 cm, abdominal segments wider than 5.5 cm, rapidly enlarging size (over 1 cm per year), or symptomatic disease. Repair should be undertaken earlier in patients with Marfan disease due to their significantly weaker aortic lumen. Thoracoabdominal aneurysms are traditionally repaired using an open approach, but recently some have used fenestrated endovascular grafts or placement of an endovascular prosthesis in combination with aortic debranching (sequential branch grafts to the renal and visceral vessels).

When open repair is necessary, a retroperitoneal approach is used, replacing the aneurysmal aorta and reimplanting the visceral and renal vessels. The celiac, SMA, and right renal artery are reimplanted as a single patch, with the left renal artery reimplanted separately. Spinal drainage and left heart bypass may be used in more extensive repairs.

2. Abdominal Aortic Aneurysm

a) Epidemiology and Etiology

Approximately 15,000 deaths annually in the United States are attributed to abdominal aortic aneurysms (AAA). Surgical treatment with replacement of the aneurysm with a prosthetic graft is the currently most established therapeutic approach with less than 5% of mortality and morbidity rated for elective cases. Endovascular repair of infrarenal aortic aneurysms is rapidly gaining favor in patients with favorable anatomy. In contrast the mortality rate is still very high for emergency repair of a ruptured abdominal aortic aneurysm of any type.

An abdominal aorta aneurysm (AAA) is now thought to be secondary to hyperactivity in matrix metalloproteases leading to a breakdown in the tunica media and adventitia. This is thought to occur from an ongoing inflammatory response in the region. Continuing inflammation and stresses leads to a mismatch in the collagen to elastin ratio and a weakening of the arterial wall. A decrease in TIMP 1 and 2 occurs followed by an increase in MMP 1 and 9, IL-1, and TNF-alpha. Other causes include cystic medial necrosis in CTD, syphilis, fungal infections, aortitis, and trauma. Expansion of the AAA over 5.5 cm heralds a significant risk of rupture, and thus a very high morbidity and mortality. A true aneurysm has a defect in all three layers of

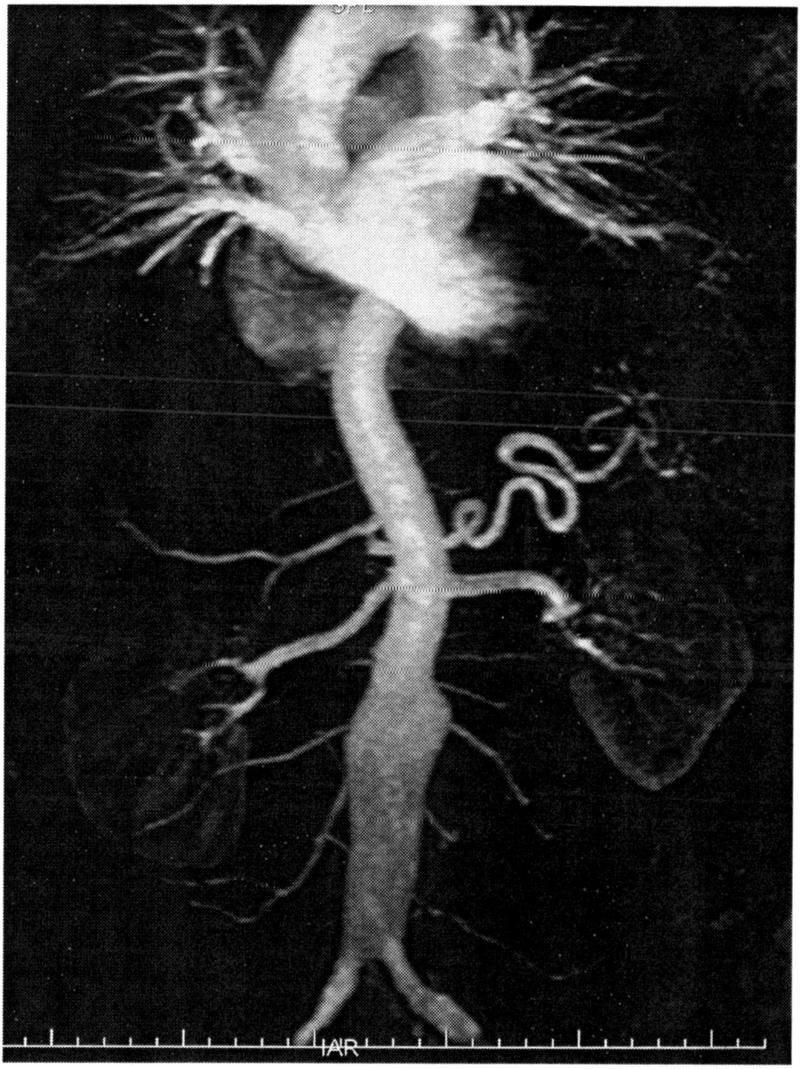

the aortic wall, while a pseudoaneurysm affects only the tunica intima and media.

The natural history of abdominal aortic aneurysms involves its progressive enlargement toward the rupture. Risk factors for rupture include size, rapid enlargement (> 0.5 cm/year), infection (mycotic aneurysm), HTN, COPD, smoking, and females of gestational age.

TABLE 9. Rates of rupture of AAA

3-5.5 cm	0.6% / year
5.6-5.9 cm	10% / year
6-6.9 cm	20% / year
7-7.9 cm	30% / year
> 8.0 cm	50% / year

b) Presentation and Diagnosis

Most patients with AAA are asymptomatic. There is typically a history of CAD. Diagnosis of AAA is by US, but CTA is preferred to demonstrate the precise dimensions of the mass. Angiogram was previously the gold standard. Complicated presentations may include thromboembolic phenomenon to the distal lower extremities and end organs, acute occlusion leading to abrupt claudication, and fistula formation with the inferior vena cava or duodenum. The former leads to high flow congestive heart failure, while the latter leads to rapid exsanguination. Rupture presents with pain, a pulsatile mass, syncope, and hypotension.

c) Treatment

Medical therapy, such as smoking cessation and cardiovascular risk factor reduction, has been demonstrated to be highly beneficial. Although the pharmacologic role of beta-blockers in limiting the expansion of the aneurysm remains controversial, their use is highly recommended for treatment of hypertension and angina.

The UK Small Aneurysm Trial randomly assigned 1,090 patients with asymptomatic AAA of 4.0-5.5 cm in diameter to early elective surgery or ultrasonographic monitoring every 6 months, deferring the repair until the aneurysm exceeded 5.5 cm in diameter, grew more than 1 cm/year, or became symptomatic. The study found an initial survival disadvantage for patients undergoing early surgery with a 30 day perioperative mortality of 5.4%. At 3 and 8 year follow up, a lower mortality rate in the surgical arm was observed (43% vs. 48%). The lower mortality with surgery may have been due to beneficial changes in lifestyle such as smoking cessation.

Further analysis of the trial data showed a median aneurysm growth of 0.33 cm/year with a risk of rupture of 1.6% in the initial follow up in the surveillance group. This increased during the last three years of follow up to a 3.2% risk of rupture per year. The risk of rupture was higher in women.

Optimal surveillance intervals were also estimated to minimize the likelihood of aneurysm growth between interval visits. It was estimated that ultrasonography should be performed at intervals of 36, 24, 12 and three months for aneurysms of 3.5, 4.0, 4.5, and 5 cm, respectively.

The United Stated ADAM trial showed essentially no difference in mortality for the repair of aneurysms with a 4.0-5.5 cm diameter. The 2005 American College of Cardiology/American Heart Association guidelines recommend surgical repair for abdominal aortic aneurysms with a diameter > 5.5 cm. Aneurysms with diameter 4.0 to 5.4 cm should be monitored by ultrasound or CT every 6 months. Aneurysms with diameter between 3.0 and 4.0 cm should be monitored with ultrasound every 2 years.

Appropriate patients selection and timing for repair is based upon the identification of individuals at high risk of rupture. Once rupture occurs, emergency repair is required. The majority of authors suggest that repair is warranted in patients with AAA > 5.5 cm in diameter.

Perioperative care, improvement of surgical technique, and the use of autologous blood donation and cell savers in the operating room have decreased the morbidity and mortality of open AAA repair. Regardless of these advances, myocardial infarction remains as the most important cause of death after surgery.

d) Endovascular vs. Open Repair

Endovascular repair (EVAR) consists of the insertion of an endoluminal graft within the aorta and exclusion of the aneurysm from the systemic flow. The choice of recommending an endovascular repair vs. an open repair of an abdominal aortic aneurysm depends on three important factors:

- **Aneurysm size.** The UK Small aneurysm Trial, the EVAR trial, and the EUROSTAR data show a clear correlation between aneurysm size and outcome (type I endoleak, mortality, conversion to open repair, and post-EVAR rupture).
- **Aneurysm morphology.** Several parameters such as neck length, diameter, angulation, parietal calcification, intraluminal thrombus, aneurysm tortuosity, iliac artery aneurysm diameter, calcification, and femoral artery diameter are considerations. Contraindications to EVAR include an infrarenal neck less than 10 mm, angulation over 45 degrees, and an insufficient landing zone at the iliac arteries.
- **Surgical risk.** This defined by the following factors: age > 60 years, AAA size > 6.5 cm, rupture, CHF, CAD, valvular heart disease, arrhythmia, COPD, and CRF (Cr > 1.8).

The Dutch DREAM trial and the EVAR 1 study have shown lower mortality rates at 30 days with endovascular repair compared to open repair. This survival benefit ceases after the first year and may have a worse long term survival compared to open repair due to graft-related complications. There are reports in the literature that indicate that the prevalence of bowel ischemia may be higher following EVAR and eliminate the cost advantage of this procedure.

Current ACC/AHA guidelines recommend endovascular repair for high-risk patients. EVAR may be considered in low risk patients but evidence of benefit is still debated. The landing zone is particularly important with an EVAR; obstruction of a single internal iliac artery is often tolerated, but the most common complaint that follows is buttock claudication.

e) Complications of EVAR

The persistence of systemic blood flow within an EVAR-excluded aneurysmal sac is called an endoleak, and is the most important complication of an EVAR. Four types of endoleak have been described as shown in the table below.

TABLE 10. EVAR endoleaks

Type I endoleak	Perigraft flow into the aneurysm sac around either the proximal or distal attachment sites.
Type II endoleak	Backbleeding due to collateral blood flow into the aneurysmal sac via patent lumbar arteries or IMA.
Type III endoleak	Leakage of blood through structural defects in the graft.
Type IV endoleak	Diffusion of blood through microscopic defects.

3. Aortic Dissection

a) Etiology

Aortic dissection is the result of a transverse tear through the intima and media of the aortic wall leading to extravasation of blood, compromise of flow to other arterial branches, and rupture with exsanguinating hemorrhage. Aortic dissection is attributable to HTN, congenital heart defects, CTD, syphilis, pregnancy, coarctation of the aorta (as in Turner syndrome), abuse of cocaine, and trauma. The Treponema pallidum organisms of syphilis cause aortic dissection through infection of the vasa vasorum with subsequent irritation by the inflammatory and immune reaction.

Aortic dissection is classified by the DeBakey system into three types: type I involves the ascending aorta and part of the distal aorta, and is the most common of the three types; type II involves only the ascending aorta; and type III involves only the descending aorta. The Stanford system classifies aortic dissections into the type A class if the ascending aorta is affected, and the type B class if the descending aorta is affected. In simpler terms, ascending dissections require surgical management to avoid aortic root rupture. Descending dissections are treated with blood pressure control via beta-blockers and hydralazine.

b) Presentation and Diagnosis

Aortic dissection presents as a tearing sensation with severe chest pain that radiates to the back. HTN is typically present, discordant pulses between extremities can be measured, and AR is typically present. Diagnosis is made by CXR that indicates loss of the aortic knob and a widened mediastinum, CT with IV contrast or TEE that demonstrates an intimal flap with extravasation of blood, and angiogram as the gold standard. A CXR should be obtained in all patients suspected of MI, as the thrombolytic therapy used in MI is absolutely contraindicated in aortic dissection. Indications for repair include compromise of blood flow, enlargement rate over 0.5 cm/year, and pain associated with dissection; these are all associated with an increase in risk of rupture.

c) Treatment

Aortic dissection is treated with blood pressure control, immediate surgical repair for type A/type II dissections, and medical management for uncomplicated type B/type III dissections. Complications of treatment include the development of MI, stroke, and tamponade. While open repair of complicated acute Type B dissections remains the gold standard, endovascular repair is rapidly gaining popularity, and several trials are underway to determine the optimal treatment of this problem.

4. Renal Artery Aneurysm

a) Assessment

Renal artery aneurysm may present with pain, hematuria, hypertension, and thromboembolism to the kidney, but most patients are asymptomatic. Causes of true aneurysm involving all three layers of the lumen include fibromuscular dysplasia and Ehlers-Danlos syndrome. False aneurysms involving the intima and media may be secondary to trauma, instrumentation, inflammation, polyarteritis nodosa, and Kawasaki disease. One in four patients present with bilateral disease, and one in three patients have multiple manifestations of disease.

Diagnostic imaging begins with ultrasound, followed by CTA or MRA for anatomic imaging and surgical planning. The latter two studies are preferred due to their improved resolving power and precise information about aneurysm size.

b) Management

Intervention is indicated in patients with symptomatic disease, women who wish to become pregnant, and size over 2 cm. Any dissection or rupture requires immediate repair. Smaller aneurysms do not require repair unless it is found in a woman who wishes to become pregnant. Emergent surgical management is required in cases of rupture or symptomatic disease and requires a midline laparotomy, cross-clamping of the aorta until control is gained over the renal artery, followed by nephrectomy. Renal artery reconstruction with interposition graft or reimplantation nephrectomy is possible if the kidney is intact and the patient is stable.

Isolated disease in a stable patient can be repaired electively. Patch angioplasty is possible with small aneurysms. Large aneurysms require exclusion and bypass or complete reconstruction via a proximal end-to-side and distal end-to-end anastomosis. Extra-anatomic bypass is possible if there is severe aortic disease. For very distal or hilar lesions, ex vivo reconstruction may be required. Finally, transplant nephrectomy is possible if there are no other readily available options. Aneurysmal disease within the renal parenchyma requires nephrectomy.

Coil embolization of small aneurysms is possible in selected patients where the aneurysm can be isolated. Stent placement with synthetic material is possible to exclude the aneurysm completely for extrarenal disease. The contralateral kidney should always be examined prior to nephrectomy.

5. Splenic Artery Aneurysm

Splenic artery aneurysm is the third most common type of abdominal aneurysm, following aortic and iliac aneurysms. The most common causes are atherosclerosis, polyarteritis nodosa, infection, and an inflammatory process such as pancreatitis. CTA provides satisfactory anatomic imaging. Repair is indicated in women who wish to become pregnant or for aneurysms over 2 cm. Percutaneous embolization is a satisfactory option in selected patients.

VII.B. Peripheral Artery Aneurysmal Disease

1. Iliac Artery Aneurysm

The majority of patients who present with iliac artery aneurysms have a diameter of about 8 cm. The majority are secondary to hypertension and cardiovascular disease. Surgical management should be instituted for any aneurysm over 4 cm in size due to the increase in risk of spontaneous rupture. Treatment involves excision of the aneurysm if the neck is very small, or bypass and exclusion. Mortality with rupture exceeds 50%, while mortality from elective repair is less than 10%.

2. Femoral Artery Aneurysm

Femoral artery aneurysms have a predisposition toward thrombosis; rupture is rare, and the vast majority of patients will have aneurysmal disease of the aorta, iliac, popliteal, or contralateral femoral arteries. Acute thrombosis of a femoral artery aneurysm presents with acute claudication and a threatened limb. Expansion of an aneurysmal sac can lead to compression of the femoral vein within the canal, leading to distal extremity edema. Femoral nerve compression leads to medial thigh paresthesia. Thromboembolic phenomenon with blue toe syndrome can occur.

Type I femoral artery aneurysms involve the common femoral artery; type II involve the profunda. Isolated SFA disease is rare. Diagnosis is by CTA. Type I disease is repaired with a Dacron interposition graft. Type II disease is treated with reimplantation or bypass. Isolated SFA disease is treated with bypass.

3. Popliteal Artery Aneurysm

Popliteal aneurysms are the most common peripheral aneurysm. The most common presentation is distal embolization. Half of all patients have bilateral disease, and 75% have additional aneurysms elsewhere (i.e. AAA). Most patients are asymptomatic at the time of diagnosis. Popliteal artery aneurysms over 2 cm should be treated with exclusion of the aneurysm followed by a bypass graft. Large, symptomatic aneurysms causing compression can also be treated with incision through the sac and interposition of a graft in the body of the sac.

VIII. Vascular Access for Hemodialysis

VIII.A. Radiocephalic Fistula

The construction of an anastomosis between the radial artery and the cephalic vein in the wrist was first described by Brescia in 1966. This is the most dependable type of hemodialysis access. A long term prospective study noted a 1 year patency rate for first time fistulas of 90% and a 4 year patency rate of 75%. At least 4-6 weeks must elapse before the fistula will be ready for hemodialysis.

VIII.B. Brachiocephalic and Brachiobasilic Fistulae

The brachiocephalic and brachiobasilic arteriovenous fistulae may be used for hemodialysis access. Their 3-year patency rate is 80%.

VIII.C. Arteriovenous Grafting

Ultimately, when all the possible autogenous HD access has been exhausted, prosthetic conduit (PTFE) to form a bridge fistula is the best alternative. PTFE can be constructed between virtually any suitably sized artery and vein. Patency at 12 months has been reported to be 70%, while at 48 months is between 43% and 60%. Thrombosis of the conduit is a relatively common complication ranging between 7% and 55%. Infection is also a risk. In 80 fistulae monitored for 30 months, the overall incidence of infection was 19%, with 67% occurring in the first 4 months of use. In the same study, the majority (67%) required excision. Pseudoaneurysm formation at the needle puncture site develops in about 5% of fistulae.

VIII.D. Complications of Fistula Formation

Venous hypertension can develop following formation of an AV fistula. Treatment is bypass of the stenosis, which has a higher patency compared to angioplasty. Excision of a fistula can be done for refractory or complex cases.

Unintended major AV fistula formation should be treated with coil embolization or surgery due to the risk of high output CHF. Large arteriovenous fistulas lead to a decrease in peripheral vascular resistance. Active pulsatile bleeding, ulceration, or a compromised arterial supply requires definitive repair. Pseudoaneurysms under 2 cm can be observed; larger ones require excision or repair. Small intimal damage of a vessel can be observed if the distal pulses are intact.

IX. Vascular Trauma

IX.A. Head and Neck Vascular Trauma

1. Etiology and Pathophysiology

Severe penetrating and blunt trauma to the head and neck may lead to compromise of the carotid circulation, along with concomitant injuries to the neurovascular structures, vertebral column, trachea, and esophagus. Morbidity is high from carotid artery disruption.

2. Presentation and Diagnosis

Severe injury to the head and neck that is sufficient to disrupt the vascular supply is also likely to cause devastating injuries to nearby vital structures. Limited injuries from stab wounds may damage vascular structures without leading to severe trauma to other major structures. The vast majority of head and neck injuries leading to vascular trauma are from penetrating trauma; however, older patients with calcified carotid arteries may suffer serious vascular compromise from blunt injuries leading to "whiplash-type" injuries.

Zone I injuries occur superior to the root of the neck (suprasternal notch) and inferior to the cricoid cartilage. The carotid, vertebral, and subclavian arteries are exposed in this region. Barring obvious damage to these structures from penetrating injury to this zone, it is usually safe to observe this type of injury.

Zone II injuries occur between the cricoid cartilage and angle of the mandible. The internal and external carotid arteries are in this zone. All zone II injuries require exploration in the operating room.

Zone III injuries occur between the angle of the mandible and the base of the skull. The infraclinoid internal carotid and vertebral arteries are located in this region. Injuries to this region may be observed unless there is obvious compromise of these structures.

Diagnosis by cerebral arteriography is indicated for most zone I and III injuries. Most zone II injuries will require arteriography in the operating room. Doppler is a satisfactory bedside imaging study for zone II injuries. CTA is a reasonable option for all stable patients.

Blunt head and neck trauma may lead to the development of a carotid artery dissection. Carotid dissection may be asymptomatic or may cause severe headache, Horner syndrome, and stroke. Late complications include aneurysmal degeneration and stroke. Management is usually anticoagulation, as surgical and endovascular therapies do not improve outcome. Diagnosis requires a high index of suspicion and is confirmed by CTA or conventional angiogram.

3. Treatment

Treatment begins with the ABCs of advanced trauma life support (ATLS). The airway must be secured, satisfactory pulmonary ventilation assured, and an intact circulatory system confirmed. Active hemorrhage must be stopped with care taken when placing a pressure dressing over the carotid vessels. Wounds should not be probed in the emergency room due to the risk of causing unstable bleeding. Any obvious vascular injury is taken to the operating room for repair. Otherwise, operative management is dictated by the zones of the neck.

Due to the complex anatomy of zone I and III injuries, attempts at interventional management should be made whenever possible. All zone II injuries should be explored in the operating room whenever there is a question of vascular compromise. Severe damage to the carotid artery may require ligation, which has a very high risk of causing thromboembolism and stroke.

A supraclavicular incision and potentially removing the head of the clavicle can be done to gain exposure to zone I neck injuries. A standard neck incision parallel to the sternocleidomastoid is the accepted approach for zone II and III injuries. Cervical incisions can be done for zone III injuries.

IX.B. Thoracoabdominal Vascular Trauma

1. Epidemiology and Etiology

Major vascular injury to the thoracoabdominal compartment is most commonly secondary to penetrating injuries, especially gunshot wounds (nearly 80%). Only 10% of major injuries are secondary to blunt trauma and stab wounds.

2. Pathophysiology

The mechanism of injury to the thoracoabdominal vasculature in blunt trauma is typically secondary to the rapid deceleration forces leading to avulsion. Crush injuries can also cause avulsion and tearing of vessels. The most commonly injured vessels are small arterial branches; severe injury to major vessels is likely to lead to immediate death with no hope for salvage (i.e. the first peak of trauma-related deaths nameable to hospital care).

3. Presentation

Penetrating injuries can lead to disruption of vessels and internal organs. Gunshot wounds in particular can rapidly lead to hypovolemic shock from hemorrhage. Combined with disruption of the bowel for abdominal injuries, sepsis can also rapidly set in. Patients with such injuries will present with severe metabolic acidosis, severe hemorrhage, and hypothermia. Impaired coagulation leading to fatal hemorrhage is imminent without aggressive resuscitation and operative management.

4. Diagnosis and Treatment

Regardless of the mechanism of injury, severe thoracoabdominal vascular injuries will quickly lead to death. Any compromise of major vessels will likely lead to exsanguination even before EMS personnel arrive. Smaller vascular injuries may provide enough time for a patient to get to a level 1 trauma center. Aggressive resuscitation and rapid transport to the operating room within the Golden Hour may make a difference in survival, provided there is a sufficiently high threshold of suspicion for intra-abdominal injury.

Blunt trauma to the thoracoabdominal aorta can lead to transection secondary to rapid deceleration. Most such injuries are located just distal to the arch, but can occur anywhere along the length of the vessel. Nearly 20% of individuals involved in a high speed motor vehicle collision will sustain this type of injury, and the vast majority will die at the scene from exsanguination. Those with incomplete transection may survive long enough to get to a hospital. The presence of a widened mediastinum, a subtle pseudoaneurysm on a CTA, or exam findings consistent with mass effect from an aneurysm upon the esophagus or trachea can be demonstrated.

All patients with aortic transection require intervention, but a growing body of evidence suggests that stable, asymptomatic patients can be monitored with serial imaging tests while other injuries are stabilized. Surgical correction remains the gold standard, but endovascular repair is gaining popularity as early data indicate a reduction in morbidity and mortality with the endovascular approach, especially in unstable patients.

Any patient with a penetrating injury to the abdomen and/or suspected intra-abdominal injury should be taken to the operating room as soon as they are stabilized. Time should not be wasted on CT scans or unnecessary procedures. Immediate exploratory laparotomy, packing of all four quadrants, and sequential evaluation of the abdomen is the key to salvaging patients with serious thoracoabdominal injuries.

If the diagnosis is not obvious, a diagnostic peritoneal lavage (DPL) and/or focused abdominal ultrasound for trauma (FAST) should be performed. A positive result requires immediate surgery. Stable patients with a low index of suspicion for intra-abdominal injury may undergo a CT scan with contrast.

Severe thoracoabdominal bleeding requires proximal compression of the aorta until control is regained over the compromised vessel. Transection of the pancreas, ligation of the celiac artery, and rapid retroperitoneal mobilization via the Kocher maneuver assist with rapid surgical exposure.

Severe superior midline bleeding is likely due to disruption of the aorta or vena cava, celiac artery, SMA, or renal arteries. Severe inferior midline bleeding can be attributed to aortic or vena cava injury or IMA. The Cattel maneuver (mobilization of the right colon and small intestine) followed by aortic clamping may be necessary. Posterior injuries to the IVC are repaired by going through the anterior wall and correcting the defect from within the IVC itself. Anterior injuries to the IVC are repaired primarily. Ligation of the IVC may be necessary but is associated with a very high mortality.

Disruption of the hepatoduodenal ligament leads to severe bleeding from the portal vein or hepatic artery. The Pringle maneuver (clamping the porta hepatis) is required. Severe injury to the portal vein or hepatic artery is treated by ligation. Staged repair may be attempted. A hepaticojejunostomy may eventually be required once the patient is stable due to disruption of the biliary tree.

Lateral bleeding is likely due to renal artery disruption and requires surgery only if there is active, symptomatic bleeding. Nephrectomy may be required but should be performed only after examining the contralateral kidney. A large number of renal artery injuries can be repaired.

Severe pelvic bleeding should be managed by stabilization of the pelvis, potential external fixation, and coil embolization by vascular interventional radiology. Continued bleeding may require surgery due to disruption of the iliac tree. Control of the aortic bifurcation should be obtained first, followed by primary repair of these vessels.

IX.C. Upper and Lower Extremity Vascular Trauma

1. Epidemiology and Etiology

Amputations for extremity trauma were once the mainstay of treatment for blunt and penetrating injuries. Advances in critical care, surgical technique, interventional radiology, and antibiotics have transformed the management of the critically injured patient. Extremity trauma is divided into blunt and penetrating injuries, and the overall management and outcomes are very different.

2. Pathophysiology

Penetrating injuries to the arms and legs are commonly secondary to gunshot wounds and knife injuries. Penetrating injuries can lead to acute disruption of the vascular system with immediate symptoms of neurovascular compromise to the extremity. Transection in conjunction with severe hemorrhage leading to hypovolemic shock can rapidly compromise an extremity and result in a critically ill patient.

Blunt trauma is most commonly due to a motor vehicle accident causing crush injury. Fractures, dislocation, and the development of compartment syndrome from myonecrosis can cause an impediment to vascular flow and lead to progressive ischemia. When coupled with injuries elsewhere in the body that lead to shock and sepsis, the already tenuous blood supply to the extremities may be entirely disrupted.

3. Presentation

Patients with acute penetrating injuries often present with an obvious wound and hemorrhage. Pulsatile bleeding may be observed from arterial disruption. Hematoma formation, bruits, palpable thrills, and in more extreme cases, a cold, pulseless arm or leg may be present. Severe blunt injury may lead to ischemic changes that worsen over time and cause neurovascular compromise to the extremity. Fractures can also lead to vascular disruption. For example, humeral head fractures can lead to a disruption of the axillary artery, and avascular necrosis can occur with femoral head fractures and scaphoid fractures.

4. Diagnosis

Expedient diagnosis is required to salvage a potentially compromised limb. Plain films are necessary as part of the initial imaging survey once the ABCs and primary survey are completed. Any fractures or dislocations should be reduced promptly. A thorough documentation of peripheral pulses is necessary, and ABIs should be completed. Significant abnormalities or discordance between two extremities implies vascular compromise unless the patient has a known history of peripheral vascular disease.

Diagnostic imaging should proceed by way of a CTA with careful evaluation of the vascular anatomy throughout the entire affected extremity. Patients who will require an operation for other reasons (i.e. open fracture, abdominal procedures) and who are reasonably stable will benefit from an intraoperative arteriography by a vascular surgeon. Contrast dye is minimized with this targeted approach and the patient is already prepared and draped for revascularization, should it be necessary. Ultrasound is also an invaluable physiologic study to document flow and distal pulses.

5. Treatment

The primary treatment for extremity trauma is surgery whenever there is a threatened extremity. However, the use of endovascularly placed covered stents is becoming more common. Patients with isolated vascular injuries and minimal disruption of the soft tissue and fascial planes are particularly good candidates for this approach. The appropriate anatomical considerations are necessary as part of the preoperative evaluation; for example, patients with traumatic arteriovenous fistula formation may be excellent candidates for endovascular repair, while those with discontinuity in a vessel will do better with an open approach.

The chance for saving a limb is greatest if revascularization proceeds within three hours of the injury. Primary end-to-end anastomosis is possible if the disrupted segment is less than 1 cm. Significantly more disruption will require a PTFE graft or vein transposition. Severe bleeding in a critically ill patient may permit only ligation and amputation. An attempt to salvage all major venous injury is recommended due to the risk of causing further damage to the extremity if the vein is simply ligated.

Blunt injury to an extremity causing vascular compromise, or following any emergency vascular reconstruction in a severely injured arm or leg, should prompt a four compartment fasciotomy to prevent compartment syndrome. Even prophylactic fasciotomy is completed for selected patients based off the mangled extremity severity score (MESS). The four criteria for the MESS score are as follows:

- Degree of soft tissue or bony injury
- Critical limb ischemia
- Shock
- Age

There are many complications for acute vascular trauma in the extremity. Among them are pseudoaneurysm formation, hemorrhage, and infection.

A variety of interventional and surgical techniques are available for treating these complications, but critically ill patients who develop severe complications may only have the option of amputation. Thrombosis of the reconstructed vascular supply should be prevented with anticoagulation when it is safe to do so in the patient.

X. Congenital Vascular Disease

X.A. Popliteal Artery Entrapment

1. Assessment

Occlusion of the popliteal artery may lead to a threatened lower extremity. Significant disease can lead to claudication, tissue loss, gangrene, and eventually necrosis, thereby necessitating amputation. In addition to aneurysm and thrombosis, popliteal entrapment syndrome may occur due to a congenital defect in the surrounding anatomy. Affecting mostly young men, the primary presentation of popliteal entrapment is claudication of the calf. Entrapment of this artery occurs due to an abnormal muscular insertion from the gastrocnemius or abnormal fibrous bands from the popliteus muscle. While physiologic studies may be normal at rest, use of the afflicted joint presents with claudication and a decrease in distal flow. Anatomic imaging should be obtained via CTA.

2. Management

The most appropriate treatment for popliteal entrapment syndrome is lysis of all fibrotic adhesions using a posterior approach. Myotomy or transection of occlusive bands can be completed if the gastrocnemius or popliteus are involved. Resection and interposition graft placement of any compromised segments may be necessary.

X.B. Vascular Anomalies

1. Epidemiology and Etiology

Vascular anomalies are the result of a derangement in ontogeny leading to a disruption in normal endothelial channel formation, and are divided into two major subgroups: proliferative (vascular tumors) and non-proliferative/

hypertrophic (vascular malformations). Hemangiomas are the most common type of vascular tumors: they present at birth and spontaneously resolve in all cases. Vascular malformations, although congenital, may present at any time in life, and are further divided into high-flow lesions and low-flow lesions. Vascular malformations never resolve spontaneously.

2. Pathophysiology

Hemangiomas are rapidly growing lesions with an alteration in angiogenesis. Vascular malformations are due to a disruption in endothelial channel formation that evolves in step with development of the patient. Vascular malformations may involve the arterial or venous blood supply, or be restricted to lymphatic channels, or involve a combination of these elements.

3. Presentation

Hemangiomata present as a punctate red vascular malformation at birth but rapidly grow to a larger defect. The majority of these will spontaneously regress by age 7. Rapid growth in the first few months of life can be distressing to parents, but involution typically begins by age 3.

Vascular malformations do not improve with time; instead, their continued growth with the child leads to a variety of complications. Several different types of vascular malformations may be evident: a purely capillary malformation presents as a port-wine stain within specific boundaries; a venous malformation is manifest with time; lymphatic malformations may be more subtle. Regardless of the type, they remain fixed relative to nearby landmarks.

4. Diagnosis

Both types of lesions may be evident on physical exam. Ultrasound is important for documenting high-flow lesions, which may be particularly present with evolving hemangiomas and large arterial malformations. Slow-flow lesions are likely to be present with venous and lymphatic malformations. The most sensitive test to differentiate a hemangioma from a vascular malformation is MRI.

5. Treatment

The majority of hemangiomas can be safely monitored as nearly 90% of them will spontaneously involute. Steroids are effective for the management of growing hemangiomas. Immunosuppressants, chemotherapy, and interferon 2α are options for clinically significant hemangiomas. Angiography may be necessary to permit coil embolization for an evolving lesion. Surgical resection is reserved for large lesions refractory to medical management, or lesions that fail to resolve by age 7.

Sclerotherapy is an option for venous malformations. Arterial malformations and more extensive venous malformations require embolization and/or surgical excision. Laser photocoagulation can be used for sensitive lesions on the face. Whenever surgery is mandated, complete excision is required due to the high rate of recurrence; simple ligation is contraindicated for the same reason. High-flow lesions may require management with both embolization and surgery due to the risk of a high-output congestive heart failure.

Regardless of the lesion type and treatment employed, vascular malformations are rarely, if ever, cured. Rather, repeated treatments throughout the individual's life may be needed to control local and systemic symptoms.

XI. Venous Disease

XI.A. Subclavian Vein Thrombosis

1. Etiology

Paget-von Schrötter syndrome, known as subclavian vein thrombosis when it occurs due to complications from an indwelling catheter, is the development of extensive clots leading to plethora of the affected extremity or face. Besides catheter placement, other causes include hypercoagulability syndromes, TPN, cancer, and the use of a hemodialysis catheter. Paget-von Schrötter syndrome is specifically of idiopathic origin and leads to effort-induced thrombosis. Specific causes of this disease include anatomic malformations such as abnormal insertions of the anterior scalene muscle, cervical rib, depression of the shoulder (as in Poland syndrome), and exercise leading to a transient hypercoagulable state.

2. Pathophysiology and Presentation

Patients with subclavian vein thrombosis typically present with peripheral nonpitting edema, distal extremity cyanosis, facial edema, and occasionally changes to the vision. Repetitive activity, especially in young males, can also lead to a similar spectrum of clinical findings and is often secondary to subclavian vein compression at the thoracic outlet.

3. Diagnosis and Treatment

In addition to a thorough hematologic workup, ultrasound and venography are necessary to evaluate the extent of the thrombus burden. Treatment is by way of physical therapy, anticoagulation, and if the cause is from Paget-von Schrötter syndrome, thrombolytic therapy.

Anatomic malformations should be surgically corrected. Catheter thrombectomy can be completed if patients present early and is a preferred approach at several centers. In the event that surgical resection of anomalous structures is necessary, a transaxillary approach is preferred with the patient in a lateral thoracotomy position.

XI.B. Deep Vein Thrombosis

1. Etiology and Pathophysiology

Venous thrombosis finds its main pathogenic moment in Virchow's triad:

- Blood flow alteration
- Vascular endothelial injury
- Hypercoagulable state

Causes of venous thrombosis can be hereditary and acquired. Inherited thrombophilia is a generic tendency towards venous thromboembolism. The most frequent causes of genetic thrombophilia are:

- **Factor V Leiden mutation.** This a genetic mutation in which factor V becomes resistant to breakdown by activated protein C. This mutation occurs in approximately 5% of people with European heritage.

The relative risk of venous thromboembolism in heterozygotes is 5-10 fold higher and 80-fold higher in homozygotes.

- **Prothrombin gene mutation.** This occurs in approximately 2% of Caucasians and is associated with a 2-3 fold increase in risk of thromboembolism.
- **Protein C and S deficiency.** This mutation leads to incomplete inactivation of factor Va and factor VIIIa. Protein C deficiency is also seen in patients with liver failure and in those who are receiving warfarin.
- **Antithrombin deficiency.** This is an autosomal dominant disorder that presents with persistent venous thromboembolism in the second decade of life. Heparin infusion or LMWH is usually effective if the antithrombin level is greater than 50%. Antithrombin concentrate has been given in patients with levels below 50%. This is typically noted in cases of insufficient anticoagulation with heparin alone.
- **Hyperhomocysteinemia.** In this disorder the plasma level of homocysteine is above the 95th percentile. Genetic and/or acquired mutations of the enzymatic pathway that converts homocysteine to cysteine, along with dietary deficiencies of vitamins B1 or B6 are common causes of hyperhomocystememia. Case control studies have shown that hyperhomocystememia is an independent risk factor for atherosclerosis. Treatment with folate and vitamin B12 is usually effective in lowering the homocysteine levels.
- **Antiphospholipid antibodies** include IgGs, IgAs, and IgMs that target antigens from the platelet and endothelial phospholipid layer. Patients with these antibodies are at risk for arterial and venous thrombosis, recurrent miscarriages, and thrombocytopenia. These antibodies may be detected in patients with autoimmune disorders such as lupus, infections such as HIV, and patients who are given particular medications such as chlorpromazine, hydralazine and dilantin. The Russell venom clotting time and anticardiolipin antibody assay confirm the diagnosis of antiphospholipid syndrome. Treatment with warfarin seems to be associated with a higher failure rate. In some cases, LMWH and antiplatelet agents may be needed (see page 49 for a detailed discussion of some of these hypercoagulable disorders).

Acquired risk factors for thrombosis include a prior thrombotic event, recent major surgery, presence of a central venous catheter, trauma, immobilization, pregnancy, use of contraceptives, myeloproliferative disorders, and neoplasms. In a recent meta-analysis of cardiovascular risks factors in patients with VTE, the top five risk factors are as follows:

- Obesity
- Hypertension
- Diabetes mellitus
- Smoking
- Hypercholesterolemia

2. Presentation and Diagnosis

Physical examination of patients with DVT may reveal a palpable cord (thrombosed vein), extremity pain, edema, erythema, and superficial vein dilation. A tender palpable cord, typically from the great saphenous vein, is a hallmark of thrombophlebitis. Homan and Brauer signs are poorly specific and sensitive in patients with DVT of lower extremity.

Phlegmasia cerulea dolens is an uncommon form of massive proximal venous thrombosis of the lower extremities, usually characterized by a high degree of morbidity from severe leg pain, swelling, cyanosis, edema, gangrene, compartment syndrome, and arterial compromise. Evolution of this disorder is followed by circulatory collapse and shock.

Diagnosis of DVT is made by duplex ultrasound, which has a positive predictive value of 94%. Venography, once the gold standard for DVT diagnosis, is now of only historical value.

3. Treatment

Anticoagulation with heparin, LMWH, or fondaparinux is the mainstay of DVT treatment. A PTT 1.5-2.5 times higher than the mean of the control value is recommended in case unfractionated heparin is administered (typical range 60-80). Once adequate anticoagulation with heparin is achieved, the patient should be bridged to warfarin with a target INR of 2.5 (range 2-3).

The duration of the treatment varies depending upon:

- Presence of a massive DVT
- Presence of a pulmonary embolism
- Risk of bleeding with anticoagulation
- Presence of additional comorbid conditions that warrant hospitalized care

Patients with their first DVT due to a reversible and time-limited risk factor, such as trauma or surgery, should receive anticoagulation for 3 months only. Recurrent DVT should be treated with six months to one year of anticoagulation. DVT / PE in a patient already being anticoagulated necessitates IVC filter placement and lifelong anticoagulation. Caval filters are recommended in case of persistence of massive DVT with pulmonary embolism, non response to medical therapy and/or increased risk of bleeding. Thrombolytic therapy and thrombectomy as DVT treatment may be considered in patients with proximal occlusive DVT with significant edema and symptoms, and has been shown to reduce the incidence of post-thrombotic syndrome.

Post-thrombotic syndrome is the incompetence of the superficial venous system due to a deep vein thrombosis. The pathogenesis is related to the incompetence of the perforating vein valves that connect the superficial with deep venous system in the lower extremity. Post-thrombotic syndrome is characterized by edema, development of secondary varicose veins, and development of venous ulcers. Elastic, graduated compressive stockings (30-40 mmHg) are recommended in these patients. Unna boots are applied in patients with ulcers. Endoscopic ligation and/or sclerofoam ablation of the incompetent perforating veins has shown improvement of symptoms and accelerated healing of the ulcer.

XI.C. Chronic Venous Insufficiency

1. Assessment

Saphenofemoral reflux disease presents with swelling, pruritus, and pain in the distal extremities. Reflux disease can lead to the formation of varicose veins and is secondary to loss of one-way valvular function within the superficial veins. Dysfunction of the superficial vein system requires shunting of blood to the deep system to permit proper oxygenation of venous blood.

Chronic venous insufficiency (CVI) is a multifactorial syndrome characterized by incompetence of superficial vein valves with development of:

- Teleangiectasias
- Varicose veins
- Skin changes, such as lipodermatosclerosis
- Venous ulcers

Reflux through incompetent vein valves is the most important hemodynamic change underlying the development venous insufficiency.

2. Management

The ligation of the saphenofemoral junction and the stripping of the great saphenous vein (GSV) or short saphenous vein (SSV) are now of historical value. The percutaneous laser and/or radiofrequency ablation of the GSV and SSV are now common treatment modalities. The injection of sclerosant agent in the venous lumen with the purpose of creating a chemical thrombosis and ablation the vein has been proposed.

XI.D. Venous Stasis Ulcers

Venous stasis ulcers develop in the lower extremity, usually at the ankle level, as a consequence of cutaneous inflammation driven by hemodynamic changes in the superficial and deep venous systems. These hemodynamic changes include high venous pressure, turbulent flow, and high shear stress. This leads to activation of a self-perpetuating inflammatory cascade causing skin changes (lipodermatosclerosis) and venous ulcer formation. Treatment of the ulcer is targeted to the correction of blood flow derangements. Compression stockings, Unna boots, and ablation of the incompetent veins are the main treatment modalities.

XII. Lymphatic Disease

XII.A. Lymphedema

1. Etiology and Pathophysiology

Lymphedema is secondary to a congenital or acquired disruption in lymphatic drainage, leading to an accumulation of lipid-rich fluid and concomitant swelling. Most cases are secondary to axillary node dissection completed as part of the treatment for breast cancer; the incidence is particularly high after radiation therapy to the axilla following surgery. Lymphedema is classified as either primary or secondary disease.

Primary lymphedema can be congenital in nature, lymphedema praecox, or lymphedema tarda. Congenital lymphedema comprises about a quarter of all primary causes and is often manifest at birth. Lymphedema praecox is the most common type and comprises about 70% of cases. This subtype is evident before the age of 35 and commonly presents as left lower extremity swelling. Lymphedema tarda presents after age 35 and is often due to a defect in the valves of the lymphatic system. Secondary lymphedema is commonly iatrogenic in nature. Of note, the brain and muscles do not have lymphatic drainage.

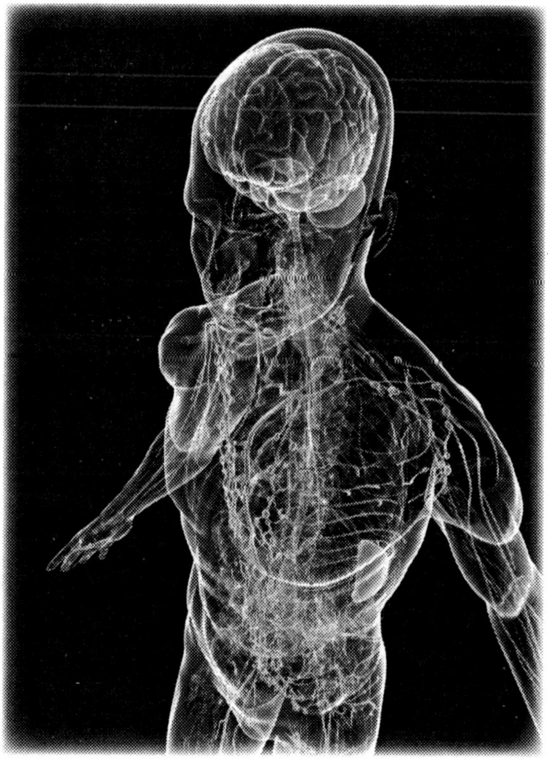

Vascular Surgery

2. Presentation and Diagnosis

Disruption of the normal lymph channels and subsequent outflow obstruction leads to a flow reversal within the lymphatic system, fibrosis, and inflammation. In extreme cases, this leads to severe dermal manifestation of disease and development of lymphangiosarcoma. Lymphangiosarcoma is typically manifest in about 10% of patients after 10 years of disease. Lymphedema following axillary lymph node dissection for breast cancer is referred to as Stewart-Treves syndrome.

Imaging via lymphoscintography and MRI indicate abnormal lymphatic channels and secondary manifestations of disease.

3. Treatment

The majority of therapy is conservative, employing compressive pressure stockings, pump compression therapy, and meticulous hygiene. Surgery is palliative and is done to reduce lymphatic volume or improve drainage. With severe cutaneous manifestations, a staged excision of the skin can be completed to entirely separate it from the lymphatic system.

XII.B. Lymphadenitis

Lymphadenitis presents as tender and enlarged lymph nodes typically secondary to a local infection. Suppurative lymphadenitis is the result of infection by gram positive cocci and presents with fever. Treatment involves a third generation cephalosporin and possible incision and drainage of the affected node if an abscess forms. In instances of chronic disease, complete excision and culture is necessary due to the risk of infection by TB or fungus. Necrotizing disease should raise the suspicion for cat-scratch disease; complete resection is required.

Vascular Surgery

GASTROINTESTINAL

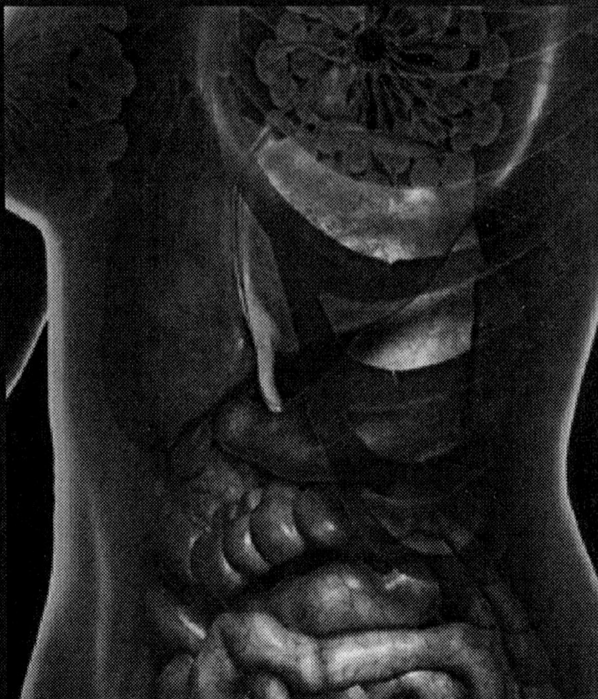

There is only one ultimate and effectual preventive for the maladies to which flesh is heir, and that is death.

Harvey Cushing
Father of Neurosurgery (1869-1939)

SURGISPHERE

GASTROINTESTINAL SURGERY

Sapan S. Desai, M.D., Ph.D., Jackie Garonzik, M.D.

I. Stomach

I.A. General Concepts

1. Anatomy

The stomach is divided into the cardia, body, fundus, and antrum. The fundus is the superior portion of the stomach above the gastroesophageal junction. The cardia is the portion along the lesser curvature at the gastroesophageal junction. The body is the continuation until the stomach abruptly arcs toward the midline at the incisura angularis. The antrum is the stomach distal to the incisura and is proximal to the pyloric sphincter. The stomach is anchored at the gastroesophageal junction and the duodenum.

The stomach is composed of three smooth muscle layers. The outer longitudinal, the middle circular, and inner oblique layers work in tandem to assist with digestion. The longitudinal layers are found along the lesser and greater curvatures. The circular muscle is found throughout the stomach, but is especially thick at the pylorus.

Three major cell types predominant the gastric mucosa. Parietal cells produce acid and intrinsic factor, the latter of which eventually binds with vitamin B12 and is absorbed in the terminal ileum. Atrophic gastritis can lead to a deficiency in this factor. Chief cells secrete pepsinogen, which is converted to pepsin by the acidic environment of the stomach and begins protein digestion. G-cells secrete gastrin (discussed on page 200). The cardiac glands secrete mucous, which protects the lining of the stomach. NSAIDs can lead to a reduction in mucous secretion and promote gastric ulcer formation in susceptible individuals.

2. Vascular Supply

The blood supply to the stomach is derived from the celiac axis. The celiac trunk divides into the left gastric, common hepatic, and splenic arteries. The common hepatic divides into the proper hepatic, right gastric, and gastroduodenal arteries. The left and right gastric arteries supply the lesser curvature. The gastroduodenal supplies the distal portion of the greater curvature, the duodenum, and gives off branches that supply the pancreas. The gastroduodenal artery (GDA) also gives off the right gastroepiploic. The splenic artery gives off the dorsal pancreatic, short gastric, and left gastroepiploic branches. The short gastric arteries are distributed to the greater curvature and fundus. The right and left gastroepiploic arteries supply the greater curvature. There is an extensive network of anastomoses between these arteries.

There are occasionally variations in the source of these arteries. The right gastric artery may occasionally arise as a branch of the GDA. Extensive collaterals to the duodenum via the GDA, right gastroepiploic, and right gastric arteries are also present. Finally, the right gastroepiploic is particular noteworthy as it is the major source of blood to the gastric pouch following an esophagogastrectomy.

3. Innervation

The vagus provides the parasympathetic innervation to the stomach through a plexus formed between the right and left vagus nerves. The left vagus nerve forms a plexus located anterior to the esophagus and primarily goes to the lesser curvature and anterior portion of the stomach. The right vagus forms a posterior network that goes primarily to the celiac plexus and posterior portion of the stomach. The sympathetic network plays a role in pain sensation and is derived from the mid-thoracic nerves.

4. Physiology

a) Gastrin

Gastrin stimulates acid production by parietal cells through histamine release and pepsin production by chief cells. Gastrin is stimulated by gastric distention, vagal stimulation, hypercalcemia, and the amino acids tryptophan and phenylalanine. Gastrin is inhibited by antral and duodenal acidification ($pH < 3$) as part of a feedback reaction. An abnormal pentagastrin stimulation test with a paradoxical rise in gastrin is diagnostic for Zollinger-Ellison syndrome. Gastrin is also elevated in atrophic gastritis and pernicious anemia due to a breakdown in feedback regulation.

b) Somatostatin

Somatostatin is a potent inhibitor of the gastrointestinal (GI) system and functions via a G-protein mechanism. Somatostatin also decreases gastric emptying, inhibits gallbladder contraction, and decreases pancreatic secretions. Somatostatin is induced by duodenal acidification, gastrin, secretin, and cholecystokinin (CCK). Somatostatin is also induced by prostaglandin E2 (PGE2) and can be inhibited by cholinergics. The synthetic form of somatostatin is octreotide, which is used as a treatment for variceal bleeding, carcinoid syndrome, and other neuroendocrine tumors.

c) Ghrelin

Ghrelin stimulates food intake through appetite induction at the hypothalamus and direct effects on the pituitary, stomach, pancreas, and small bowel. Ghrelin functions via a G-protein receptor. Elimination of ghrelin is hypothesized as one of the mechanisms of weight loss achieved via bariatric surgery.

d) Secretin

Secretin leads to the release of bicarbonate-rich and chloride-poor fluid from the pancreas. This is due to the exchange of bicarbonate for chloride; the effect is neutralization of the acidic contents entering into the duodenum from the stomach. Secretin stimulates pepsin release and the inhibits gastrin release, and mediates its effects through the second messenger cAMP. Without stimulation, the normal constituents of pancreatic fluid are sodium and potassium at a concentration iso-osmolar to that found in the serum.

e) Cholecystokinin

Cholecystokinin (CCK) is a 33 amino acid peptide hormone that stimulates fat and protein digestion. It is produced by the I-cells of the duodenum, and also leads to the secretion of digestive enzymes by the pancreas and bile through gallbladder contraction. CCK suppresses hunger and has recently been implicated in playing a role in drug tolerance to opioids. CCK may be involved in the hypersensitivity to pain experienced during opioid withdrawal. CCK also relaxes the sphincter of Oddi, stimulates secretin release, and stimulates intestinal motility. CCK production is stimulated by long-chain lipids entering the duodenum. Trypsin inactivates CCK.

f) Motilin

Motilin is a polypeptide hormone secreted by M cells in the duodenum and jejunum. Motilin stimulates gastrointestinal motility by inducing the migrating myoelectric complex via erythromycin receptors. Motilin also stimulates pepsin production. Alkaline pH in the duodenum stimulates release. At low pH, motilin inhibits gastric motor activity; at high pH motilin stimulates gastric motor activity. Small bowel motility is inhibited by the neuropeptide substance P.

g) Acid Production

Gastric acid is produced by the parietal cells in the stomach. Parietal cells release bicarbonate into the blood stream, known as the alkaline tide, during this process. Carbonate anhydrase catalyzes the formation of carbonic acid from CO_2 and H_2O. Gastric acid secretion has three phases - the cephalic phase that releases 30% of the total acid in anticipation of eating, the gastric phase that releases 60% of the total acid during digestion, and the intestinal phase that releases 10% of the acid during the secretion of chyme into the small intestine. Acid production is induced by the acetylcholine, gastrin, and histamine receptors found on parietal cells. Acetylcholine stimulates parietal cells via M3 muscarinic receptors and subsequent calcium release. Gastrin leads to activation of the IP3 / DAG pathway. Histamine functions with the H2 receptor to induce cAMP; histamine release is induced by gastrin.

h) Digestion

Saliva, gastric acid, and small intestine fluid have very high levels of potassium. Overall, saliva has the highest amount of potassium at 1170 mg/L, followed by gastric acid at 1120 mg/L. Centroacinar cells of the pancreas secrete bicarbonate and are stimulated by secretin. Basophilic cells of the exocrine pancreas secrete pancreatic amylase, lipase, trypsinogen, chymotrypsinogen, and other digestive enzymes. These cells are stimulated by CCK. Trypsinogen is activated by enterokinase, an enzyme found in the intestinal brush border.

Trypsin is the active form of trypsinogen, and activates pancreatic enzymes in the duodenum. High flow pancreatic duct secretions tend to be low in chloride due to secretin stimulation. Amylase and lipase are secreted in active forms by the pancreas. Amylase hydrolyzes carbohydrates in the jejunum. It is cleared rapidly by the kidneys when found in the serum.

i) Absorption

Fat, water, sodium, folic acid, proteins, and calcium are absorbed by the jejunum. Protein absorption is an active process that uses sodium cotransporters. Proteins are absorbed throughout the duodenum and jejunum. The ileum plays only a small role in protein absorption.

Nutrients and fluid are absorbed by the ascending colon. Colonocytes receive their energy from short length free fatty acids like butyrate. Long chain fatty acids are absorbed as chylomicrons by central lacteals. Medium chain fatty acids are absorbed via portal venous blood. Lipids are not directly converted to carbohydrates as acetyl CoA cannot be reversed to create pyruvate. Micelles are composed of lecithin and cholesterol. Steatorrhea following ileal resection is typically due to the loss of bile absorption at the ileum.

j) Migrating Myoelectric Complex

The MMC is composed of cyclic waves of activity that regularly sweep through the intestines during a fasting state. The MMC triggers peristaltic waves, starting in the stomach once every 90 minutes between meals. The MMC is partially regulated by motilin, starting in the stomach as a response to vagal stimulation. The MMC is independent of other extrinsic nerve activity. The MMC starts in the distal esophagus and goes through the entire small intestine. The MMC is dependent upon Na-K-ATPases.

TABLE 1. Gastrointestinal agents.

DRUG	INDICATIONS	MECHANISM OF ACTION	CONTRAINDICATIONS
Diphenhydramine (H1 antihistamine)	Sedative Allergic reactions	H1 receptor blocker; reduces smooth muscle contraction	Severe muscarinic acetylcholine antagonism that may lead to MI in overdose
Promethazine (H1 antihistamine)	Antiemetic Sedative	H1 receptor blocker	Closed angle glaucoma, alcohol, hypotension, coma, hepatic disease, BPH
Ranitidine (H2 blocker)	GERD, PUD	H2 receptor antagonist to prevent stomach acid production	Hepatic disease
Omeprazole (Proton pump inhibitor)	GERD, PUD ZE syndrome H. pylori infection	Proton pump inhibitor that prevents hydrochloric acid secretion from parietal cells	Do not give with antacids due to decreased absorption Prevent antifungal absorption
Metoclopramide (Motility agent)	Gastroparesis N/V	Antidopaminergic effect increases GI motility Prokinetic agent to empty stomach	Sedation, diarrhea, EPS including PD and TD, dystonia
Mannitol (Osmotic agent)	Reduce ICP Oliguric renal failure	Hypertonic solution to increase water and salt excretion in distal tubule Opens BBB through shrinking the endothelial cells	Rare
Lactulose (Osmotic agent)	Constipation Hepatic encephalopathy	Produces ammonia by bacterial flora to reduce body ammonia levels Osmotic reaction draws fluids into the lumen and leads to bowel movements	Diarrhea à dehydration Hypernatremia

I.B. Morphologic Disorders

1. Gastric Volvulus

a) Assessment

Gastric volvulus is torsion of the stomach leading to gastric outlet obstruction and potential ischemia of the stomach. The combination of epigastric pain, retching, and inability to pass a nasogastric tube was first described by Borchardt and is specific to gastric volvulus. A closed loop obstruction is present. One of two types can occur: type I volvulus is the most common and is due to overly flexible anchoring gastric ligaments; type II is more common in children and is due to a congenital defect leading to increased gastric mobility.

b) Management

Surgical reduction of the volvulus followed by anterior gastropexy is necessary. Gastrectomy may be done if there is gastric necrosis.

2. Gastric Outlet Obstruction

a) Assessment

Gastric outlet obstruction presents with a hypochloremic, hypokalemic metabolic alkalosis leading to dehydration. Due to worsening dehydration, sodium conservation occurs with the kidney, leading to a renal tubular acidosis with subsequent aciduria. Causes include peptic ulcer disease, pyloric stenosis, and cancer.

b) Management

Resection of frank tumor may be required if cancer is the cause of the obstruction. Antrectomy, vagotomy, and a Billroth I procedure can be done for functional obstructions.

I.C. Metabolic Disorders

1. Peptic Ulcer Disease

a) Etiology and Epidemiology

Peptic ulcer disease is the formation of mucosal erosion within the gastrointestinal tract. It is divided into gastric ulcers and duodenal ulcers. Peptic ulcer disease occurs secondary to a breakdown in the homeostasis between acid production and the protective mucosal barrier. This disruption has a number of causes, but is most commonly attributed to H. pylori infection. As a result, the primary method of treatment involves antibiotic therapy to eradicate H. pylori infection. Refractory or severe cases require surgical management. Other causes include NSAIDs, burns (i.e. Curling ulcers), head injury (i.e. Cushing ulcers), stress ("type A" personality), alcohol abuse, and smoking. Longstanding gastritis is commonly present. The most common type of peptic ulcer is a duodenal ulcer. About 5% of gastric ulcers are associated with underlying malignancy.

b) Pathophysiology

H. pylori is the most commonly implicated cause of gastric ulcer disease and leads to 70% of all cases. The remainder are due to NSAIDs. H. pylori also plays a role in the development of duodenal ulcers; however, the major predisposing causes are excess gastric acid secretion and breakdown of the mucosal barrier through NSAIDs and inhibition of prostaglandin E (PGE). Elevated gastric acid production in Zollinger-Ellison (ZE) syndrome can also lead to duodenal ulcer formation. Twenty percent of patients with H. pylori develop symptomatic PUD, while 90% of patients with ZE syndrome develop PUD.

Chronic H. pylori infection has also been tied to the development of mucosa-associated lymphoid tissue (MALT) lymphoma. Chronic superficial gastritis and atrophic gastritis can occur. The latter condition can lead gastric adenocarcinoma. Eradication of H. pylori is acceptable management of a low-grade MALToma.

c) Presentation

Gastric ulcers present with sharp, burning pain in the epigastrium shortly following food consumption. The lag time is typically between 10-30 minutes, during which time the stomach increases acid production and additional insult occurs to the protective barrier of the stomach and the epithelium. Gastric ulcers lead to nausea and vomiting, and the pain may lead to weight loss and anorexia. Nearly one-quarter of all individuals with gastric ulcers will experience significant hemorrhaging. As a result, gastric ulcers carry a significantly higher risk of complications and death than do duodenal ulcers.

Duodenal ulcers become symptomatic several hours after ingesting a meal. Patients may awaken at night with severe epigastric pain and burning. Duodenal ulcers are relieved by ingesting additional food, which causes the acidic gastric contents to be retained within the stomach and gives bicarbonate within the proximal duodenum a chance to neutralize the high level of acid.

d) Diagnosis

Diagnosis of gastric ulcer is by endoscopy and biopsy. Multiple biopsies are important in gastric ulcer disease due to the association with stomach cancer; biopsies should also be taken at the corpus and antrum as part of a search for H. pylori. The presence of H. pylori can also be detected using noninvasive tests such as a urease breath test and serology, while invasive tests such as a rapid urease test, biopsy, and culture can be utilized as confirmatory tests. Gastric ulcers likely to bleed have a visible vessel 50% of the time on endoscopy.

Diagnosis of duodenal ulcer is made through endoscopy. Due to the diminished risk of malignancy, biopsy is usually not performed. H. pylori infection in duodenal ulcers is diagnosed via a urease breath test that detects carbon isotopes after ingesting radiolabeled urea.

e) Classification

Gastric ulcers are divided into five major types. Type I ulcers occur on the lesser curvature of the stomach and are associated with type A blood. Type II ulcers occur along the lesser curvature and in the duodenum. Type III ulcers are prepyloric. Type IV ulcers are located cranially on the lesser curvature. Type V ulcers can occur anywhere along the body of the stomach and are associated with NSAID abuse. Benign gastric ulcers are usually located along the greater curvature.

f) Medical Treatment

Treatment options for gastric ulcers involve the eradication of H. pylori using bismuth salts, amoxicillin, metronidazole, and a proton pump inhibitor for a period of 10 days. For individuals allergic to penicillin, amoxicillin can be substituted with clarithromycin. Prostaglandin E in the form of misoprostol or sucralfate buttress the mucosal barrier. Symptoms can also be reduced through lifestyle changes such as discontinuing alcohol use, smoking cessation, and reducing the use of NSAIDs and steroids.

The treatment for duodenal ulcers is similar to that for gastric ulcers.

g) Surgical Treatment

Severe gastric ulcer disease that is refractory to medical management may require a surgical intervention to curtail acid production by the stomach. The most common options include truncal vagotomy with pyloroplasty, truncal vagotomy with antrectomy, and proximal gastric vagotomy. Truncal vagotomy eliminates vagal stimulation of the fundus and dramatically reduces acid production. However, the MMC is disrupted in the stomach and can lead to functional gastroparesis. This is the impetus for completing a Heineke-Mikulicz pyloroplasty or antrectomy. A Heineke-Mikulicz pyloroplasty makes a relaxing longitudinal incision in the muscular layer of the pyloric sphincter; this is a treatment similar to that used for pyloric stenosis in children. Antrectomy amplifies the effects of a truncal vagotomy by reducing G cells and gastrin production in the stomach; this procedure involves resection of the antrum of the stomach above the incisura toward the pylorus. A

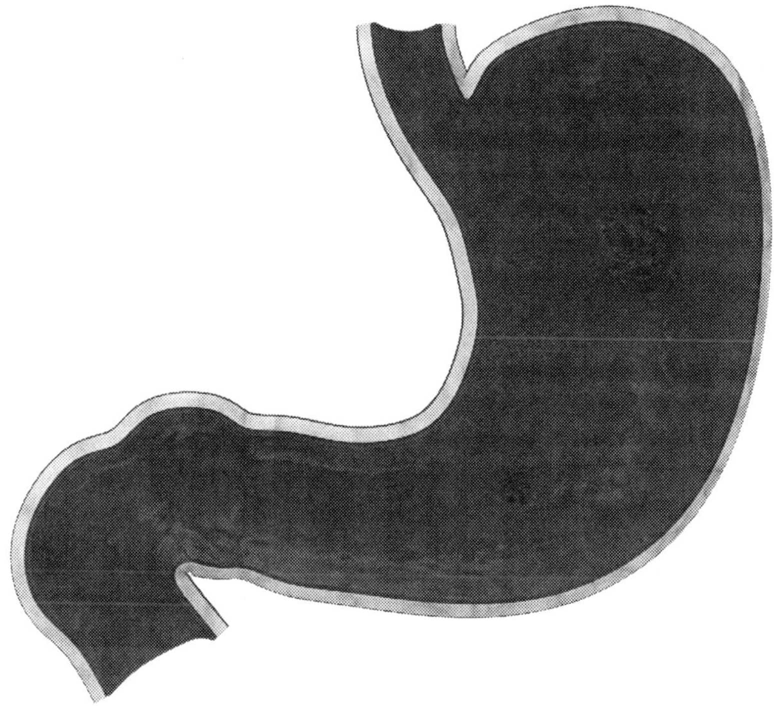

gastroduodenostomy (Billroth I) or gastrojejunostomy (Billroth II) follows to complete the circuit. A proximal vagotomy eliminates only the innervations to the parietal cells and does not need a drainage procedure as the stomach function usually remains intact.

The most significant complications of surgery include a hypergastrinemic state. Antrectomy with truncal vagotomy prevents this. Truncal vagotomy with pyloroplasty will lead to increased emptying of liquids and solids. Gastric emptying of liquids is accelerated after proximal vagotomy. Emptying of solid foods is typically unchanged. Dumping syndrome may occur but most patients will have spontaneous resolution within several months. Symptoms of dumping syndrome include pain, diaphoresis, lightheadedness, weakness, and diarrhea after ingesting a meal. This is presumably due to the high osmotic load reaching the duodenum and leading to rapid shifts in electrolytes and fluids. Dumping syndrome is more common after a truncal vagotomy. Dumping syndrome is treated by decreasing fluid intake to smaller amounts throughout the day. Fatty foods and simple sugars should be avoided, and meals should be smaller in size.

Surgery is the best option for duodenal ulcers when the ulcer is refractory to medical management after three months, or there is hemorrhage, obstruction, or perforation. Perforation of a duodenal ulcer requires prompt surgical attention and is repaired via a Graham patch procedure in which omentum is used to cover the defect. The presence of duodenal ulcers does not imply the same risk of a concomitant cancer as it does for gastric ulcers.

h) Complications

Severe gastric ulcer disease can lead to fatal hemorrhage. If suspected, diagnosis by an upper GI endoscopy is immediately mandated, followed by surgical intervention if hemostasis is not expeditiously achieved (either via endoscopy or vascular interventional procedures). Unstable patients should be managed surgically.

Complications may arise as side effects of treatment. Cimetidine is an H2 blocker that can cause testicular degeneration and gynecomastia, and should be avoided in patients on warfarin, phenytoin, or theophylline due to its inhibition of cytochrome P450.

2. Gastroparesis

a) Assessment

Gastroparesis occurs when there is a delay in the normal emptying of the stomach, leading to food being present in the stomach for prolonged periods of time and diminished gastric digestive function. Gastroparesis presents with early satiety, nausea, and vomiting and is due to degeneration of the vagus nerve innervation to the stomach. This degeneration may be attributed to diabetic neuropathy in patients with longstanding diabetes.

b) Management

Diagnosis of gastroparesis is made through radiolabeled studies that gauge the digestive function of the gastrointestinal tract. Metoclopramide to minimize the symptoms of nausea and vomiting is the treatment of choice.

3. Morbid Obesity

a) Assessment

Morbid obesity is defined as a body mass index (BMI) greater than 40. Obesity is a BMI over 30, while overweight is a BMI over 25. BMI is calculated as the weight in kilograms divided by the height in meters squared. Obesity is an epidemic and has major ramifications on health. Patients with morbid obesity have a significant risk of dysfunction of multiple systems and a reduction in life span by nearly 25%. Multiple causes of obesity have been elucidated and both genetic and environmental causes likely play an effect in affected patients.

b) Medical Management

Morbidly obese patients should be managed with an aggressive change in diet and exercise, and amelioration of all co-existing diseases (i.e. diabetes, heart failure, etc.). Patients refractory to medical management are candidates for surgery if they have a BMI over 40 without other comorbid conditions, or a BMI over 35 with comorbid conditions.

c) Surgical Management

Four major surgical interventions are favored by bariatric surgeons. Vertical gastric banding involves the creation of an opening near the gastroesophageal junction. A band is placed around this, thereby extending the conduit from the GE junction. The area between the opening and the cardia is stapled off, leading to one way flow of solid and liquids from the esophagus, through the band, and then to the remainder of the stomach. This band can be adjusted. Vertical banding has a variable success rate but as many as 30% can have a normal weight and another 50% will experience therapeutic weight loss.

A sleeve gastrectomy involves resection of the stomach along the greater curvature. Only about 15% of the stomach remains and leads to a significant reduction in the ability to tolerate large oral intake. Very large patients are candidates for sleeve gastrectomy given its reduced operating time and ability to initiate weight loss. A second stage procedure by way of a Roux-en-Y gastric bypass or duodenal switch can be completed if additional weight loss is necessary.

A Roux-en-Y gastric bypass combines the two approaches above and leads to both a restriction on oral intake and a decrease in absorption. It is more successful than either of the two approaches in patients who can tolerate the procedure, but can lead to a higher incidence of marginal ulcer formation, B12 deficiency, and iron-deficiency anemia. Laparoscopic Roux-en-Y gastric bypass (LRYGB) reduces hospital stays and improves patient comfort.

A less common procedure is a biliopancreatic diversion that involves a distal gastrectomy and anastomosis of the gastric remnant with the distal small bowel. Only a small amount of the oral intake is thereby absorbed. However, this leads to a high excretion of fat, causing foul-smelling diarrhea. Significant vitamin and protein deficiencies also occur.

d) Complications of Gastric Bypass

The most significant complication of Roux-en-Y bypass surgery is the development of an anastomotic leak at the gastrojejunal junction. Early signs include a grossly dilated stomach, tachycardia, increasing white count, fever, and hiccupping. An upper GI study with gastrograffin contrast can identify a leak; however, all patients with a high enough suspicion for leak should be taken back to the operating room for a diagnostic laparoscopy. Wide drainage and distal feeding are sufficient in patients who are not otherwise compromised.

B1 deficiency occurs in gastric bypass patients and presents as emesis, thigh numbness, and paresthesia that may progress to axonal degeneration with paralysis. B12 deficiency occurs months or years after surgery and presents with anemia, glossitis, and paresthesias. Iron deficiency is common and presents as anemia with brittle nails.

Other complications following bypass is the development of cholecystitis approximately six months following surgery and development of a marginal ulcer. Standard management is endoscopy for all patients with clinically significant complaints. Due to the presence of the Roux limb, open endoscopy may be necessary when it becomes important to instrument the biliary tree. Stomal stenosis can occur occasionally and is treated with bougie dilation.

Internal hernias may rarely occur following a Roux-en-Y gastric bypass. Most internal hernias are due to congenital or iatrogenic defects within the intraperitoneal anatomy. Herniation into various soft tissue foramina (i.e. foramen of Winslow), herniation through defects in the mesentery, and herniation around artificially fixed structures (i.e. mesocolic hernia) can occur. Incomplete closure of the mesentery after a bowel resection can lead to mesenteric hernia formation. Internal hernia formation after a Roux-en-Y is a surgical emergency. Internal hernias are more common with LRYGB compared to an open procedure due to defects at the jejunojejunal anastomosis, the opening for the retrocolic Roux limb, and behind the Roux limb. Internal hernias have a high risk of incarceration and strangulation leading to rapid bowel compromise and necrosis.

4. Ménétrier Disease

a) Assessment

Ménétrier disease is enlargement of the rugae and increased secretion of mucus by the stomach, leading to hypoalbuminemia and ulceration. It may be secondary to CMV, H. pylori, or overexpression of TGF-alpha. It typically presents with cachexia, postprandial abdominal pain, ascites, and anemia. There is an elevated risk of gastric adenocarcinoma.

b) Management

Hyperplasic hypersecretory gastropathy is treated by a high protein diet and gastrectomy if symptomatic management fails.

I.D. Cancer

1. Gastric Adenocarcinoma

a) Etiology

Gastric adenocarcinoma is the second leading cause of cancer-related death around the world. The majority of individuals with gastric cancer have metastatic disease at the time of diagnosis. Six month survival hovers between 10-50% depending on the extent of disease. There is a 2% risk of cancer as the underlying etiology in patients who present with clinically-significant indigestion. Acanthosis nigricans and seborrheic keratosis are associated with gastric cancer.

b) Pathophysiology and Presentation

Contributing factors include gastritis, H. pylori infection, smoking, and genetic transmission. Presenting signs include indigestion, loss of appetite, abdominal pain, anorexia, and bleeding. Patients with adenomatous polyps over 2 cm in size have a nearly 20% risk of developing cancer. These premalignant lesions have a significant risk of harboring carcinoma-in-situ and should be removed endoscopically. Lesions over 2 cm may require operative management for excision.

Two distinct types of adenocarcinoma may occur: a polypoid form generally occurs in males and spreads hematogenously. A diffuse form spreads via lymphatics and occurs in younger patients; the prognosis with this diffuse form is poor. Mutations in HER-2/neu and K-ras are commonly found with gastric adenocarcinoma.

c) Diagnosis

Gastric adenocarcinoma is diagnosed by endoscopy, upper GI swallow study, and CT scan. Suspicious polyps should be biopsied. Ulcers with an irregular, necrotic border are particularly worrisome. Evaluation for H. pylori is necessary so that antibiotic therapy can be started. Diagnostic imaging studies include CT scanning and air/barium contrast studies. However, direct visualization with endoscopy remains the gold standard as CT scanning and contrast studies have a limited sensitivity and specificity. Infiltrative gastric cancers are difficult to diagnose by any of these three means and may best be imaged and biopsied with endoscopic ultrasound. Metastatic spread is present nearly 20% of the time at the time of diagnosis.

d) Treatment

Following diagnosis and imaging, a surgical plan should be formulated. All potentially resectable tumors should be approached via a diagnostic laparoscopy. This modality offers a superior method for directly visualizing the main tumor, along with any potentially metastatic lesions to the liver and omentum. Satisfactory staging with identification of unresectable disease may change the surgical plan and lead to either a palliative total gastrectomy with Roux-en-Y or palliative chemoradiation. Resectable disease is typically treated with conversion to a laparotomy. Focal tumors can be treated with distal gastrectomy if it involves the antrum; proximal disease typically requires a total gastrectomy. High lesions may be treated with an esophagogastrectomy. More extensive tumor may be treated with en bloc resection of affected organs.

2. Gastric Lymphoma

a) Etiology

Primary gastric lymphoma composes about 10% of gastric malignancies and about 2% of all lymphomas; however, many lymphomas may eventually metastasize to the stomach. Primary gastric lymphoma is most common among the elderly and presents with epigastric pain, early satiety, weight loss, and malaise.

b) Pathophysiology and Presentation

MALT lymphoma is a form of non-Hodgkin lymphoma (NHL) that involves the mucosa-associated lymphoid tissue (MALT), typically of the stomach. High-grade MALTomas are cancers originating from B cells in the marginal zone of the MALT. Gastric MALToma is associated with chronic inflammation due to H. pylori infection. Pain and anorexia are the most common symptoms.

c) Diagnosis

Diagnosis via biopsy during an esophagogastroduodenoscopy typically clinches the diagnosis. CT helps to stage the disease, while LDH levels can be monitored for prognosis. Findings on imaging studies are similar to that for gastric adenocarcinoma.

d) Treatment

Chemotherapy is equivalent to surgery for the treatment of gastric lymphoma. The preferred regimen is CHOP and rituximab. Surgery is reserved for cases that have significant comorbidities, such as gastric outlet obstruction. A subtotal gastrectomy can be completed for these patients.

3. Gastrointestinal Stromal Tumor

a) Etiology and Epidemiology

Gastrointestinal stromal tumors (GIST) comprise less than 5% of all gastric cancers and are more common in the elderly.

b) Pathophysiology

GISTs are connective tissue tumors that occur in the stomach or small intestine. These slow-growing tumors may arise from the autonomic nervous system of the GI system, specifically from the interstitial cells of Cajal. The most common mutation is in the tyrosine kinase receptor gene c-kit. Concomitant mutations in PDGFR-alpha is also common. Spread is by direct extension.

c) Presentation and Diagnosis

GISTs present with abdominal pain and a palpable mass in thin patients. Diagnosis is made by CT scan that indicates a large, fleshy tumor with internal necrosis. Spindle cells that stain for CD117 (c-kit) are typically seen on histology.

d) Treatment

Treatment for GISTs is by way of complete resection whenever possible. Some control over the tumor can be had with imatinib, a tyrosine kinase inhibitor against c-kit. GISTs affect some 1 in 100,000 patients. Radiation has little impact in these oxygen-starved tumors.

II. Small Intestine

II.A. General Concepts

1. Anatomy

The layers of the small intestine from inside to out are the mucosa, submucosa, muscularis propria, and the serosa. The nerve plexuses throughout the GI tract include the subserosal Auerbach plexus and the submucosal Meissner plexus. The duodenum begins at the pylorus and continues to the ligament of Treitz, where it becomes the jejunum. The portal triad lies posterior to the first portion of the duodenum. The duodenum becomes retroperitoneal at D2 just after it crosses the gastroduodenal artery; hence, posterior ulcers of the duodenum can lead to major bleeding issues if they ulcerate into this artery. The Kocher maneuver is used to mobilize the duodenum and expose the pancreas. The third and fourth portion of the duodenum overlie the aorta and are proximal to the hepatic flexure. The jejunum and ileum comprise the remainder of the small intestine and are about 7-8 meters in length. The ileocecal valve separates the small intestine from the colon and functions as a sphincter.

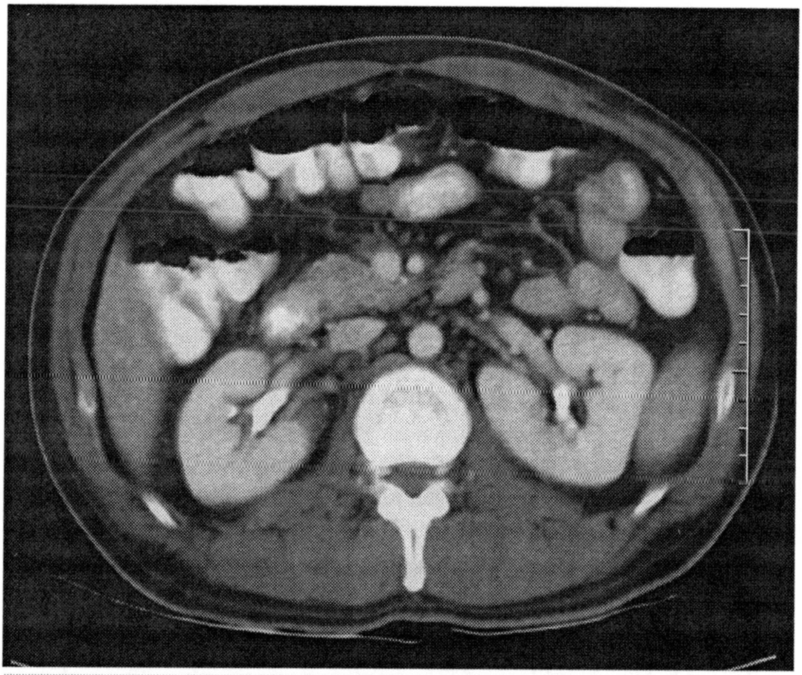

2. Vascular and Biliary Anatomy

The vascular supply to the duodenum emanates from the gastroduodenal artery, the superior pancreaticoduodenal arteries (via the gastroduodenal artery) and the inferior pancreaticoduodenal arteries (via the superior mesenteric artery). The superior mesenteric artery (SMA) also gives rise to the jejunal perforators and forms arcades that supply the entire small bowel. The end arteries are known as the vasa recta and become shorter and more branched along the distal small bowel.

The hepatoduodenal ligament contains the porta hepatis: portal vein, hepatic artery, and common bile duct. The Pringle maneuver is used to clamp this ligament in the event of injury to the right hepatic artery during a cholecystectomy. The common bile duct is approximately 8 cm long within this ligament and is located to the right of the hepatic artery and anterior to the portal vein.

3. Physiology

Peyer's patches are located within the small intestine and are the source of IgA production. They are an important part of maintaining immunity and this is one reason to aggressively feed postoperative patients. Some studies have shown that this helps to promote an overall immune system response and may play a role in promoting resistance to overall infection. The most common bacteria within the colon are B. fragilis, E. coli and Enterococcus spp.

Neurotransmitters that function within the nervous system of the intestine include acetylcholine, serotonin, nitric oxide, VIP, substance P, somatostatin, and neurokinin A.

Of the 10-12 L of fluid that arrives at the small intestine over a 24 hour period, only 2 L is oral intake; the remainder is generated by the body. About 8 L of this fluid is absorbed by the small bowel; the rest is absorbed by the ascending colon. Most electrolyte absorption also takes place within the small bowel.

II.B. Morphologic Disorders

1. Diverticulosis

a) Assessment

Diverticular disease of the small bowel is secondary to abnormal peristalsis and high pressure zones leading to outpouchings along the mesenteric border. Diverticulae within the duodenum are more common than elsewhere in the small bowel, and the majority are asymptomatic. Inflammation can lead to diverticulitis, bleeding, small bowel obstruction, and perforation. Diagnosis is made by CT scan with contrast and enteroclysis. Endoscopy can also be completed.

b) Management

Clinically symptomatic patients with complications related to diverticular disease are typically treated with antibiotics, bowel rest, and IV hydration. Bleeding can be managed via coil embolization or endoscopy. Serious disease refractory to medical management requires a small bowel resection with primary reanastomosis. A single troublesome diverticulum can be managed by simple diverticulectomy. Patients with diverticular disease within the C-loop of the duodenum may require a choledochoduodenostomy.

2. Meckel Diverticulum

a) Assessment

A Meckel diverticulum is a common congenital defect of the small intestine located approximately 2 feet from the ileocecal valve, affecting 2% of the population, has 2 types of tissue (gastric and pancreatic), is about 2 inches in length, manifests by age 2, and is symptomatic 2% of the time. Presentation is similar to small bowel diverticular disease with similar complications. The most common symptom is painless rectal bleeding. Diagnosis is made by technetium-99m scanning, which can detect ectopic gastric mucosa. A colonoscopy may be necessary if the Meckel scan fails. Severe bleeding may necessitate angiography and potential coil embolization.

b) Management

Grossly symptomatic disease is treated with surgical resection. The simple presence of a wide base or other factors in the setting of asymptomatic disease are insufficient findings to indicate surgery..

3. Intussusception

a) Assessment

Intussusception in adults is likely due to the presence of cancer (i.e. colon cancer or metastatic melanoma). A partial or complete SBO typically ensues, along with cramping abdominal pain and, occasionally, bloody diarrhea. Intussusception presents with nausea, bilious emesis, rectal bleeding with currant jelly stools, and abdominal pain. A palpable mass may be present in thinner patients. Intussusception can be complicated by ischemia and necrotic bowel.

b) Management

Diagnosis by ultrasound or CT scan is sufficient. Air contrast or barium enema can be both diagnostic and therapeutic. Patients who have a successful reduction should be monitored overnight due to the 10% recurrence rate. Intussusception in adults is typically managed by a diagnostic laparoscopy due to its strong link with cancer. A small bowel resection with end-to-end anastomosis may be required.

4. Afferent Limb Obstruction

a) Assessment

Afferent limb obstruction (also known as blind loop syndrome) is a complication associated with a Billroth II procedure in which a distal gastric resection followed by a gastrojejunal anastomosis is formed. Afferent limb obstruction is typically due to ulcer formation or technical error. The location of the obstruction is at the limb associated with the gastric remnant going to the duodenum. It presents as severe epigastric pain following eating and leads to a bilious emesis without food.

b) Management

Definitive treatment involves conversion of the Billroth II to a Roux-en-Y gastric bypass. A Billroth II procedure does not delay emptying, unlike a Roux-en-Y gastric bypass.

5. Ileus

a) Assessment

Ileus develops following inflammation, manipulation, or surgery to the small bowel and presents with intestinal paralysis. Peristalsis is inhibited and constipation occurs. Nausea and vomiting may occur with continued PO intake.

b) Management

Ileus is best treated with conservative management with bowel rest, IV hydration, and stimulation of the GI tract. Decompression via nasogastric tube placement can also be done. TPN can be used in prolonged cases. Patients with disease refractory to this management may require an exploratory laparotomy with lysis of adhesions and decompression. Electrolyte derangements should also be corrected.

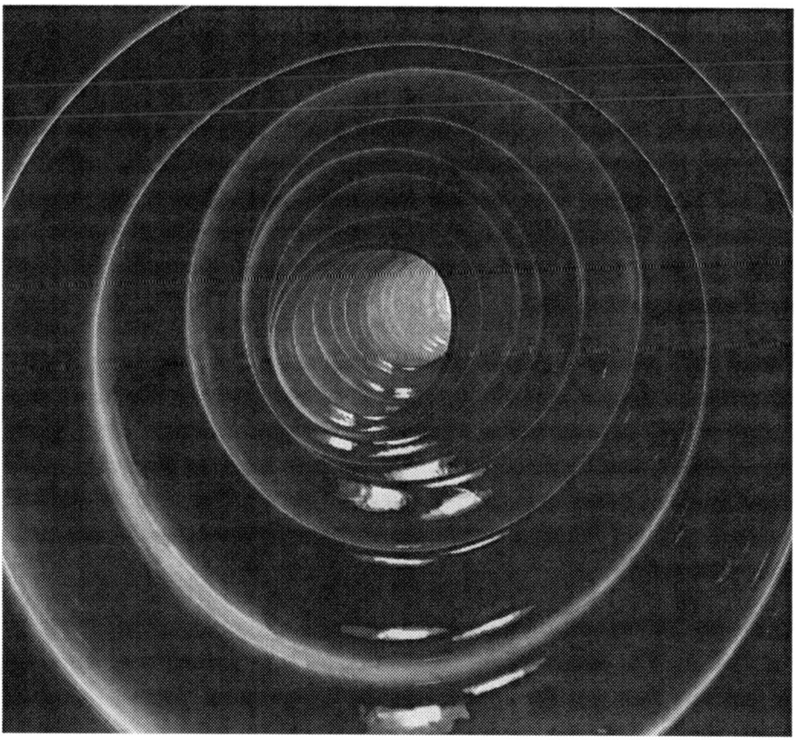

6. Small Bowel Obstruction

a) Etiology

Small bowel obstructions (SBO) are characterized by whether anterograde intestinal flow is permissible (partial vs. complete bowel obstruction), whether retrograde intestinal flow is possible (open vs. closed loop obstruction), whether obstruction has lead to vascular compromise (strangulated obstruction), whether the obstruction is close to the stomach and duodenum (proximal) or the colon (distal), and whether the defect is mechanical (i.e. structural) or functional (i.e. neurogenic) in nature. The region where the obstruction has occurred is referred to as the transition point.

SBO has a wide variety of causes, ranging from various anatomic defects (i.e. hernia or volvulus), to inflammatory diseases (i.e. Crohn disease and diverticulitis), trauma (i.e. duodenal hematoma), and carcinogenic (i.e. small bowel adenocarcinoma, metastatic melanoma).

b) Pathophysiology

SBO prevents forward transit of intestinal flow. This creates a pressure head at the site of obstruction, stasis of intestinal contents, proliferation of bacteria, and local edema from vascular compromise secondary to the pressure and swelling. Typically, the longer these processes are permitted to go on, the worse the prognosis. A number of considerations guide the medical and surgical management of SBO.

Partial SBO permits a greater freedom with medical management. Partial obstructions do not typically generate the same pressure elevations as a complete SBO as some transit of intestinal contents continues distal to the site of obstruction. Proximal loops of bowel may not be as distended, while distal loops of bowel may contain intestinal matter. Due to some residual continuing bowel function, symptoms are typically not as severe as a complete obstruction.

Complete SBO presents with severe symptoms out of proportion to physical findings. The nature of the obstruction leads to a continuous build up of pressure that steadily causes vascular compromise, permits bacterial proliferation with release of toxins, and breaks down host defenses. Without urgent intervention, a complete obstruction may lead to perforation and sepsis.

c) Presentation

Depending on the length of time and nature of the obstruction, a variety of symptoms may be present. Nausea, vomiting, abdominal pain, and abdominal distention are nearly universal findings. Slow but progressive symptoms with diminishing bowel function may signal the transition from a partial obstruction to a complete blockade. Acute and severe symptoms may signal a closed loop obstruction. The onset of fevers, rising WBC count, peritoneal signs, and sepsis strongly indicate perforation and/or bowel necrosis.

d) Diagnosis

Small bowel obstruction may be diagnosed by history and physical examination. However, the location and nature of the obstruction is best characterized by CT scan. Plain abdominal films assist with early diagnosis and may lead to early operation in the presence of free air that indicates perforation. Dilated loops of small bowel (> 3-4 cm) and colon (10 cm) may be evident on imaging studies. If the specific location of the obstruction is not clearly elucidated, a diagnostic and potentially therapeutic study can be completed by way of a small bowel follow through (SBFT) study.

e) Medical Treatment

Patients with SBO are approached with proximal and distal decompression to reduce the pressure build up at the transition point. Nasogastric tube (NGT) placement with low continuous wall suction (LCWS), nil per os (NPO) status, intravenous fluid (IVF) hydration, and symptomatic treatment of nausea and pain are the essentials. If the patient is expected to be without nutrition for over 7 days, supplementation with TPN and / or PPN is indicated. Such treatment for a partial SBO may lead to resolution in over 80% of patients. Progressive symptoms or a bowel obstruction that has failed to resolve with medical management may require surgery.

f) Surgical Management

A variety of surgical options exist for the management of SBO. The traditional approach is a midline laparotomy, lysis of adhesions, and possible resection of bowel at the transition point if it is in questionable health or the blockade cannot be readily cleared. Any clearly compromised bowel should be resected and a primary reanastomosis attempted. In some cases, a diverting loop ileostomy may be necessary to permit a distal anastomosis to heal.

Surgery for SBO is complicated by the potential for enterotomies, enterocutaneous fistula formation, inability to close the abdomen, short bowel syndrome, and diverting ostomy should access to the affected region prove impossible. Prior abdominal procedures may make surgery challenging due to adhesive bands and a "frozen" abdomen. Patience must be exercised in these cases to avoid bowel injury and potential short bowel syndrome.

A small bowel resection can cause significant morbidity depending on the area and length that is resected. Resection of the terminal ileum decreases conjugated bile salt absorption (unconjugated bile salts are absorbed in the jejunum), causing a decrease in water absorption by the colon and subsequent diarrhea. Megaloblastic anemia can occur from lack of vitamin B12 absorption in the ileum. Decreased binding of oxalate in the small intestine increases oxalate absorption in the colon and subsequent oxalate stone deposition in the kidney and gallbladder. Oxalate normally binds to calcium in the bowel to form calcium oxalate, which is excreted with feces. However, the precipitation of fatty acids with calcium in the colon following resection of the terminal ileum leads to net absorption.

7. Enterocutaneous Fistula

An enterocutaneous fistula (ECF) is the result of an enterotomy leading to leakage of toxic gastrointestinal contents into the abdomen. Through containment of the abscess, the body naturally shunts this content to the outside by the development of a fistula between the small intestine and skin. Treatment is to remove all foreign bodies, minimize the effects of inflammatory bowel surgery (i.e. infliximab therapy), resolve any distal obstructions, stabilize the patient, and start TPN. Octreotide may also have some benefit.

8. Short Bowel Syndrome

Resection of the small intestine to with less than 100 cm remaining causes short bowel syndrome. Unless congenital in origin, most cases are iatrogenic. Although compensatory changes occur in the small intestine, including expansion of villi, an increase in bowel diameter, and a decrease in the rate of peristalsis, extensive resection leads to lifelong dependence on TPN due to the inability to absorb sufficient nutrients enterally. Only70% of patients on lifelong TPN do well after just 2 years. Due to the increased morbidity and mortality, selected patients may be eligible for an intestinal transplant – a procedure that itself carries enormous morbidity and mortality and has a 4 year survival of only 60%. Step procedures exist at specialized institutions where duplication of the small intestine can be attempted – the overall success is controversial.

II.C. Metabolic Disorders

1. Malabsorption Syndromes

a) Etiology

Derangements in the small bowel may lead to selective deficiencies in various nutrients and minerals. Malabsorption syndromes commonly occur due to defects in digestion, poor distribution of emulsifying bile acids, changes to the anatomy of the bowel, obstruction to the lymphatic drainage of the bowel, decreased function or surface area available for absorption, alterations in hormones, and infection.

b) Pathophysiology – Carbohydrates

Defects in absorption related to monosaccharides involve the entire small bowel. Only monosaccharides are absorbed due to defects in the degradation of complex carbohydrates, poor transport with the sodium cotransporter due to low amounts of sodium in meals, or excess fructose in the diet that overwhelms the fructose transporters and causes an osmotic diarrhea.

c) Pathophysiology – Lactose Intolerance

Lactose is a sugar in dairy products, but some patients have an inherent deficiency in lactase that worsens with age. It is common in adult patients from Africa, Asians, and a minority of Caucasians. This congenital defect in lactase leads to symptoms including abdominal cramps, flatus, and diarrhea.

d) Pathophysiology – Lipids

The absorption of lipids and lipid-soluble vitamins such as vitamins D, E, K, and A occurs within the ileum. Lipase hydrolyzes triglycerides; bile salts emulsify fats and form micelles; and digestive products must be reabsorbed in the ileum. Micelles permit absorption of the fat-soluble vitamins.

e) Pathophysiology – Amino Acids and Nucleic Acids

The absorption of amino acids occurs in the jejunum. Protein digestion relies on pancreatic enzymes such as trypsin, chymotrypsin, and elastase. Cotransport of most amino acids requires sodium, but there are also sodium-independent transporters available for amino acids. Nucleic acid transport occurs throughout the small intestine and requires pancreatic nucleases to cleave nucleic acids into pentoses for passive transport through diffusion.

f) Pathophysiology – Fluids

Fluids are absorbed mostly in the jejunum, followed by the ileum and ascending colon. The small intestine secretes an additional 7 L to the 2 L ingested daily, with only 200 mL remaining for defecation after absorption by the intestines. Water moves parallel to the osmotic gradients, and thus any defect in fluid absorption requires a search for shifts in these gradients.

g) Pathophysiology – Vitamins and Bile Salts

The transport of water-soluble vitamins occurs in the duodenum through passive diffusion. Vitamin B12 requires intrinsic factor made by parietal cells in the stomach for absorption in the terminal ileum. Bile salts are reabsorbed through an active transport process in the ileum for enterohepatic circulation.

h) Pathophysiology – Electrolytes

Sodium, potassium, chloride, calcium, and iron ions are absorbed and secreted throughout much of the small intestine. The majority of chloride, calcium, and iron transport occurs in the duodenum. Sodium ions are absorbed through an active and a passive mechanism, while secretion of sodium ions into the intestinal lumen occurs through the Na+-K+-ATPase transport system. Potassium ions are absorbed in the small intestine, and secreted in the colon. Chloride ions are secreted in small amounts, but absorbed in the duodenum. Calcium ions are actively transported with the assistance of 1,2,5-dihydroxycholecalciferol and protein absorption. A diet high in phosphates or oxalates inhibits calcium ion transport. Iron ion transport is generally poor and is best done when iron is reduced by stomach acid into the Fe2+ form, as this ferrous form freely diffuses through the mucosa and binds to the iron storage molecule apoferritin. The iron then moves from apoferritin to the transport protein transferrin.

i) Presentation

The signs and symptoms of malabsorption syndromes are numerous and depend on the particular etiology of the disorder. Generally, malabsorption syndromes present with steatorrhea, deficiencies in one or more vitamins and/or minerals, weight loss, bloating and abdominal pain, osteoporosis with poor calcium absorption, diarrhea, flatus, amenorrhea, anemia and platelet defects leading to easy bruising, and neuropathy.

j) Diagnosis and Treatment

Diagnosis of malabsorption syndromes is made using a Sudan stain to confirm the presence of steatorrhea and doing a biopsy of the small bowel to determine the presence of certain malabsorptive diseases. Treatment for is accomplished by correcting deficits through replacement of particular nutrients or replacing pancreatic enzymes. All malabsorptive syndromes require vitamin replacement due to normal losses experienced with the diarrhea. Lactose intolerance is treated by avoiding dairy products and administering lactase supplements.

II.D. Inflammatory and Infectious Diseases

1. Diarrhea

a) Etiology

Diarrhea may be due to a number of disparate causes, including infectious, medication-induced, inflammatory, osmotic, secretory, and altered intestinal motility etiologies. The most common causes of infectious diarrhea include E. coli (ETEC), Vibrio cholerae, E. coli (O157:H7), Giardia lamblia, rotavirus, Norwalk agent, Salmonella, and Clostridium difficile. The most common causes of bloody diarrhea are Campylobacter, E. coli (EHEC), E. histolytica, Salmonella, and Shigella. Inflammatory diarrhea is secondary to inflammatory bowel disease and infections from AIDS. Osmotic diarrhea is due to lactase deficiency and celiac sprue disease. Secretory diarrhea may occur from carcinoid syndrome and gastrinoma. Altered intestinal motility leading to diarrhea may be secondary to irritable bowel syndrome.

b) Pathophysiology

Diarrhea is defined as increase in stool weight over 200 grams per day or abnormally frequent passage of stools. Nine of the 10 liters of fluids that enter the gastrointestinal tract are absorbed in the small intestine, and only about 1 liter passes into the large intestine. Of that liter, about 4/5's of it are reabsorbed by the ascending colon and the remainder goes towards stool formation. Most cases of diarrhea lasting less than two weeks are infectious in etiology, while chronic diarrhea lasting more than a few weeks is typically due to lactase deficiency.

c) Infectious Diarrhea

Infectious diarrhea from E. coli may be enterotoxigenic (ETEC) such as traveler's diarrhea, enteroinvasive (EIEC) or enterohemorrhagic (EHEC) and present with fever and bloody diarrhea. The most common bacterial diarrhea in North America is Campylobacter, which may also lead to reactive arthritis. Diarrhea in day care centers that is commonly transmitted through impure food or water is commonly due to Shigella. Salmonella is a cause of diarrhea in patients who consumed improperly prepared poultry or dairy products. Diarrhea that presents similar to appendicitis but with joint pain and a skin rash should lead to a clinical suspicion for Yersinea. Poorly cooked beef and unpasteurized dairy products may lead to poisoning with E. coli O157:H7 and concomitant thrombotic thrombocytopenic purpura (TTP) or hemolytic uremic syndrome (HUS).

Diarrhea from viral agents are very common, especially Norwalk agent on cruise ships and rotavirus through oral-fecal infection. Shigella infection leads to diarrhea after several hours or days. Staphylococcus aureus infection leads to rapid diarrhea within a few hours. Most infectious diarrhea occurs within one day. Common microorganisms found in diarrhea in immunocompromised individuals include Mycobacterium avium, Cryptosporidium, and Isosporium.

d) Iatrogenic Diarrhea

Diarrhea may be induced through the consumption of a number of medications. These include laxatives, antibiotics such as penicillins, cephalosporins, ciprofloxacin, clindamycin, and tetracycline, antacids that contain magnesium, colchicine, beta blockers such as propranolol, quinidine, theophylline, diuretics such as furosemide or thiazide diuretics, angiotensin-converting enzyme (ACE) inhibitors, and antidepressants such as fluoxetine and sertraline. Diarrhea following digoxin and lithium is typically an early sign of toxicity, and diarrhea following consumption of medications is typically a sign that the offending drug should be stopped.

e) Inflammatory Diarrhea

Inflammatory diarrhea is associated with intestinal changes in inflammatory bowel disease such as Crohn disease and ulcerative colitis, and in infections associated with AIDS. Ulcerative colitis tends to present with a bloody diarrhea, while Crohn disease tends to present with a diarrhea that contains more mucus and pus, and smaller amounts of blood.

f) Osmotic Diarrhea

TABLE 2. Osmotic Diarrhea

Cause	Indigestible solutes and high carbohydrate content (mannitol, sorbitol, and fructose).
Presentation	Watery diarrhea which abates after expulsion of offending solute.
Treatment	Eliminate offending nutrient(s).

g) Secretory Diarrhea

Secretory diarrhea is often a result of gastrinoma. High levels of vasoactive intestinal peptide (VIP) from pancreatic adenomas and irritation from laxatives (such as phenolphthalein) may lead to secretory diarrhea. Secretory diarrhea tends to be very high in volume, and resolves with treatment of the underlying disorder or cessation of the offending medication. Secretory diarrhea is the diagnosis if the stool osmotic gap is negative. A positive osmotic gap indicates malabsorptive diarrhea.

$$\text{Stool Osmotic Gap} = 2\ Na^{+} + K^{+} - \text{Osmolality}$$

h) Villous Adenoma

Villous adenomas of the small bowel are more rare, but can become quite large with a malignant potential of about 50% at 5 cm. Villous adenomas may present with watery diarrhea. A villous adenoma may present with a decrease in bicarbonate, a drop in urine pH.

2. Appendicitis

a) Etiology and Pathophysiology

In most people, the appendix is a retrocecal 10 cm appendage of the cecum that is located at the junction of the three taeniae coli. On colonoscopy, it is near the "crow's foot", itself an indication of the confluence of the taeniae. The mesoappendix contains the appendiceal artery, which is a branch of the ileocolic artery.

In patients with appendicitis, the most common cause is obstruction and bacterial overgrowth. This swelling leads to vascular compromise and results in a gangrenous appendix – appendicitis. Perforation will typically occur within 24 hours as the gangrene proceeds to necrosis. In younger patients, the most common cause of appendiceal obstruction is from lymphoid hyperplasia; fecalith is more common in older patients. Other less common causes include carcinoid and adenocarcinoma; carcinoid is the most common tumor-related cause of appendicitis.

b) Presentation and Diagnosis

Early signs of appendicitis include periumbilical pain and malaise. As symptoms proceed, the pain becomes better localized to the right lower quadrant. Nausea, occasional vomiting, and some loss of appetite occur. Fever and an elevated WBC count present, and the patient is typically tender over McBurney's point. Other physical exam findings include a positive Rovsing sign (palpation over the left lower quadrant leads to peritoneal irritation and pain in the right lower quadrant), obturator sign (internal rotation of the leg exacerbates symptoms of an appendix located near the pelvic brim), and an iliopsoas sign (extension of the right hip leads to pain and implies a retrocecal appendix).

A clinical diagnosis is sufficient to take a patient to the OR for an appendectomy. When the diagnosis may be not be clear (i.e. young woman), a CT scan can be invaluable in confirming the diagnosis, precisely determining the location of the appendix, and evaluating for perforation. Periappendiceal fat stranding, incomplete filling of the appendix, gross dilation over 6 mm, wall thickening, and enhancement with IV contrast are CT findings for appendicitis. Ultrasound may be used to make the diagnosis in young children.

c) Treatment

Treatment of appendicitis is by open or laparoscopic appendectomy. The laparoscopic approach uses a periumbilical incision and two ports spaced apart in a triangular configuration on the left side of the abdomen. Open approaches consist of making an oblique incision near McBurney's point.

A normal appendix but abnormal ovarian cyst on laparoscopic examination is treated by removing the appendix and treating the cyst afterwards to prevent confusion regarding the status of the appendix in the future should the right lower quadrant pain recur. Terminal ileitis in the setting of a normal cecum and appendix should also prompt removal of the appendix. A cystic mass at the base of the appendix is likely a cystadenocarcinoma and should be treated by a right hemicolectomy. Due diligence is required to avoid spilling the contents as seeding of the tumor will occur. The presence of a walled-off abscess can be treated with a CT-guided drain placement followed by interval appendectomy.

3. Intra-Abdominal Abscess

a) Assessment

The presence of an infected collection of fluid or pus requires removal in order for the nidus of infection to resolve. The body is unable to clear significant collections, regardless of antibiotic therapy. Abscesses may be the result of surgical diseases like appendicitis or diverticulitis, or may be iatrogenic following particularly contaminated procedures. The extent of abscess formation is best gauged by CT scan. The clinical status of the patient should also be assessed and the WBC and vital signs should be monitored.

b) Management

Abscesses are separated into either contained or open collections. Small contained perforations are amenable to conservative management and may be safely observed if a CT-guided drain placement is not feasible. All other collections need to be drained. Difficulty with drain placement requires an open intervention with drain placement. Most contaminated or dirty cases will automatically result in drain placement to avoid coming back to the OR or going to radiology for postoperative drainage of new collections.

4. Pneumatosis Intestinalis

a) Assessment

Pneumatosis intestinalis is a nonspecific finding often seen on CT. In isolation, it may be secondary to various pulmonary diseases, lupus, or from medications. In conjunction with abdominal pain, it may be secondary to ileus, bowel obstruction, ulcers, gastroenteritis, or diverticular disease. In critically-ill patients, pneumatosis may be a sign of ischemia or toxic megacolon. Air may permeate the bowel wall via the mediastinum from airway disease or from translocation of gas-producing bacteria that translocate across the bowel wall.

b) Management

Asymptomatic pneumatosis is managed expectantly and often requires no therapy at all. Pneumatosis with abdominal pain is often treated with bowel rest and TPN with serial examinations. A specific region with disease may be resected if the pain fails to resolve or there is progression of disease. Critically-ill patients with pneumatosis often require emergent operation for necrotic bowel or toxic megacolon with a prolonged period of postoperative bowel rest.

5. Radiation Enteritis

Radiation enteritis is small bowel injury due to radiotherapy leading to inflammation, edema, and decreased bowel function. Nausea, vomiting, anorexia, and ileus may result. The most appropriate therapy is IV hydration, bowel rest, and octreotide for severe symptoms. If a focal area is especially affected, surgical resection is possible; however, in most cases, there is no definitive cure for chronic disease.

II F. Trauma

1. Duodenal Hematoma

a) Assessment

A duodenal hematoma is the result of blunt abdominal trauma and presents with nausea, vomiting, and a right upper quadrant mass. It is diagnosed by an upper GI study that indicates filling of the duodenal lumen with a coiled spring sign in the second and third portions due to compression from the hematoma. Symptoms may not become apparent for up to 24 hours following the initial injury. Amylase tends to be elevated.

b) Management

Treatment is to make the patient NPO, insert an NG tube, and start TPN. Drainage of the hematoma can be successfully done after seven days if the patient does not improve clinically.

II.F. Cancer

1. Carcinoid

a) Etiology and Epidemiology

Carcinoid syndrome is the result of a neuroendocrine tumor that secretes hormones or neurotransmitters that have an effect on the gastrointestinal system. These active compounds can include serotonin (5-HT), adrenocorticotrophic hormone (ACTH), histamine, dopamine, tryptophan, substance P, and bradykinin. It is part of the MEN type I disorder, and the incidence of carcinoid syndrome is greater in patients who have Gardner syndrome or Crohn disease.

b) Pathophysiology

The majority of carcinoids are in the appendix, but the endocrine cells in this location tend not to have any effect. The majority of carcinoids in the ileum are secreting, as are those found in the lung. Carcinoid typically causes most of its effects through the conversion of tryptophan to serotonin, and the unchecked production of serotonin may lead to symptoms of niacin deficiency and subsequent pellagra.

c) Presentation

Many carcinoids are asymptomatic and discovered only incidentally. Those located in the appendix may create symptoms of appendicitis, and carcinoid in the small intestine may lead to obstruction or diarrhea. The classic triad includes flushing due to excessive bradykinin production, diarrhea from excessive serotonin release, and valvular heart disease that primarily affects the mitral valve from excess serotonin. Other classic symptoms include anorexia, hypotension, tachycardia, and alcohol intolerance. Carcinoid may metastasize to the liver and cause right upper quadrant (RUQ) pain and elevated liver function tests (LFTs), and the lung to cause wheezing, obstructed bronchus, and pneumonia.

d) Diagnosis

Diagnosis of carcinoid syndrome is with a 24 hour 5-hydroxyindolacetic acid (5-HIAA) collection; elevated titers are 100% specific for carcinoid. Point collections through serum or urine samples may also be done. 5-HIAA is the metabolite of serotonin when it is broken down by monoamine oxidase (MAO) and then by aldehyde dehydrogenase. CT of the lung and abdomen are compulsory to detect metastasis. The most common location for carcinoid is in the appendix (50%), followed by the ileum (25%) and rectum (20%). Ileal carcinoid has the highest potential for metastasis; appendiceal carcinoid has the lowest potential for metastasis. Appendiceal carcinoid is the second most common type of appendiceal cancer; mucinous adenocarcinoma is the most common. Mucinous adenocarcinoma of the appendix requires a right hemicolectomy.

e) Treatment

Carcinoid syndrome is treated with surgical resection and radiation therapy. With metastasis to the liver, embolization and alpha interferon therapy are used with resection. Symptomatic control of carcinoid can be achieved with the somatostatin analog octreotide. Survival after diagnosis of active carcinoid syndrome is typically 3 years. Carcinoid of the appendix has a good prognosis, while disease outside of the appendix has a 50% 5 year survival.

Appendiceal carcinoids less than 2 centimeters at the distal end can be treated by appendectomy. Carcinoids over 2 centimeters or those at the base require a right hemicolectomy. A rectal carcinoid less than 1 cm can be treated by endoscopic excision; carcinoid between 1 to 2 cm requires transanal excision; carcinoid over 2 cm requires an LAR. Invasive carcinoid requires an LAR or APR. Most rectal carcinoids over 2 cm have metastasis to the liver on presentation, and the vast majority have metastasized to local lymph nodes. The presence of a gastric carcinoid receives local excision if less than 1 cm; subtotal gastrectomy with omentectomy may be required for carcinoid larger than 1 cm.

2. Mucinous Cystadenoma

a) Assessment

Mucinous cystadenoma is the benign version that produces excess mucus, typically from within the appendix. Dissemination of this tumor throughout the abdomen can lead to pseudomyxoma peritonei. The most common cancer of the appendix is mucinous cystadenocarcinoma and comprises over ⅓ of all appendiceal malignancies. This fast-growing, invasive tumor is more likely to lead to pseudomyxoma peritonei. Early symptoms include appendicitis, abdominal distention, and hernia formation.

b) Management

Treatment for mucinous cystadenoma with disease restricted to the appendix should be treated by appendectomy with care taken to avoid rupture. Mucinous cystadenocarcinoma requires a right hemicolectomy. If the diagnosis is made after appendectomy, a completion right hemicolectomy should be done. Patients with pseudomyxoma peritonei should have gross debulking and intraoperative hyperthermic peritoneal chemotherapy. Postoperative chemotherapy is necessary if the etiology is cystadenocarcinoma. Five year survival with mucinous cystadenoma is near 80%. Five year survival is near 50% for metastatic mucinous cystadenocarcinoma.

3. Adenocarcinoma

a) Assessment

Nearly ⅓ of all small bowel tumors manifest as adenocarcinoma. The most common location is the duodenum, and Crohn disease and polyposis are major risk factors. Early signs of cancer include obstruction, weight loss, and pain. Tumors located near the ampulla may lead to biliary obstruction and pancreatitis. Diagnosis is made by CT or MRI. Upper GI endoscopy is valuable for proximal tumors.

b) Management

Early identification of these tumors permits a potentially curative resection of the entire mass. Masses that affect the proximal duodenum may be treated with a pancreaticoduodenectomy, while tumors that affect the distal duodenum may be amenable to duodenectomy alone. If unresectable disease is found, palliation with duodenal stent placement and/or chemoradiation may be indicated. Metastatic disease to the ovaries is common. Five year survival varies between 50-80% depending on the extent of the tumor burden.

c) Signet Ring Adenocarcinoma

Signet ring adenocarcinoma can occur throughout the small intestine, stomach and lungs. Early, extensive metastasis is common leading to perforated appendicitis, ascites, abdominal distention, and seeding throughout the peritoneum and ovaries. Treatment requires a right hemicolectomy, intraoperative intraperitoneal chemotherapy with cytoreduction, and postoperative FOLFOX therapy. Five year survival is less than 20%.

III. Large Intestine

III.A. Anatomy

1. Surgical Anatomy

The large intestine begins at the cecum and ends five feet later at the rectum. Haustra, taeniae coli, and epiploic appendages differentiate the large intestine from the small intestine. The hepatic flexure is somewhat more inferior compared to the splenic flexure due to the extent of the liver. The phrenocolic and splenocolic ligaments must be transected in order to mobilize the left colon. The peritoneal fold that anchors the transverse colon is known as the transverse mesocolon. The sigmoid colon is mobile and can lead to volvulus in some patients. The left ureter travels near the sigmoid colon and crosses the pelvic brim just anterior to the junction of the external and internal iliac arteries with the common iliac artery. The rectum begins at the sacral promontory near S3.

a) Anal Verge

The anal verge, also known as the pectinate line or anorectal junction, is the junction of the hindgut and proctodeum and separates the upper ⅔s of the anal canal from the lower ⅓. There are differences in lymphatic drainage,

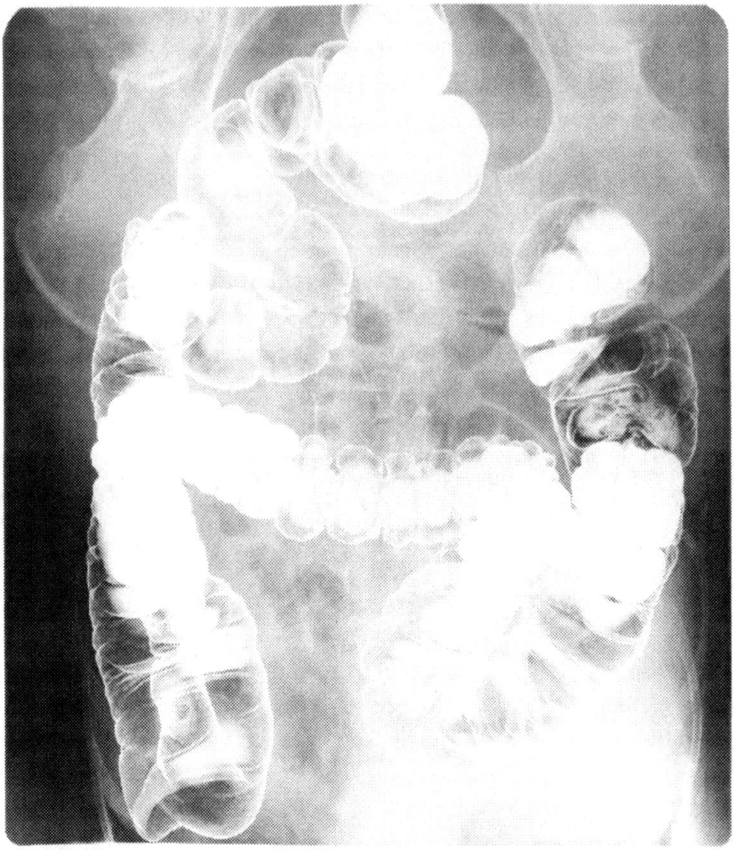

epithelial layers, embryologic origin, vascular supply, and innervations between the anal canal (below the pectinate line) and the rectum. The anal canal is typically about 3 cm in length.

Above the pectinate line (i.e. rectum), the lymphatic drainage is to the internal iliac and inferior mesenteric nodes; the anal canal drains into the superficial inguinal nodes. Columnar epithelium dominates above, while squamous epithelium is found below. The endoderm is the embryologic origin of tissue above the pectinate line, while ectoderm is the main source below. The blood supply to the rectum is mostly from the superior rectal artery and vein, while the inferior rectal artery and vein supply the anal canal. The inferior hypogastric plexus supplies the tissues cranially, while the inferior rectal nerves are found caudally. A somewhat arbitrary distinction is that internal hemorrhoids are found above the pectinate line and tend to be less painful than external hemorrhoids, found below the pectinate line.

2. Vascular Supply

The right colic artery arises from the SMA and supplies the ascending colon. It anastomosis with the middle colic artery, also a branch of the SMA. The middle colic supplies the transverse colon. The middle colic artery anastomosis with the left colic artery, a branch of the IMA. Another anastomosis between the SMA and IMA occurs via the marginal artery of Drummond that travels within the mesentery and close to the bowel. A meandering mesenteric artery (arc of Riolan) is a similar vessel that travels near the root of the mesentery. The sigmoid and superior rectal branches emanate from the IMA to supply the sigmoid colon and rectum, respectively. The middle and inferior rectal arteries come from the hypogastric artery. Lymphatic drainage above the dentate line of the anal canal goes to the inferior mesenteric nodes, while drainage below the dentate line goes to the internal iliac lymph nodes.

3. Physiology

a) Fluid Balance

The ascending colon absorbs the majority of the fluid that reaches it and leaves only about 200 mL to aid in the formation of stool. Sodium chloride is absorbed via an active process, while potassium and bicarbonate are secreted. Butyrate serves as the primary energy source for the colon; this short chain fatty acid is produced by local flora.

III.B. Morphologic Disease

1. Diverticulosis

a) Etiology

Diverticulosis is the development of a sac-like outpouching of the colon that herniates between the taeniae coli. Diverticulosis is the most common cause of significant bleeding from the lower gastrointestinal tract in elderly patients. The outpouchings of diverticulosis generally occur in the sigmoid colon, likely due to the higher pressures experienced in this section of the gastrointestinal tract. Diverticulosis is more common in patients who have a diet poor in fiber, and generally affects a majority of the elderly population. The majority tend to occur after the age of 85. Twenty percent of patients with diverticulosis will develop diverticulitis. Complications occur in 1/5 of patients.

b) Pathophysiology and Presentation

Diverticulosis can cause inflammation of the mucosa and erosion into an intestinal artery, leading to painless hemorrhage and bright red blood per rectum. The majority of bleeds occur with right-sided diverticulae, and tend to resolve spontaneously. Most cases of diverticulosis tend to be painless, but abdominal pain relieved by defecation can occur.

c) Diagnosis

Diagnosis of diverticulosis is made through colonoscopy that detects the outpouching. A more sensitive test is barium enema, which is also a safer test as the colonoscopy can lead to perforation of the sac. A nuclear medicine scan with tagged red blood cell or angiography can be used to assess the cause of the lower gastrointestinal bleed; coil embolization with angiography can also and potentially stop the bleeding.

d) Treatment

Diverticulosis is treated by correcting the cause of the lower gastrointestinal bleeding. A complication of diverticulosis is the inflammation of the outpouching, leading to diverticulitis. Significant bleeding that is not halted by endoscopy or coil embolization may require a hemicolectomy for definitive cure.

2. Diverticulitis

a) Pathophysiology and Presentation

Diverticulitis is inflammation of colon outpouchings due to fecalith formation and proliferation of bacteria within the diverticulum. Diverticulitis typically presents with left lower quadrant abdominal pain. Right lower quadrant pain is typically due to Meckel diverticulitis. Irritation from the diverticulum can lead to urinary urgency and constipation. As the disease progresses, fever and peritoneal signs can develop. A sigmoid mass may be present upon physical examination in the event of a perforation.

b) Diagnosis

Diagnosis of diverticulitis requires blood cultures positive for infection, leukocytosis, and a CT scan confirming the diagnosis. In diverticulitis, invasive tests such as barium enema and colonoscopy are contraindicated due to the increased risk of perforation and subsequent peritonitis and sepsis, especially in the acute phase of diverticulitis.

c) Treatment

Treatment of diverticulitis is with bowel rest, hydration, antibiotics to cover bowel flora, and pain control. An interval sigmoidectomy is done electively to reduce the 25% chance of recurrent disease. A screening colonoscopy should be done once the acute phase has resolved. A contained abscess is treated with CT-guided drain placement and antibiotics, while gross perforation requires a Hartmann's procedure.

3. Cecal Volvulus

a) Assessment

Cecal volvulus occurs in the setting of a partial malrotation and leads to a closed loop obstruction with ischemia and necrosis. Diagnosis is by exam and plain films that indicate a dilated loop of bowel with a bird beak sign pointing to the LUQ. Pneumatosis intestinalis, fat stranding, and distal decompression of the colon are found on CT. Cecal volvulus is associated with colon cancer and diverticulitis, and can occur along its axial plane or transverse plane. Axial torsion has a higher morbidity due to earlier vascular compromise, while the cecal bascule-type torsion along the transverse plane may be associated with a congenital defect. Cecal volvulus presents with a surgical abdomen.

b) Management

Early diagnosis is the key to reducing the extensive morbidity and mortality that can occur with cecal volvulus. Early imaging with plain films and resuscitation are important. Patients who are benign and stable can have an attempt at reduction via barium enema. If this fails, or the patient has compromised bowel, a right hemicolectomy is necessary.

4. Sigmoid Volvulus

a) Assessment

Among the types of volvulus that can affect the GI tract, sigmoid volvulus is the most common, especially among the elderly. It is due to an anatomic defect leading to redundant sigmoid colon with insufficient anchoring to the mesentery. Sigmoid volvulus presents with distention, obstipation, fever, and peritoneal signs. Mesenteric rotation is likely to lead to vascular compromise, while axial rotation may be asymptomatic. Diagnosis by exam and plain films is made. A bird's beak sign, thumbprinting, distention of the sigmoid colon, and corkscrewing are all signs of sigmoid volvulus on plain films and CT scan.

b) Management

Treatment of sigmoid volvulus is by rectal tube placement, sigmoidoscopy, or barium enema. Patients with intestinal compromise or who fail conservative management require sigmoidectomy and a Hartmann's procedure. While some practitioners may due a primary anastomosis, this is not the board answer.

5. Colonic Pseudo-obstruction

a) Assessment

Ogilvie syndrome is bowel distention leading to atonic obstruction. It may occur after non-abdominal procedures, especially following cardiac surgery. It is thought to be due to neurologic dysfunction, abnormalities in electrolytes, and advanced age.

b) Management

Ogilvie syndrome is treated with nasogastric tube decompression and intravenous neostigmine to stimulate the parasympathetic system. Atropine should be on hand in the event of significant bradycardia. Decompression with colonoscopy has a 90% success rate but a 40% recurrence rate. In the worst circumstances, an exploratory laparotomy with bowel resection or cecostomy is required. The cecum is at the greatest risk of perforation.

6. Constipation

a) Presentation and Diagnosis

Constipation is abnormal passage of stools less than 3 times every 7 days. Constipation can be secondary to a low fiber diet with dehydration, due to diabetes-related complications, iatrogenic causes, obstruction, pregnancy, Hirschsprung disease, Chagas disease, or hypothyroidism. Narcotics, anticholinergics, iron, and calcium-channel blockers can cause constipation.

b) Treatment

Constipation is treated by hydration. A high fiber diet with up to 30 grams per day avoids constipation. Laxatives that lead to increased bulk and emollient laxatives may also be prescribed.

7. Hemorrhoids

a) Etiology and Pathophysiology

Hemorrhoids occur due to a defect in the structural supports of the anal canal. External hemorrhoids occur with prolapse of this soft tissue distal to the dentate line. Internal hemorrhoids are classified by various degrees of prolapsed but are typically painless due to the lack of anoderm covering. External hemorrhoids are painful only with thrombosis.

b) Presentation and Diagnosis

First degree internal hemorrhoids present with bleeding but no prolapse. Second degree hemorrhoids have prolapse with bleeding, but reduce spontaneously. Third degree internal hemorrhoids require manual reduction, while fourth degree hemorrhoids cannot be reduced and are strangulated.

c) Treatment

The majority of hemorrhoidal disease can be treated with dietary modification, laxatives, emollients, and avoiding straining. Clinically-significant disease can be treated with band ligation. The presence of pain or fever following band ligation requires immediate surgical evaluation due to the risk of perineal sepsis and death.

Hemorrhoidectomy is typically done for prolapsed or strangulated hemorrhoids. Closed procedures can be used for either type of hemorrhoid and involves sharp resection down to the anal sphincter. Open resection can be done to reduce pain. A stapled hemorrhoidopexy with hemorrhoidectomy can be done with an EEA stapler. The biggest complication of surgical interventions is anal stenosis if excess anoderm is resected.

8. Anal Fissure

a) Pathophysiology

Anal fissures are linear tears in the anal mucosa that typically occur in the posterior midline unless there are contravening factors. Inflammatory bowel disease, HIV, or other immunocompromised states can lead to fissure formation along a different plane.

b) Presentation and Diagnosis

Anal fissures are painful and may bleed, especially upon defecation. Delayed diagnosis by managing the disease medically and awaiting resolution of the immediate pain syndrome is prudent.

c) Treatment

Medical management of anal fissure is with Sitz baths and stool softeners. Lateral internal sphincterotomy can be completed if symptoms are refractory to medical management after three weeks. Botox injections have not been shown to be efficacious. Complications of sphincterotomy include fecal incontinence, urinary retention, fistula formation, and abscess.

9. Fistula-in-Ano

a) Assessment

Sepsis of the anal canal can lead to fistula formation. There are four types of fistulae. Intersphincteric fistulae are the most common and is located between the external and internal anal sphincters. Trans-sphincteric fistulae travels through the external anal sphincter and invades the ischiorectal space. Suprasphincteric fistulae travels through the levator ani by passing over the external anal sphincter; these fistulae are rare. Extrasphincteric fistulae travel from the rectum to perineum outside of the sphincters and is commonly secondary to trauma. Anterior fistulae connect with the rectum linearly, while posterior fistulae curve into an internal opening with the rectum.

b) Management

Treatment of fistulae requires careful diagnosis by probing without generating artificial tracts, completing an anoscopy to identify the internal opening, and draining the infection. Superficial disease can be treated with fistulotomy or Seton placement. Setons are especially preferred in anterior fistulae in women or with significant disease. Sitz baths should be used.

10. Procidentia

Procidentia is diagnosed by the presence of prolapsed concentric folds of rectum. It is more common in women who have given birth. Symptoms include constipation, incontinence, and prolapse. Rectopexy against the presacral fascia or resection of redundant rectosigmoid intestine are the treatments; the former is preferred for patients with numerous comorbidities, while the latter is optimal for patients with significant issues with defecation. Resection has a better outcome.

11. Rectovaginal Fistula

The development of an abnormal connection between the vagina and rectum can lead to output of gas or fecal matter from the vagina. There are multiple causes and treatment involves reduction of underlying etiologies followed by an endorectal advancement flap or sphincteroplasty. Transperineal repair can be used to completely excise the fistula but is typically used when other options have failed. Very proximal disease requires an exploratory laparotomy with a layered closure of the rectum and vagina after separating the two. Patients with rectovaginal fistula in the setting of Crohn disease do well with a primary repair.

12. Fecal Incontinence

Fecal incontinence can lead to total loss of control over defecation and is commonly due to defects in the sphincter complex or damage to the pudendal nerve during delivery. Management via Kegel exercises to strengthen the pelvic floor, enemas to control bowel movements, or repair of the sphincter complex can be done. An end colostomy can also be done in extenuating circumstances. Artificial sphincters have also been used.

13. Rectocele

Rectocele is the prolapsed of the rectum into the vagina leading to constipation and disruption of intercourse. Patients with significant disease who require manual defecation should be treated with surgery. Treatment is via a transperineal or transanal mucosal flap formation with rectopexy.

III.C. Infectious and Inflammatory Disease

1. Pilonidal Disease

a) Assessment

Pilonidal disease, also known as Jeep's disease, is infection of the sacrococcygeal region with ingrown hair seeding an infectious nidus. Abscess formation develops, and extensive disease can occur. Recurrent disease is a hallmark of pilonidal disease unless there is complete resection of the infectious nodule.

b) Management

Treatment of pilonidal cyst disease requires excision of the infectious nodule seeding the abscess cavity with drainage of pus. Initial management via a simple I&D to permit maximum resolution of inflammation is acceptable, followed by operative resection. Primary total excision can also be done for smaller cysts. The wound is left open in all cases. Marsupialization of the skin is another permissible technique. Primary excision and marsupialization have the lowest recurrence rates.

2. Hidradenitis Suppurativa

Hidradenitis is an apocrine gland infection leading to abscess formation. It presents with gross inflammation with purulent drainage. Treatment involves drainage of the abscess cavities, biopsies to check for malignancy, and antibiotic therapy. Opening the fistulae tracts can also be done. Extensive disease may require a skin graft.

3. Proctitis and Anusitis

a) Assessment

Inflammation of the rectum and anus can occur from inflammatory bowel disease, Clostridium difficile, Salmonella, Shigella, or radiation therapy. Inflammation of the epithelial lining leads to rectal bleeding, change in bowel habits, tenesmus, fecal urgency, constipation, and abdominal cramping. Stool cultures, anorectal swabs, and other studies are done for diagnosis.

b) Management

Proctitis due to IBD is treated with sulfasalazine, 5-ASA, steroids, immunosuppressants, and antibiotics. Salmonella, Shigella, Yersinia, and Campylobacter infections are self-limited. E. histolytica is treated with metronidazole and iodoquinol. C. difficile is treated with vancomycin or metronidazole. Pain control, steroids, and 6-mercaptopurine or azathioprine are used for radiation-induced proctitis.

4. Irritable Bowel Syndrome

a) Etiology and Epidemiology

Irritable bowel syndrome is the most common outpatient gastrointestinal complaint. IBS causes alteration in bowel habits from a change in intestinal motility. Irritable bowel syndrome is most common in young adults and affects females twice as much as males.

b) Presentation and Diagnosis

Irritable bowel syndrome presents as alternating diarrhea and constipation with abdominal pain, bloating, and distention relieved by defecation. Diagnosis is made by the presence of intermittent symptoms for more than three months with no night time symptoms. The lack of systemic symptoms and the presence of stress typically clinch the diagnosis. The symptoms must include two elements from the Rome criteria, which are altered passage of stool, abnormal frequency, change in consistency, mucus in stool, and abdominal distention. The differential diagnosis of irritable bowel syndrome includes Giardia infection, inflammatory bowel disease, lactase deficiency, hypothyroidism, and colon cancer. Irritable bowel syndrome is associated with fibromyalgia, interstitial cystitis, fatigue, and depression.

c) Treatment

Irritable bowel syndrome is treated with a high-fiber, low-fat diet to promote proper passage of intestinal contents. All gas-forming foods should be eliminated. One of the following medications may also be used in severe cases: psyllium, antispasmodics, anticholinergics, antidiarrheals, tricyclic antidepressants, anxiolytics, or osmotic laxatives.

5. Pseudomembranous Colitis

a) Etiology and Pathophysiology

Pseudomembranous colitis is diarrhea caused by Clostridium difficile that overgrows within the colon and disrupts the normal bacterial flora, leading to impaired absorption. C. difficile releases a toxin that may lead to damage to the mucosa and further contributes to the diarrhea. Pseudomembranous colitis commonly occurs between a week and a month after stopping antibiotics, and the most commonly implicated antibiotics are clindamycin, vancomycin, ciprofloxacin, and cephalosporins.

b) Presentation and Diagnosis

Pseudomembranous colitis presents with watery diarrhea that contains scant blood, abdominal cramping, fever, and leukocytosis. Diagnosis is made by searching for the C. difficile toxin in stool samples. The majority of patients with actual C. difficile infection will have a positive test after testing three separate stool samples. Sigmoidoscopy or colonoscopy is sometimes used to visualize yellow membranous plaques on the mucosa.

c) Treatment

Treatment of C. difficile requires metronidazole or vancomycin. Oral metronidazole is preferred unless the strain is resistant, then oral or IV vancomycin becomes the preferred regimen. Toxin can be bound with cholestyramine. Inhibitors of motility such as loperamide should be avoided. Treatment for up to two weeks is necessary. If treatment is not started in a timely manner, severe inflammation and infection can occur throughout all layers of the colonic epithelium, leading to severe diarrhea, sepsis, and toxic megacolon. Plain films of the abdomen demonstrate long loops of colon with signs of edema in the bowel wall (known as a positive "thumbprinting" sign). Colectomy may be necessary in this event.

6. Crohn Disease

a) Etiology and Epidemiology

Inflammatory bowel disease is significantly more common in the Ashkenazi Jewish and Caucasian populations, and tends to affect young adults up to the age of 35 but may also affect individuals over 60 years of age. There is a strong pattern of family inheritance. Crohn disease has an incidence of approximately 5 in 100,000 individuals, and is more common in men. Crohn disease is three times more likely to cause colon cancer, with the risk increasing over time. Although the precise cause remains unknown, antibodies to alpha-Saccharyomyces cerevesiae as predictive of disease development.

b) Pathophysiology

Crohn disease leads to inflammation of the intestines. It affects all of the layers of the bowel, leading to the formation of fistulas and abscesses. Crohn disease spares the rectum in about half of all patients, but may be found in any location of the gastrointestinal tract. Discontinuous, skipping lesions are present with normal bowel located between stretches of diseased bowel. Thickening of the submucosal layer in the diseased region also leads to a cobblestone appearance that alternates with regions of ulceration of the submucosal layer. The most commonly affected regions of the gastrointestinal tract are the terminal ileum (⅓ of all cases), the colon (⅓ of all cases), or both regions (⅓ of all cases).

c) Presentation

Crohn disease presents with nonbloody diarrhea, unless there is involvement of the rectum. Crampy abdominal pain, weight loss, fever, malaise, and a tender right lower quadrant are signs and symptoms. Up to 1 in 5 patients with Crohn disease may have extraintestinal manifestations such as arthritis, uveitis, iritis, erythema nodosum, and pyoderma gangrenosum. Calcium oxalate stones may be present in the kidney.

d) Diagnosis

Crohn disease is diagnosed through colonoscopy (skip lesions, cobblestoning, abscess formation, and fistulas may be pathognomonic). Histology demonstrates granulomas.

e) Treatment

The cornerstone of treatment is to reduce inflammation, which is achieved by sulfasalazine and corticosteroids. Sulfasalazine is a combination of sulfapyridine and 5-aminosalicylic acid (5-ASA). Immunosuppressive therapy can be used in lieu of corticosteroids, and may include the use of 6-mercaptopurine, infliximab, methotrexate, and azathioprine. If Crohn disease affects the small intestine, sulfasalazine is replaced with 5-ASA. Metronidazole and ciprofloxacin should be used if the disease is complicated by fistula formation. Experimental therapies with antibodies or cytokines against tumor necrosis factor (TNF) such as remicade or infliximab have also success. Infliximab is an IgG targeted against TNF. Pretreatment with 6-MP reduces antibody formation against infliximab. Surgical treatment for duodenal Crohn disease is gastrojejunostomy and vagotomy.

f) Supportive Therapy

Supportive therapy for Crohn disease includes the use of antidiarrheals such as loperamide or diphenoxylate for diarrhea due to fatty acids, or cholestyramine for those with other causes of diarrhea. Antidiarrheals are absolutely contraindicated in individuals with toxic megacolon or those with severe colitis that may lead to toxic megacolon. Anticholinergics are used to reduce the symptoms of inflammatory bowel disease, including abdominal cramping and urgency. Diarrhea following ileocecectomy can occur from a paucity of bile salts and can be alleviated by exogenous bile salts administration. The most effective acute treatment for perirectal fistula secondary to Crohn disease is infliximab. A stricturoplasty is preferred in young patients with multiple, short Crohn's related strictures.

7. Ulcerative Colitis

a) Etiology and Epidemiology

Ulcerative colitis is approximately equal to Crohn disease in incidence. Ulcerative colitis affects the same populations and age groups, but is more common in women. There is a 30 fold increase in the risk of colon cancer with ulcerative colitis. In 1 out of 10 persons, ulcerative colitis spontaneously remits. In ¾, symptoms are intermittent. In 1/10, the symptoms are continuous, and in ½0, death results due to complications.

b) Pathophysiology

Ulcerative colitis tends to have continuous lesions that are restricted to the mucosa. This leads to rectal discharge of mucus, blood, and pus. Ulcerative colitis begins with rectal involvement, and lesions in the majority of patients extend from the rectum into adjacent gastrointestinal structures. A positive ANCA is associated with ulcerative colitis.

c) Presentation and Diagnosis

Bloody diarrhea and rectal pain herald ulcerative colitis. Colonoscopy demonstrates continuous lesions emanating from the rectum, and a lead pipe colon secondary to scarring from chronic damage. Granulomas are not present.

d) Treatment

Treatment of ulcerative colitis is similar to that of Crohn disease, including the use of sulfasalazine, azathioprine, 6-mercaptopurine, and corticosteroids for management of the inflammation. Colectomy is mandatory after 15 years of symptoms to minimize the risk of colon cancer; this is typically curative. The presence of toxic megacolon with ulcerative colitis is treated with fluid resuscitation, high dose steroids, electrolytes, and total proctocolectomy with ileal pouch-anal anastomosis. Other surgical interventions include TPC with continent ileostomy, and TPC with end ileostomy. Other indications for surgery include hemorrhage, obstruction, perforation, worsening clinical course, and prophylaxis.

e) Intestinal Complications

Complications of ulcerative colitis include perforation, stricture formation, hemorrhage, and toxic megacolon. Toxic megacolon is especially likely to occur with severe inflammation leading to bowel dilation. Hypotension and sepsis may then ensue.

f) Extraintestinal Complications

Both Crohn disease and ulcerative colitis may be complicated with a number of extraintestinal symptoms. Those that affect the eye include episcleritis and uveitis. Uveitis is more common in Crohn disease. Episcleritis presents with uveitis, erythema nodosum, and colitic arthritis. Dermatologic symptoms include erythema nodosum (especially in Crohn disease), pyoderma gangrenosum (ulcerative colitis), and aphthous ulcers (Crohn disease). Colitic arthritis is more common in Crohn disease, and ankylosing spondylitis is often an epiphenomenon of ulcerative colitis. Primary sclerosing cholangitis is more common in ulcerative colitis, while primary biliary cirrhosis is associated with Crohn disease. Renal failure due to amyloidosis can occur in Crohn disease. All forms of inflammatory bowel disease may be complicated with anemia, thromboembolic disorders, steatohepatitis, and cholelithiasis.

III.D. CANCER

1. Colorectal Cancer

a) Epidemiology and Etiology

Colorectal cancer is the second most common cause of cancer-related death in men and women in the United States. Worldwide, colon cancer ranks behind lung cancer and gastric cancer. A combination of genetic and environmental causes play a role in the development of colon cancer. The lifetime risk of colon cancer is about 5%, with risk increasing as a function of age.

Colon cancer risk can be two or three times the baseline risk when it is part of familial syndromes, such as FAP and HNPCC. Cancer risk increases rapidly with the number of affected first degree relatives, especially if they were diagnosed under the age of 50. Polyps and second degree relatives with cancer can increase the risk between 50% and 300%. Other risk factors include inherited or acquired genetic defects and ulcerative colitis. Environmental risk factors include a diet rich in red meat, low fiber, or high fat; exposure to carcinogens; smoking; and chronic infection by S. bovis. Other independent risk factors include age over 40, a history of radiation exposure to the pelvis, and a familial or personal history of colorectal cancer.

b) Pathophysiology

The two hit hypothesis guides the mutagenesis that occurs behind the development and progression of colorectal cancer. An initial insult to the genome causes a mutation in the DNA sequence, traditionally described as mutations in p53, APC, DCC, and dozens of other loci. This is followed by a series of steps that facilitate cell division and eventually, uncontrolled proliferation of carcinogenic cells. Mutations in tumor suppressor genes, oncogenes, and mismatch repair genes all contribute to the development of cancer. Only one oncogene must be mutated to start the oncogenic process, while both tumor suppressor gene alleles must be changed to promote tumorigenesis.

Adenomatous polyposis coli (APC) (5q21) is a tumor suppressor gene mutated in familial adenomatous polyposis (FAP). This defect is one of the first to occur in the tumorigenesis of colorectal cancer. FAP, discussed in more detail on page 262, leads to the development of thousands of adenomatous polyps in the colon, which together lead to a great risk of carcinogenesis (n.b. the increase in risk comes from the increase in number of polyps). A mutation in APC leads to a rise in beta-catenin and induction of cellular proliferation.

One of the most common mutations occurs in the tumor suppressor gene p53 on chromosome 17p. Defects in this gene contributes to the development of colorectal cancer in nearly 75% of patients and are commonly found as part of the adenoma to carcinoma transition. Li-Fraumeni syndrome is an inherited defect in p53; perhaps one reason why this syndrome does not present with colorectal cancer is due to the lack of other mutations earlier in the carcinogenic process.

The deleted in colorectal cancer (DCC) gene on chromosome 18q21 is a tumor suppressor gene that may play a role in the adenoma to carcinoma sequence. Mutations in other genes on this locus have been found to play a role in the development of pancreatic cancer (DPC4). DCC is deleted in about 70% of colorectal cancers. SMAD2 is also located at this location and leads to alterations in transforming growth factor (TGF) beta signal transduction.

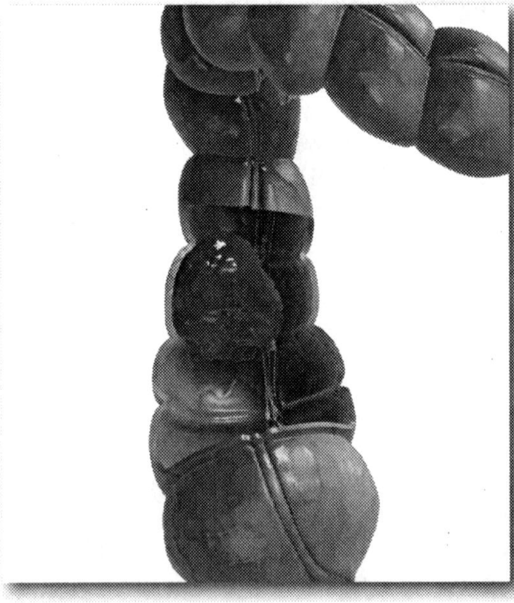

Defects in the ras family of oncogenes leads to alterations in G protein-mediated signal transduction. Mutations in K-ras and other members of the ras family are found in about half of all patients with colorectal cancer. The end result is bringing formerly quiescent cells out of the G0 resting phase and to induce cell proliferation.

Mutations in mismatch repair genes also contribute to the development of colorectal cancer. Mismatch repair genes function to repair DNA mutations, and defects in these genes lead to an accumulation of defects and a higher risk for carcinogenesis. Microsatellite instability occurs, and this is the hallmark of hereditary nonpolyposis colorectal cancer (HNPCC). Among the defects found in this syndrome include hMSH2, hMSH3, hMSH6, hMLH1, hPMS1, and hPMS2. Defects in these enzymes lead to hypermethylation, base-pair insertions, and base-pair deletions.

c) Presentation

There are two types of polyps that may be present in the colon. Benign polyps may be local areas of swelling from inflammation, or a hamartomatous tissue growth. Juvenile polyps are another type of benign polyps and have no malignant potential. Potentially malignant polyps are adenomas and have potential to start the adenoma to carcinoma sequence. Adenomatous polyps have a nearly 10 fold increase in colon cancer risk. Multiple polyps amplify this risk.

There are three types of adenomatous polyps: pure villous (10% of all polyps), tubulovillous (20%), and tubular (70%). Villous adenomas have the highest risk of becoming cancerous (about 40%), followed by tubulovillous (20%), and tubular (5%). Polyps over 2 cm in size have a greater potential for malignancy; villous polyps over 2 cm have over a 50% chance of harboring malignancy. Villous adenomas larger than 4 cm with induration have a 90% risk of being cancerous. This adenomatous-carcinomatosis sequence is thought to occur over 10 years. Smaller polyps may lead to cancer in less than a quarter of patients over 20 years. Villous adenomas are more likely to be sessile than the other two types.

d) Presentation

Colon cancer may present with bright red blood if located in the left colon, or tarry stools if present in the right colon; this rule has numerous exceptions. For example, a briskly bleeding polyp in the right colon may also present with hematochezia. Constipation accompanies left-sided tumors, while right-sided tumors may have melena. Sigmoid tumors may present with diverticulitis-like symptoms. Fistula formation may be a sign of underlying malignancy. Weight loss, cachexia, and abdominal pain are other nonspecific signs of cancer. Circumferential growth of a tumor may lead to an obstructing mass, leading to signs and symptoms of bowel obstruction.

e) Screening

Colon cancer screening guidelines are proposed by the American Cancer Society, which recommends annual digital rectal exam in all individuals age 40 and over. Occult blood tests with the stool (FOBT) are recommended in individuals over the age of 50. In asymptomatic individuals with no risk factors for colon cancer, colonoscopy is done every 10 years starting at the age of 50. Digital rectal exam may find up to half of all colon cancers.

TABLE 3. Colon cancer screening.

Annual digital rectal exam in all over 40.
FOBT in all over 50.
Flexible sigmoidoscopy every 5 years over 50.
Colonoscopy for those with risk factors.

f) Diagnostic Imaging

Imaging via a double contrast barium enema provides an adjunctive means of evaluating the colon, especially in patients in whom a colonoscopy is very difficult to complete. Barium enema is able to evaluate the right colon, whereas making the turn around the hepatic flexure cannot be completed in over 5% of colonoscopies.

CT imaging is a vital part of the workup for any patient with a suspected colorectal cancer. CT scanning will provide information about the location and dimensions of the mass, indicate the potential for resection by identifying extension of the tumor to nearby regions, search for evidence of metastatic disease – particularly to the liver, and also give anatomic information about the abdomen that may affect surgical decision-making.

g) Colonoscopy

Colonoscopy is a superior diagnostic test compared to FOBT, sigmoidoscopy, and barium enema. Colonoscopy has a higher sensitivity and specificity, and also permits the chance for a curative endoscopic resection for any suspicious lesion. Unlike the other approaches, colonoscopy has a 1% risk of perforation and 2% risk for hemorrhage. Significant free perforation may need surgical intervention to achieve either primary repair or proximal diverting colostomy / ileostomy. Flexible sigmoidoscopy can be used in lieu of colonoscopy if it is combined with a double contrast barium enema. This combination should be repeated every 5 years, while a colonoscopy should be done every 10 years. High risk patients should have a colonoscopy every 5 years; suspicious findings may mandate screening even sooner.

Every attempt should be made to completely remove a polyp via colonoscopy; failure to do so requires an operative intervention for a colectomy. Tubular polyps can often be removed via a snare. Sessile polyps may require surgical intervention due to the risk of perforation. Pathologic examination is important for all collected specimens – if there is evidence of cancer invading through the submucosa, surgical resection of the affected region (i.e. hemicolectomy) may be necessary. Masses over 4 cm cannot be treated endoscopically due to the high potential for invasive disease; they require surgical intervention and resection.

The finding of a single adenoma less than 1 cm in size that is fully resected should be followed up with a repeat colonoscopy in 5 years. An adenoma over 1 cm in size that is fully resected should have a repeat colonoscopy in 3 years. Patients who have had a history of cancer that has been surgically resected should have a colonoscopy within 1 year of surgery, repeated again in 2-3 years, then completed every 5 years.

h) Staging

Following the diagnosis of colon cancer, classification into one of four Duke's stages is done to determine the prognosis. In stage A disease, the cancer is limited to the mucosa and submucosa, and carries a greater than 90% 5 year survival. In stage B disease, the cancer has invaded the muscularis propria, with a 70% 5 year survival. Stage C disease has invasion into local lymph nodes, with a 30% 5 year survival. Stage D disease has distant metastases with limited survival after a few years. R0 resections have negative margins with total tumor removal; R1 resections have microscopically-positive margins; and R2 resections have gross positive margins. Duke's staging is correlated to the AJCC TNM classification, as indicated in the table below. The AJCC TNM criteria are in the table on the facing page. The AJCC staging criteria are on the following table, and are now the preferred criteria for staging for colorectal cancer. The discrepancy between stage IIIA survival being slightly greater than stage IIB survival (85% vs. 80%) may reflect insufficient lymph node samples being collected during resection. At least 12 lymph nodes should be collected for an adequate sample to be evaluated for staging.

Table 4. Staging of Colon Cancer—Duke's Stages

Stage A	Cancer limited to mucosa and submucosa. 90% 5 year survival. Colonoscopy after 1 year, then 5 year intervals if normal. CEA every 3 months for 2 years.	T1N0 T2N0
Stage B	Cancer invades the muscularis propria. 70% 5 year survival. Questionable benefit with adjuvant chemotherapy. 5-FU is indicated with T4 lesions and lymph node sample with less than 12 nodes. Regardless, most centers will start FOLFOX. CEA is monitored every 3-6 months, then annually after 5 years. Annual CT scans are done for 3 years.	T3N0 T4N0
Stage C	Invasion of local lymph nodes. 30% 5 year survival rate. The optimal treatment is FOLFOX adjuvant chemotherapy. Monitoring is done in a similar manner as stage 2 disease.	TXN1 TXN2
Stage D	Distant metastases. Limited survival. Palliative therapy with FOLFOX and newer agents is done. Avastin (anti-VEGF monoclonal antibody) and Erbitux (anti-EGFR monoclonal antibody) can be used.	TXNXM1

Table 5. TNM Classification of Colorectal Cancer

T0	No tumor	N0	No nodes affected
Tis	Carcinoma in situ	N1	1-3 regional nodes positive
T1	Invasion of the submucosa	N2	4+ regional nodes positive
T2	Invasion of the muscularis propria	N3	Central node invasion
T3	Invasion into the serosa and/or pericolic fat	M0	No metastasis
T4	Invasion to adjacent structures and/or peritoneal cavity	M1	Metastasis present (most commonly to the liver)

Table 6. AJCC Staging for Colorectal Cancer

Stage	T	N	M	Survival	Treatment
0	Tis	N0	M0	~100%	Endoscopic resection
I	T1, T2	N0	M0	95%	Surgical resection
IIA	T3	N0	M0	70-80%	Surgical resection Role for chemotherapy and radiation in certain patients
IIB	T4	N0	M0		
IIIA	T1, T2	N1	M0	40-85%	Surgical resection Adjuvant chemotherapy and radiation therapy
IIIB	T3, T4	N1	M0		
IIIC	T*	N2	M0		
IV	T*	N*	M1	8%	Palliative therapy Surgical diversion in symptomatic patients

The most common site of metastatic disease from colon cancer is the liver. Lower colon cancers and rectal cancers can also spread to the lung via the vena cava (inferior hemorrhoidal veins) and bone via the posterior vertebral venous plexus.

Table 7. Metastatic Colon Cancer

Hepatic metastasis	25% 5-year survival once resected; up to 3mm metastases can be detected by intraoperative ultrasound
Pulmonary metastasis	20% 5-year survival once resected
Common sites of metastasis	Prostate, breast, lung, kidney, thyroid, and bone (least likely)

i) Surgical Management

Anatomy directs surgery. The location of the mass determines the optimal surgical approach. A right hemicolectomy requires ligation of the distal branches of the middle colic, the right colic, and ileocolic arteries. It removes the cecum and ascending colon. An extended right hemicolectomy is a modified approach that takes all of the branches of the middle colic and extends the resection farther along the transverse colon.

A transverse colectomy ligates the middle colic artery only and removes the majority of the transverse colon from the hepatic to the splenic flexure.

A left hemicolectomy resects the colon from the distal ⅓ of the transverse colon to the sigmoid colon with ligation of the inferior mesenteric artery. A sigmoid colectomy ligates the sigmoid arteries. 5 cm margins are necessary for adequate resection, but it is believed that tumor typically does not spread more than 2 cm from the grossly visible mass.

Tumors that affect the middle ⅓ of the rectum, or approximately 5-10 cm from the anal verge, may be treated with a low anterior resection (LAR), APR, coloanal resection, wide local excision, or neoadjuvant chemoradiation. Tumors that affect the lower ⅓ of the rectum, defined as 0-5 cm from the anal verge, may be treated with neoadjuvant chemoradiation (i.e. Nigro protocol), transanal excision, or abdominoperineal resection (APR).

A transanal excision is permissible if the tumor is limited to the submucosa, has no evidence of lymph node involvement, is less than 4 cm in size, and is located within 5 cm of the anal verge. An endorectal ultrasound and/or MRI are necessary for appropriate staging. In properly selected patients, outcomes can be similar to APR. More advanced tumors in this region can be treated with neoadjuvant chemoradiation via the Nigro protocol in an attempt to shrink the tumor so that a transanal excision is possible. Tumors that involve the sphincter complex or recurrent tumors at the site of a prior LAR should be treated with an APR.

A low anterior resection resections the colon from the peritoneal reflection to the sigmoid. A total mesorectal excision (TME) is completed by mobilizing the colon and resecting the soft tissue from the presacral fascia.

An abdominoperineal resection completely removes the anus and rectum and typically needs an end colostomy. An APR is completed in patients that have resectable disease, due to the high morbidity associated with this approach. Besides a transanal excision and LAR as an alternative to an APR, it is also possible to complete a coloanal anastomosis for patients that do not have involvement of the sphincter complex. A low anterior proctosigmoidectomy with colorectal anastomosis and colonic J pouch spares the anal sphincter complex and prevents frequent bowel movements following surgery.

Most patients are treated with a preoperative bowel preparation to clear the intestinal contents of fecal matter. While there is little evidence supporting this practice, it does make the operating field easier to manage. Laparoscopic colon resection is similar in efficacy to open approaches, but has a shorter hospital stay (c.f. COST Study Group results).

Following any of these procedures, if there is concern regarding the strength of the anastomosis, a diverting loop ileostomy is completed to divert intestinal flow long enough to permit healing. The ileostomy can be reversed within 3 months.

j) Neoadjuvant Therapy

Colon cancer that falls into stage I and II disease is highly amenable to surgery, and wide resection of the colon is typically done along with sampling of nearby lymph nodes to rule out higher stages of disease. Stage III disease is often treated with a combination of surgery and chemotherapy, including agents such as 5-fluorouracil (5-FU), leucovorin, and oxaliplatin (FOLFOX). Stage IV disease is treated only with palliation, but the formation of a diverting ostomy can be completed in patients with obstructing symptoms.

Radiation therapy is often used for stage II and III disease, and chemotherapy is sometimes employed in stage IIB disease.

Preoperative chemoradiation is beneficial for any patient diagnosed with rectal cancer and can change the surgical procedure to preserve the anal sphincters. Postoperative chemoradiation can lead to further improvement in survival and shrink R1/R2 tumors.

Following resection, most practitioners will monitor CEA levels as an early, sensitive indicator for recurrent disease. While an insufficient screening tool, CEA is a prognostic indicator for survival in patients that have had a rise in CEA after initially experiencing a drop after surgery. Colonoscopy used in conjunction with CEA monitoring is sufficient screening in postoperative patients.

k) Complications

Mild anastomotic leaks leading to low grade fever and some discomfort can be treated with antibiotics (i.e. ciprofloxacin and metronidazole). The presence of a contained abscess larger than 5 cm can be drained by a CT-guided procedure. The presence of a multiloculated abscess or clinical deterioration requires a Hartmann's procedure. Radiation proctitis is a side effect and tends to occur 8-12 months after radiotherapy. Formalin is a therapy for radiation proctitis.

2. Inherited Neoplasias

a) Familial Adenomatous Polyposis

Colon cancer develops over approximately a decade of having large villous or tubulovillous adenomatous polyps. The presence of familial adenomatous polyposis (FAP) syndromes from an autosomal dominant gene is a certain predictor of malignancy. FAP is due to a deletion on chromosome 5q21, and requires total colectomy to avoid colon cancer from the hundreds or thousands of polyps that inevitably form by the age of 25. Without treatment colon cancer occurs in nearly all individuals by the age of 40.

FAP is due to loss of the APC tumor suppressor gene. APC regulates beta-catenin, which is a regulator of c-myc; APC also affects Wnt to stimulate the cell cycle via induction of cyclin D1. APC is one of the first genes to be disrupted as part of the carcinomatosis sequence. FAP has left-sided tumors and is virtually guaranteed to lead to cancer by the mid-30s. Celecoxib and sulindac can be used to decrease the growth of polyps but a total procto-colectomy with ileal pouch-anal anastomosis and construction of a J-pouch is required.

The most significant risk of this procedure is damage to the pelvic nerves leading to incontinence and impotence. Patients who receive a total abdominal colectomy with ileorectal anastomosis have a 25% chance of developing rectal cancer after 20 years.

FAP also requires surveillance for cancer throughout the gastrointestinal tract. While polyps within the stomach are typically benign, those within the small intestine near the ampulla are likely malignant. Treatment is via a pancreatoduodenectomy. Otherwise, all polyps should be removed by endoscopy. Mesenteric desmoid tumor formation may lead to bowel compromise or hamper a surgeon's ability to perform a bowel resection. There is also the risk of thyroid cancer, gastric cancer, and pancreatic cancer with FAP.

In a variant of FAP, Gardner syndrome may develop with fibrous dysplasia of the skull, osteomas, desmoid tumors, and extra teeth. Gardner syndrome typically evolves into colon cancer along the FAP adenoma-carcinoma sequence. Another variant of FAP is the I1307 mutation in Ashkenazi Jews, leading to a radical increase in colorectal cancer in this population.

Turcot syndrome is the formation of polyps and tumors within the central nervous system (CNS). It presents a significant risk for colon cancer.

b) Hereditary Nonpolyposis Colon Cancer

(1) *Assessment*

Hereditary nonpolyposis colon cancer (HNPCC) is transmitted via an autosomal dominant mechanism leading to microsatellite instability in a DNA mismatch repair gene (hMSH2, hMSH3, hMSH6, hMLH1, hPMS1, and hPMS2). There is a strong risk of developing other cancers within the family. HNPCC is a strong predictor of future colon cancer development in the patient, and is the most common hereditary colon cancer. In this disorder, also known as Lynch syndrome, the cancer arises spontaneously from the mucosa, and is a strong predictor of future ovarian or endometrial cancer. Lynch I is typically a right sided colon cancer that develops in the early 40s. Lynch II leads to colon cancer and increases the risk of ovarian, bladder, small intestine, and gastric cancer. Endometrial cancers are associated with HNPCC. The presence of microsatellite instability is likely to present in later stages and therefore has a worse prognosis.

The modified Amsterdam criteria are used to assess the risk of HNPCC-related colorectal cancer development. There must be at least three relatives who have had colorectal cancer with one person a first-degree relative, cancer across two generations, and one person diagnosed with an HNPCC-related cancer prior to age 50. FAP must specifically be excluded prior to making this diagnosis. Diagnosis of HNPCC can also occur de novo as a substantial number of patients will present with a spontaneous mutation.

(2) *Management*

Colonoscopy should be conducted every 2 years starting at age 20 and annually after the age of 35 due to acceleration of the typical adenomatous-carcinoma sequence. A total abdominal colectomy with ileorectal anastomosis is required for Lynch I and Lynch II. Prophylactic TAHBSO may be required for Lynch II. CA-125 levels should be tracked for individuals with Lynch II. Proctoscopy must be done every year and disease here may require a total proctocolectomy with ileal pouch-anal anastomosis.

c) Peutz-Jegher Syndrome

Peutz-Jegher syndrome has 5% risk of leading to colon cancer and is due to a defect in STK11, an autosomal dominant gene that codes for a serine/threonine kinase. Many benign hamartomas develop within the small and large intestine, but all polyps should be removed by colonoscopy whenever possible. Peutz-Jeghers syndrome leads to pigmentation of the skin and mucosa. While the risk of colon cancer is low, Peutz-Jeghers requires surveillance for any gastrointestinal cancer, breast cancer, ovarian cancer, cervical cancer, lung cancer, thyroid cancer, biliary or pancreatic cancer, and testicular cancer. Other associated hamartomatous diseases include Cowden disease (polyps with facial epithelial lesions and breast cancer) and Cronkite-Canada syndrome (polyps with diarrhea, alopecia, and hyperpigmentation). Colonoscopy every 2 years is indicated.

d) Juvenile Polyposis Syndrome

Juvenile polyposis syndrome is an insignificant cause of colon cancer, with polyps occurring as a result of benign hamartomas within the intestines. Peutz-Jeghers and juvenile polyposis syndrome are worth keeping on the differential diagnosis of any polyposis syndrome as rapid diagnosis of these two varieties may avoid costly and invasive tests and obviate the need for prophylactic colon resection.

e) Multiple Polyposis Coli

Multiple polyposis coli is associated with numerous polyps that can lead to bleeding or intussusceptions. Mutations in the TGF-beta control element SMAD4 is present and can lead to carcinomatosis. Total abdominal colectomy with ileorectal anastomosis with rectal surveillance is the standard of care for patients with clinically-significant disease. If there is involvement of the rectum, a total proctocolectomy with ileal pouch anal anastomosis should be done.

Table 8. Other Colonic Syndromes

Gardner syndrome	Numerous polyps due to autosomal dominant disorder. Evolves into colon cancer.
Turcot syndrome	Polyps and tumors in CNS. High risk for colon cancer.
Peutz-Jeghers synd.	Many polyps in SI and LI , low cancer risk.
Juvenile Polyposis	Benign hamartomas in intestines.

3. Anal Cancer

a) Bowen Disease

Bowen disease is carcinoma in situ due to HPV 16 or 18. It is typically located above the dentate line and has an increased risk of transforming into frank squamous cell carcinoma, especially in immunocompromised patients. Bowen disease presents similar to actinic keratosis and requires a wide local excision. Surveillance is required due to the high recurrence rate.

b) Condyloma Acuminatum

Condyloma acuminatum is the development of invasive and expanding anal warts due to HPV infection. HPV-16 and 18 are associated with squamous cell cancer. Diagnosis is made by pathology. The best treatment is with wide local excision and topical electrocauterization. Involvement of the sphincter complex requires an APR. A complication of this disease is the formation of fistula with surrounding organs and tissues.

c) Squamous Cell Carcinoma

(1) *Perianal Disease*

Perianal squamous cell cancer has its prognosis determined by size. Risk factors include STDs and Bowen disease. Wide local excision is possible for microinvasive disease, but patients with more advanced disease will require chemoradiation and cisplatin followed by an APR. Advanced disease substantially drops 5-year survival.

(2) *Anal Canal Disease*

Squamous cell cancer of the anal canal is the culmination of longstanding inflammation and irritation of the anal canal. A fixed lesion is present on digital rectal examination and endorectal ultrasound can be used to stage the tumor. Tumor located above the dentate line drains into the inferior mesenteric nodes, internal iliac nodes, and along the superior rectal artery. Drainage at the dentate line is into the internal pudendal and obturator nodes. Drainage below the dentate line is to the inguinal nodes and internal iliac nodes. The size of the tumor predicts the likelihood of metastatic disease; tumors less than 2 cm are less likely to have metastasis to nodes.

Treatment of anal canal squamous cell cancer is by way of the Nigro protocol, which involves neoadjuvant 5-FU, mitomycin C, and radiation. Biopsy and possible wide local excision follow. This has relegated the role of APR to recurrent disease or disease refractory to chemoradiation.

d) Paget Disease

Extramammary Paget disease is development of an apocrine neoplasia that may develop into an adenocarcinoma. It presents as an eczematous rash and can involve the entire outer anal canal. Biopsy reveals hyperchromatic cells. Wide local excision with V-Y skin flaps is necessary for localized disease. An APR with node dissection and radiation is necessary for advanced disease. Tumor is likely to metastasize to the liver and bone.

e) Basal Cell Carcinoma

Basal cell carcinoma is characterized by ulcerated, superficial lesions leading to pruritus and bleeding. Wide local excision is necessary, but recurrent disease is likely. Large lesions are treated with APR.

f) Melanoma

Melanoma of the anal canal tends to occur at the dentate line and presents with bleeding. Melanoma is treated with a wide local excision but has an overall survival of less than 20%. WLE has the same survival as an APR.

g) Adenocarcinoma

Adenocarcinoma of the anal canal may present as the rectal form above the dentate line and is similar to adenocarcinoma of the rectum. The anal form presents within the anal canal with mucoepidermoid cells that do not involve the epithelial cells. Treatment for limited disease is wide local excision; invasive disease requires an APR. Neoadjuvant therapy with the Nigro protocol is beneficial.

Table 9. Tumors of the Anal Margin

Bowen disease	Squamous cell carcinoma	Wide local excision
Paget disease	Intraepithelial adenocarcinoma	Non-invasive: wide local excision Invasive to sphincter: APR
Basal cell	Basal cell epithelial cancer	Wide local excision
Squamous cell carcinoma	Squamous cell carcinoma	Wide local excision vs. APR
Verrucous carcinoma		Wide local excision
Kaposi sarcoma	Secondary to HIV	Wide local excision with chemoradiation

IV. Gastrointestinal Bleeding

IV.A. Procedures

1. Tagged RBC Scan

Technetium-labeled red blood cell scan is a nuclear medicine study that is used to identify the source of a slow gastrointestinal bleed. It is more sensitive than an arteriogram and will find bleeding that is no faster than 0.1 ml/min. If a slow bleed is suspected and prior attempts at localization have been futile, this is the test of choice.

2. Mesenteric Arteriogram

An arteriogram is an interventional radiology procedure that weaves a catheter into the vasculature of the gastrointestinal system and selectively injects contrast along specific vessels. The presence of a blush indicates a perforated vessel and bleeding. An arteriogram can detect bleeding as slow as 0.5 ml/min but may be as sensitive as a tagged RBC study in the right hands. While arteriogram permits coil embolization of the bleeding vessel, the major limitations are nephropathy from the contrast load and potential ischemia following therapy.

IV.B. Upper Gastrointestinal Bleed

1. Overview

a) Pathophysiology

Upper gastrointestinal (GI) bleeds are located proximal to the ligament of Treitz. Upper GI bleeds can occur at any level between the oral mucosa and the proximal portion of the duodenum, and include causes such as epistaxis, esophageal varices, esophageal tears or ruptures, gastric erosion, PUD, arteriovenous malformations (AVMs) and tumors. A posteriorly located duodenal ulcer may lead to bleeding by erosion into the gastroduodenal artery.

b) Presentation

Upper GI bleeds present with a variety of symptoms, depending on the severity of the blood loss. Minor bleeding is often asymptomatic, but may lead to nausea and hematemesis. Severe bleeding leads to melena with black, tar-like stools, hypotension, and tachycardia from the decrease in blood volume. Very brisk bleeds may lead to hypovolemic shock and bright red blood per rectum (BRBPR). Breakdown of blood by intestinal flora may lead to elevations in blood urea nitrogen (BUN), leading to false positive kidney function tests. Chronic bleeding may lead to iron deficiency anemia.

c) Diagnosis

Diagnosis is confirmed by blood present on a nasogastric lavage. A rectal exam with hemoccult testing is performed. Bleeding sites can often be directly assessed and sometimes immediately corrected via endoscopy. Active bleeding is often identified using tagged red blood cells (RBCs) or arteriography. Endoscopy is the standard of care in all upper GI bleeds.

d) Treatment

Treatment for upper GI bleeds is often carried out using an esophagogastroduodenoscopy (EGD), which permits the clinician to carry out a number of procedures to ameliorate the hemorrhage. EGD permits electrocoagulation, sclerotherapy, ligation of ruptured varices, and balloon tamponade.

Total bowel immobilization to minimize blood flow to the gastrointestinal system may be done with somatostatin. Recurrent bleeds due to PUD may be reduced through the use of proton pump inhibitors such as omeprazole. Hemorrhage that is significant enough can be localized with a tagged red blood cell study to permit finer control and ligation of bleeding vessels in the operating room. Alternatively, arteriography with coil embolization can be completed to quell brisk bleeding. Inability to localize or otherwise control severe gastric bleeding may necessitate a subtotal or total gastrectomy.

2. Vascular Ectasia

Gastric antral vascular ectasia is a cause for GI bleed from small, dilated blood vessels in the antrum that become ulcerated. It may be secondary to longstanding portal hypertension, renal failure, and scleroderma. Treatment is electrocauterization via EGD. Correction of the underlying causes is also therapeutic.

3. Dieulafoy Lesion

Dieulafoy lesion is the development of a tortuous aneurismal formation within the submucosa of the stomach leading to gastric bleeding. The majority of these lesions are located within 6 cm of the gastroesophageal junction along the lesser curvature. Treatment of a Dieulafoy lesion is by endoscopic ablation or angiography with coil embolization.

4. Esophageal and Gastric Varices

Dilated submucosal veins of the esophagus and stomach may lead to a brisk upper GI bleed and are typically found in portal hypertension or splenic vein thrombosis. Splenic vein thrombosis may be secondary to pancreatitis and leads to increased pressure in the gastric venous system through loss of the short gastric veins. Treatment is with a transjugular intrahepatic portosystemic shunt (TIPS) placement to shunt blood away from the stomach. Splenectomy and liver transplantation are other options. Medical management with octreotide is also successful. Gastric variceal obliteration can be done via endoscopy if the bleeding vessel is evident.

A TIPS procedure decreases the resistance across the liver and relieves the pressure heads causing varix formation. A shunt is placed between the hepatic vein and portal vein to create a bypass tract.

IV.C. Lower Gastrointestinal Bleed

1. Overview

a) Pathophysiology

Lower GI bleeds occur distal to the suspensory ligament of the duodenum and are located anywhere between the duodenum and the anus. The most common cause of lower GI bleed in the elderly is due to diverticulosis, but all GI bleeds should be suspected of heralding gastrointestinal cancer until ruled out. Younger patients are more likely to have lower GI bleeding from hemorrhoids, but this particular etiology is commonly managed by the patient and not seen in a clinical setting unless very severe or troublesome. Other causes of lower GI bleeds include inflammatory bowel disease, mesenteric ischemia, arteriovenous malformation (AVM) such as angiodysplasia, and infections. AVMs may present as part of a hereditary conditions that predispose to angiodysplasias, such as Osler-Rendu-Weber syndrome. The most common cause in adults is from diverticulosis. The most common cause in children is from Meckel diverticulum.

b) Presentation

Lower GI bleeds present with BRBPR, and such bleeding should begin an investigation of lower GI causes. However, not all incidents of BRBPR are due to lower GI bleeds – a particularly brisk upper GI bleed may also lead to fresh blood expressed from the rectum. Laboratory tests for occult bleeding are positive, and other systemic symptoms such as tachycardia and hypovolemia may present in a manner similar to upper GI bleeds.

c) Diagnosis

Diagnosis of lower GI bleeds is made after ruling out causes of upper GI bleed (through NG lavage and endoscopy). A digital rectal exam is mandatory to test for occult bleeding, followed by a colonoscopy in an attempt to directly visualize and potentially correct obvious sources of bleeding. As per upper GI bleeds, a tagged RBC scan and arteriography are often done. The most common cause of a lower GI bleed is an upper GI bleed.

d) Treatment

Treatment for a lower GI bleed is similar to that for upper GI bleed. All patients with GI bleeds should receive two large bore IV lines in preparation for significant volume resuscitation. A type and cross should be ordered should emergent use of blood products become necessary. Severe cases of bleeding from the lower GI tract are sometimes treated with colectomy. Moderate bleeding can be isolated with a tagged red blood cell nuclear scan or angiography. Bleeding can sometimes be stopped with angiography and coil embolization. Failure to do so requires surgical intervention and segmental resection. If the bleed cannot be localized, a total abdominal colectomy is required.

2. Angiodysplasia

Vascular malformations of the intestine may be an infrequent cause of gastrointestinal bleeding affecting the cecum and ascending colon. Confirmation of the lesion is made by colonoscopy or pill enteroscopy. The telangiectatic lesion can also be identified by a tagged RBC study or arteriography. Treatment is via electrocautery, argon plasma coagulation, coil embolization, or surgical resection (i.e. right hemicolectomy).

3. Mesenteric Ischemia

Insufficient blood flow to the small intestine from a low flow state due to shock or a thromboembolic event leads to small bowel compromise. Acute compromise presents with severe abdominal pain out of proportion to exam, ileus, and shock. Chronic disease presents with pain upon oral intake, weight loss, nausea, and vomiting. Early symptoms from thrombosis may be mild for several days. Patients with atrial fibrillation are at particularly high risk. Digitalis and diuretics may lead to a flow-limited state causing mesenteric ischemia. CT scans are specific but not very sensitive for diagnosis; signs include bowel wall thickening, pneumatosis, stranding, dilated bowel, and mesenteric edema. Treatment includes directed thrombolysis and surgical revascularization.

4. Ischemic Colitis

Bowel ischemia is typically secondary to acute thromboembolism or other vascular compromise of the blood supply to the intestine. Severe abdominal pain, bloody stools, nausea, vomiting, distention, and sepsis occur with necrosis of the intestine. Plain films may detect free air, while CT scan will identify paucity of contrast, a swirling sign in the mesentery, bowel wall thickening with pneumatosis, and even a free perforation. Angiography can be used in stable patients in an attempt to lyse the clot, while patients who have progressed to sepsis require an exploratory laparotomy with resection of the necrotic bowel. Total bowel necrosis is incompatible with life.

V. Abdominal Wall

V.A. General Concepts

1. Surgical Anatomy

The nine layers of the abdominal wall are the skin, subcutaneous tissue and fascia composed of Camper's and Scarpa's layers, external oblique muscle and aponeurosis, internal oblique muscle and aponeurosis, transversus abdominis muscle, transversalis fascia, preperitoneal fat, and peritoneum. Camper's fascia is superficial, while the deeper Scarpa's layer is more fibrotic.

The spermatic cord travels upon a cord formed by the external oblique aponeurosis; this layer eventually forms the inguinal ligament. Also known as Poupart's ligament, the femoral vessels and a potential femoral hernia pass posterior to this ligament; inguinal hernias pass anterior and superior. The internal oblique aponeurosis envelops the rectus abdominis superior to the semicircular line, then travels anterior to the rectus below this demarcation. Fibers of the internal oblique eventually become the cremaster muscle.

The margins of Hesselbach's triangle include the inguinal ligament (inferior), rectus sheath (medial), and inferior epigastric vessels (lateral). The floor is the transversalis fascia. A defect in this layer leads to hernia formation. The epigastric vessels travel within the preperitoneal space and form the lateral umbilical ligaments. The medial ligaments are the remnant of the umbilical arteries, while the median ligament is a remnant of the urachus.

2. Vascular Supply

The major vascular supply to the abdomen is derived from the intercostal and lumbar arteries and the superior and inferior epigastric vessels. The superior epigastric artery is the continuation of the internal mammary artery after it gives off the musculophrenic artery. The internal epigastric artery emanates from the external iliac artery and joins with the superior epigastric.

The gonadal artery is a direct branch of the aorta just below the renal arteries. These paired arteries become retroperitoneal and lie upon the psoas major muscle. They cross over the ureter and penetrate the deep inguinal ring to join the spermatic cord.

3. Innervation

The ilioinguinal nerve is a branch of the first lumbar nerve and accompanies the spermatic cord through the superficial inguinal ring. This sensory nerve receives sensation from the anteromedial thigh, upper scrotum, and root of the penis / mons pubis. This nerve does not pass through the deep inguinal ring. The iliohypogastric nerve is a branch of T12 and L1 and is sensory from the lateral gluteal folds and suprapubic region, and motor to the internal abdominal oblique and transversus abdominis. The genitofemoral nerve is a branch of L1 and L2 and is responsible for the cremaster reflex. The femoral branch supplies the femoral triangle, while the genital branch accompanies the spermatic cord and supplies the scrotum and cremaster.

V.B. Morphologic Conditions

1. Ventral Hernia

Ventral hernias may be acquired following surgery, which makes them known as incisional hernias. Natural defects leading to hernia formation may occur due to congenital anatomic weaknesses such as diastasis recti. Diagnosis is made by physical exam and palpation of the hernia; CT imaging can be helpful in identifying the precise defect and planning a surgical approach. The general approach to repair for small defects is primary repair without mesh; defects over 2 cm are repaired with mesh. Depending on the size and location of the defect, an anterior or laparoscopic approach may be used.

2. Umbilical Hernia

Umbilical hernias may arise from a congenital weakness within the umbilical ring or secondary to various causes. The majority of infantile hernias are self-limited and resolve within a few years. Acquired umbilical hernias may be secondary to obesity, pregnancy, or from surgical procedures that lead to a weakness at the umbilical ring. Acquired umbilical hernias may incarcerate and lead to strangulation. The most appropriate treatment for symptomatic or otherwise bothersome umbilical hernias is simple primary repair. Mesh can be used for larger defects. Umbilical hernia repair in cirrhotic patients is associated with a high morbidity and mortality due to poor tissue healing and the risk of spontaneous bacterial peritonitis. Repair should only be undertaken for incarcerated hernias and when there is frank leakage of ascites.

3. Epigastric Hernia

An epigastric hernia occurs with perforation of peritoneal contents through the linea alba. For example, perforation of small amounts of mesenteric fat through the linea alba can lead to fat incarceration and severe pain. Treatment is symptomatic management unless bowel is involved.

4. Spigelian Hernia

Spigelian hernias are located at the semilunar line. These unique hernias involve intra-abdominal contents passing through the linea semilunaris and remain deep to the external abdominal oblique. Clinical diagnosis is difficult and CT imaging is often necessary to identify and demarcate the defect. Primary repair and closure of the defect is required due to the high risk of entrapment and bowel compromise.

5. Parastomal Hernia

Parastomal hernias are a late complication of stoma placement. Serious hernia formation can lead to compromise of the bowel. Parastomal hernias can be observed until symptoms develop. Clinically-significant parastomal hernias may require relocation of the stoma if the hernia cannot be primarily repaired; alternatively, reinforcement of the fascia can be completed with mesh.

6. Inguinal Hernia

a) Epidemiology and Etiology

Groin hernias will affect about 7% of the population, and the majority are right-sided indirect inguinal hernias in men. Men are more likely than women to have a direct inguinal hernia, but indirect inguinal hernias are the most common overall for both genders.

b) Presentation and Diagnosis

Diagnosis is made by physical exam. Ultrasound and CT can be used when the diagnosis is unclear or a complicated hernia is suspected. Indirect inguinal hernias pass through the deep inguinal ring, are lateral to the inferior epigastric vessels, are covered by the internal spermatic fascia, and are congenital in nature due to failure of the internal inguinal ring to close after the testicle and spermatic cord pass through during ontogeny. Direct hernias are medial to the ring and inferior epigastric vessels and are acquired from a weakness in the abdominal floor. They are located medial to the inferior epigastric vessels and are not covered by the internal spermatic fascia. The combination of direct and indirect hernias on the same constitutes a pantaloon hernia.

c) Treatment

Based on patient preference, it is acceptable to monitor asymptomatic inguinal hernias so long as they are educated on the warning signs of incarceration. The presence of pain or a change in patient desire are sufficient indications for elective repair. Any difficulty with reduction of a potentially incarcerated hernia requires immediate repair. Patients with suspected bowel compromise can be approached via anterior incision with the understanding that an exploratory laparotomy may be necessary to examine the entire bowel and to complete a satisfactory resection in the event that necrotic bowel is found. In a similar fashion, patients who develop bowel obstruction or signs of bowel compromise after an inguinal hernia repair will also require surgical exploration of the abdomen.

d) Surgical Approaches

Anterior inguinal hernia repairs start with an oblique incision midway between the anterior superior iliac spine and the pubic tubercle. The incision is carried through the superficial tissues, Camper's and Scarpa's layers, and to the external abdominal oblique aponeurosis. This is incised via the external inguinal ring and the inguinal canal isolated. Care is taken to identify the ilioinguinal and iliohypogastric nerves; the former may be voluntarily sacrificed by some practitioners. The cremasteric fibers are separated to permit isolation of the hernia sac from the spermatic cord. The sac may be opened to ensure fidelity of the bowel. The sac is then mobilized, a high ligation completed, and a plug may be placed to seal the opening through the transversalis fascia. Cord lipomas should be excised.

In dirty cases that involve strangulated hernias and dead bowel, a primary repair without mesh is necessary. Bassini, McVay, and Shouldice repairs are all options. The Bassini repair joins the internal abdominal oblique aponeurosis, transversus abdominis, and conjoined tendon to reinforce the floor of the inguinal triangle under tension. The McVay repair can be used for any type of direct inguinal, indirect inguinal, or femoral hernia. The McVay repair apposes the transversus abdominis aponeurosis to the pectineal ligament, which is an extension of the lacunar ligament. A relaxing incision is made through the anterior rectus sheath. The Shouldice repair uses a running multilevel suture to appose the transversus abdominis and internal abdominal oblique muscles to the iliopubic tract.

A tension-free mesh repair of inguinal hernias can be done in several ways. In the Lichtenstein repair, a flat mesh is secured over the defect using nonabsorbable suture. A plug and patch uses a plug inserted into the posterior defect with an overlying mesh to further reinforce the defect and stabilize the plug. A patch can also be placed via a transabdominal preperitoneal (TAPP) approach into the defect in the transversalis and secured using tacks. A totally extraperitoneal (TEP) repair can be accomplished without violating the peritoneal cavity at all. TEP has faster dissection of the preperitoneal space and uses a balloon to dilate the space and is safer for the patient. Relative contraindications to laparoscopic inguinal hernia repair include a history of a radical retropubic prostatectomy and those with multiple prior abdominal procedures.

e) Complications of Hernia Repair

The presence of oliguria following laparoscopic hernia repair may be due to ureteral injury. The most common nerve injured in the TAPP (transabdominal preperitoneal) approach to hernia repair is the genitofemoral nerve (2%) of the time. This is closely followed by the ilioinguinal nerve (1.1%) and lateral cutaneous nerve of the thigh (1.1%). The ilioinguinal, iliohypogastric, and genitofemoral nerves also go through the region and are often transected intentionally or accidentally. Damage to the genital branch of the genitofemoral nerve leads to loss of the cremaster reflex and loss of sensation to the penis and scrotum. The femoral branch of the genitofemoral nerve provides sensation to the proximal medial thigh. The ilioinguinal provides redundant sensation to this region.

Another complication includes hemorrhage from the obturator artery, deep circumflex iliac artery, external iliac artery, cremaster artery, or inferior epigastric vessels. Constriction of the femoral vein is possible in certain repairs, leading to DVT and possible PE postoperatively. Intentional or accidental transection of the spermatic cord leads to swelling in the testes followed by atrophy in about ⅓ of patients. Orchiectomy is not required following transection of the spermatic cord. Damage to the vas deferens should be repaired primarily.

Damage to the intestines is also possible during a high ligation of the hernia sac, and care must be taken to open the hernia sac and deliberately reduce the contents of the sac prior to ligation. This is more likely to occur with an indirect hernia. Damage to the bladder wall can occasionally occur with a direct hernia, and closure in two layers is required along with Foley catheter drainage. Recurrence following indirect or direct inguinal hernia repair is about 5% per year.

7. Sliding Hernia

Sliding hernias occur when the wall of the hernia sac is an abdominal organ, such as intestine or bladder. Reduction of this component should be done; the danger is accidental high ligation of a piece of bladder or bowel.

8. Femoral Hernia

Inguinal hernias are above and medial to the pubic tubercle, while femoral hernias are inferior and lateral to the pubic tubercle. The femoral canal is bounded by the inguinal ligament anteriorly, the pectineal ligament posteriorly, the lacunar ligament medially, and the femoral vein laterally. The canal typically consists of empty space or rare lymphatics; therefore, femoral hernias are located medial to the femoral vessels. A node is occasionally located within the femoral canal, known as Cloquet's node. Femoral hernias occur when abdominal contents pass through the femoral canal. Femoral hernias are more common in women than in men; these hernias require immediate operation due to the high risk of strangulation. A McVay repair can be done to treat a femoral hernia. Division of the lacunar ligament is possible if reduction of the hernia is difficult.

9. Obturator Hernia

Obturator hernias occur through the obturator foramen, a natural defect created by the ischium and pubis through which the obturator vessels and nerve pass. Due to the gynecoid pelvis in females, they are more likely than males to develop this type of hernia. The risk of incarceration and bowel obstruction is high. Diagnosis is made by medial rotation and adduction of the thigh leading to compression of the obturator nerve and pain throughout the medial thigh and knee; this is a positive Howship-Romberg sign. Surgical reduction is required. Obturator hernias comprise only 1 in 1000 hernias; repair is taken by a transabdominal approach and repair with mesh. Mortality has been rated at 25%.

10. Lumbar Hernia

Lumbar hernias occur within the lumbar triangle, the bounds of which include the external abdominal oblique, iliac crest, and latissimus dorsi. The majority are secondary to trauma or after a nephrectomy. Hernia through the inferior triangle is known as a Petit hernia; if through the superior lumbar triangle, it is known as a Grynfeltt hernia. Repair with transabdominal mesh placement and laparoscopic transabdominal extraperitoneal repair have both been described.

11. Perineal Hernia

Perineal hernias occur through the pelvic floor and is secondary to tenesmus and constipation. Prior perineal surgery can weaken the pelvic floor and be conducive to hernia development. Repair involves mesh with appropriate anchoring or a gluteus maximus muscle flap.

12. Cystic Disease

Omental cysts are typically due to blockage of lymphatic channels and may expand to become a palpable abdominal mass. Treatment is via surgical excision and is necessary to avoid complications related to rupture, torsion, or bowel obstruction. Mesenteric cysts typically present with an abdominal mass that contains chylous fluid. Diagnosis is confirmed by CT scan and removal of the cyst is sufficient therapy. Neither of these cysts should be treated with aspiration due to the high rate of recurrence.

V.C. Degenerative Conditions

1. Ascites

a) Assessment

Ascites is commonly secondary to cirrhosis and increases the morbidity and mortality significantly due to spontaneous bacterial peritonitis. Less commonly, cancer, CHF, and nephrotic syndrome can also lead to ascites. In cirrhotics, portal hypertension and sodium retention overcome the ability of the lymphatics to clear the fluid, leading to shunting into the peritoneal cavity. Ascites is fundamentally a failure at the capillary level to maintain throughput, either due to a decrease in intracapillary oncotic pressure or increased pressure on the outflow side. Diseases of the portal vein or outflow system of the liver will lead to changes in the pressure gradient and also lead to increased exudation from capillaries.

Chylous ascites occur with lymphatic disruption, secondary to cancer or trauma. Lymphoma, GI tumors, and carcinoid are the most common malignant causes for chylous ascites. Disruption of the thoracic duct during AAA repair can also lead to this syndrome.

b) Management

Evaluation of ascites starts with paracentesis to help determine the etiology and nature of the collection. The serum-ascites albumin gradient is used to differentiate among various causes; portal hypertension would have a SAAG over 1.1, while nephrotic syndrome would be less than 1.1. Treatment for ascites is with sodium restriction, diuretics, paracentesis, albumin administration in patients refractory to medical management, TIPS, and liver transplantation.

Treatment for chylous ascites is supplemented by a low-fat diet, aggressive nutritional supplementation, and the addition of medium-chain fatty acids (which travel via the portal system to the liver) in lieu of long-chain fatty acids (which travel via lymphatics). Portovenous shunting and surgical options are limited.

2. Retroperitoneal Fibrosis

The majority of instances of retroperitoneal fibrosis are secondary to spontaneous disease, dopaminergics, or inflammation to the area. Patients with clinically-significant disease have involvement of their ureters, aorta, and inferior vena cava with the syndrome starting at the aortic bifurcation and moving superiorly. Diagnosis is confirmed by CT or MRI. CT-guided biopsy is necessary to rule out malignant causes. To avoid post renal failure, ureteral stenting or covering the ureters by an omentum (like a Graham patch repair) is completed. Chemotherapy agents such as azathioprine and tamoxifen are beneficial.

V.D. Trauma

1. Rectus Sheath Hematoma

Hematoma formation of the rectus sheath presents with a palpable mass and severe pain, and is most likely to occur in patients on anticoagulant therapy and in pregnant women. There is a positive Cullen sign and Grey Turner sign. Diagnosis is confirmed by CT scan. Treatment is symptomatic and reversal of the anticoagulation whenever possible. Continued expansion of the hematoma should be treated with arteriography and coil embolization.

2. Retroperitoneal Hematoma

Retroperitoneal hematomas are divided into zone I-III injuries. Penetrating central hematomas are zone I injuries and may occur as a result of trauma to the duodenum, pancreas, and major vessels; all such patients require exploration. Any patient who has had blunt trauma and is in shock requires operative intervention. Zone II hematomas are lateral; exploration is required only for expanding hematomas or injury to major structures. Zone III hematomas are pelvic; penetrating injury requires exploration due to risk of damage to major vascular structures. Blunt injuries should not be explored due to the risk of losing the tamponade effect.

V.E. Cancer

1. Desmoid Tumor

Desmoid tumors are common with FAP and emanate from muscle or fascia. Deeper tumors tend to expand rapidly and have a high recurrence rate but low rate of metastasis. Diagnosis is by MRI but a tissue sample is required to demonstrate the presence of spindle cells. Optimal treatment is resection and radiation.

2. Sarcoma

Sarcoma of the abdominal wall may include liposarcomas, rhabdomyosarcomas, leiomyosarcomas, fibrosarcomas, and malignant fibrous histiocytomas. A fixed, expanding, painless mass is evident and confirmed via MRI. A core needle biopsy is necessary for diagnosis. Longitudinal wide local excision may be curative. Retroperitoneal sarcoma is associated with retinoblastoma and p53 derangements. Prognostic decisions are based on tumor size and grade (histology). Survival is improved after en bloc resection; radiation has little role due to the location of the tumor.

HEPATOPANCREATOBILIARY

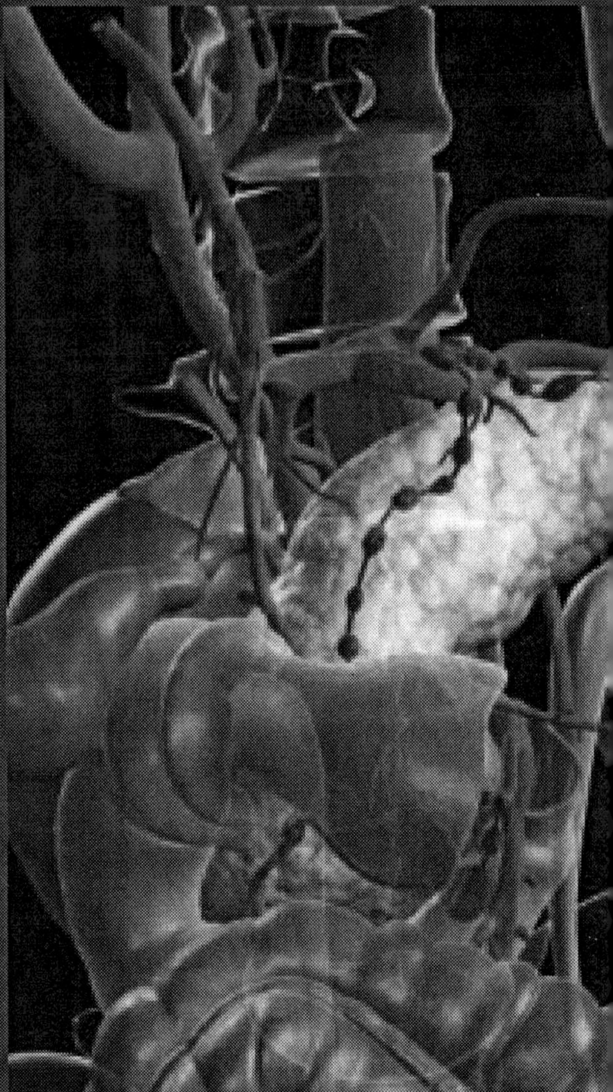

The very interesting medical career of Walther Kausch, student of Johannes Mikulicz-Radecki, is portrayed. The first successful pancreatoduodenectomy of the world in 1909 was his great surgical feat.

Specht and Stinshoff on Walther Kausch
Inventor of the Whipple Procedure (1867-1928)

HEPATOPANCREATOBILIARY SURGERY

Immanuel Turner, M.D. and Sapan S. Desai, M.D., Ph.D.

I. Introduction

An enormous body of knowledge is included in hepatopancreatobiliary surgery, and it is impossible to do justice to all of the topics that a surgeon must master. There is no substitute for practical experience gained by seeing patients and performing cases. We encourage you to review the key reference textbooks in the field and review the latest research on a routine basis. The following survey of key topics is meant to provide a broad overview of important concepts and commonly tested facts.

II. Liver

II.A. General Concepts

1. Anatomy

The liver is a three pound, cone-shaped organ that lies in the right upper quadrant. It is divided into two main lobes, each composed of thousands of lobules. It constitutes approximately 2% of adult body weight and receives 25% cardiac output. The ducts within each of the lobules coalesce to eventually form the hepatic duct, which transports bile produced by the liver to the gallbladder, and then to the duodenum. The liver receives 70% of blood supply from the portal vein and

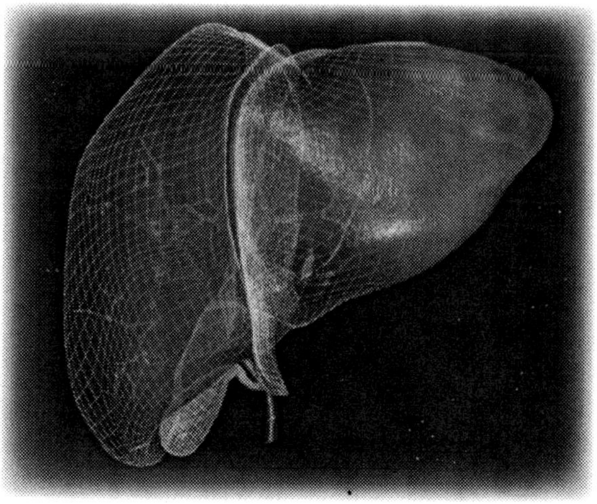

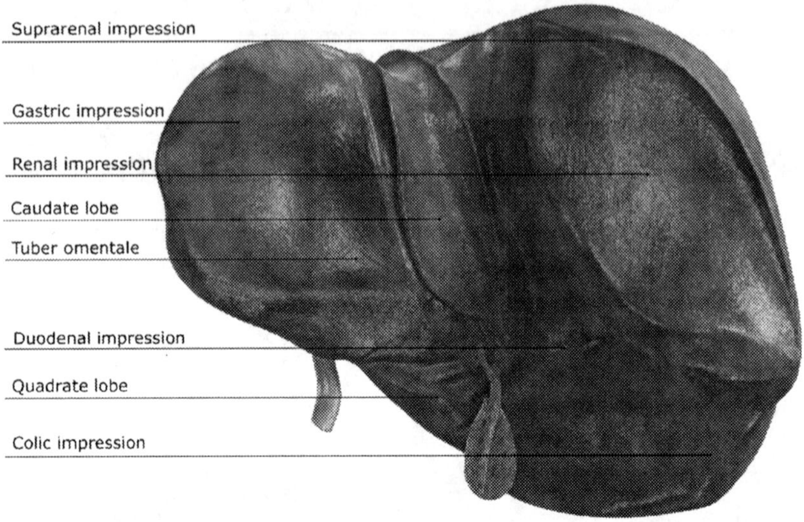

30% from hepatic artery. At any particular time, the liver contains over 10% of the body's total blood volume. Nearly ¾ of the liver can be destroyed before it is unable to carry out its functions.

The liver can be described in terms of its surface anatomy and in terms of its surgical anatomy. The surface anatomy uses various external ligaments and markers to divide the liver into several divisions. Cantlie's line divides the liver into the right and left lobes and corresponds to the imaginary line between the gallbladder and inferior vena cava. This generally corresponds to the true division between the right and left lobes, demarcated as the line between the middle hepatic vein and the inferior vena cava.

The falciform ligament divides the left lobe of the liver into a left medial and left lateral section. The falciform ligament has the ligamentum teres at its distal end, which contains the obliterated umbilical vein. The caudate lobe is located posterior to the gastrohepatic ligament, which helps to form the lesser sac.

Couinaud's description of the liver separates the liver into eight segments. Segment I is the caudate lobe and is posteriorly located between the portal vein and the inferior vena cava. Segments II and III compose the left lateral section of the liver, while segment IV composes the left medial portion.

Segment IV is often divided into the superiorly located part IVa and inferiorly located part IVb. In a clockwise manner, segments V, VI, VII, and VIII compose the right half of the liver with segments VI and VII located posteriorly and segments V and VIII located anteriorly. The division between the anterior and posterior planes is created by an imaginary line between the right hepatic vein and inferior vena cava.

Each of these segments is supplied by branches of the portal vein and hepatic artery, and drained by sectoral biliary ducts and hepatic veins. Segment IV is unique in that portions of the right and left hepatic artery provide inflow. The caudate lobe is unique in that it drains directly into the vena cava.

2. Vascular Supply

With regard to the inflow and outflow to the liver, there are several major structures. The hepatic artery provides 25% of the inflow. This artery arises from the celiac artery as the common hepatic artery (the other two major branches are the left gastric and splenic arteries). The common hepatic artery gives off the gastroduodenal and right gastric arteries and then becomes the proper hepatic artery. The proper hepatic artery travels within the hepatoduodenal ligament along with the common bile duct and portal vein. The artery is located medially, the biliary duct laterally, and the portal vein posteriorly. The proper hepatic artery splits into the right and left hepatic arteries. The right hepatic artery gives off the cystic artery in 70% of people; the cystic artery can also occasionally be a branch of the left hepatic artery or proper hepatic artery. It can also arise from a replaced right or left hepatic artery.

A replaced right hepatic artery typically arises as a direct branch of the superior mesenteric artery. A replaced left hepatic artery arises as a direct branch of the left gastric artery, travels within the lesser sac and gastrohepatic ligament, and then supplies the liver. It is for this reason that care must be taken when dissecting the caudate lobe free, as careless mobilization of the gastrohepatic ligament and lesser sac to gain access to the caudate lobe can lead to trauma to a replaced left hepatic artery. About 50% of patients will also have a middle hepatic artery branch from the proper hepatic artery.

The portal vein supplies 75% of the inflow to the liver. The portal vein is the confluence of the splenic vein and superior mesenteric vein (SMV). The inferior mesenteric vein (IMV) often empties into the splenic vein prior to its junction with the SMV.

There are three hepatic veins – the large right hepatic vein, a middle hepatic vein, and a left hepatic vein. The right hepatic vein typically empties directly into the inferior vena cava, while the middle and left hepatic veins form a common trunk before emptying into the vena cava in about 67% of patients. Other patients may have each vein emptying directly into the inferior vena cava.

The hepatic ducts follow a similar pattern as the portal vein and coalesce to form the common hepatic duct. It receives drainage from the gallbladder via the cystic duct to become the common bile duct. The common bile duct then travels into the head of the pancreas, joins with the pancreatic duct to form the common duct, then empties into the duodenum at the ampulla of Vater. There are eight major variations of the cystic duct that are described – many of them are permutations on the length of the duct and the precise location on the hepatic duct that it empties into, but one of the variations is notable as the cystic duct empties directly into the right hepatic duct. The critical view that is achieved during a laparoscopic cholecystectomy consists of the cystic duct, cystic artery, and common hepatic duct – careful dissection once this view is achieved minimizes the risk of injury to nearby structures, including the common hepatic duct.

3. Surgical Resections

The terminology related to liver resections has been revised and updated. A right hepatectomy (or hemihepatectomy) refers to resection of segments V, VI, VII, and VIII. A left hepatectomy refers to resection of segments I, II, III, and IV. A left medial hepatectomy is resection of segment IV, while a left lateral hepatectomy refers to resection of segments II and III. A left medial hepatectomy can be referred to as a segmentectomy as only one liver segment is resected. A left lateral hepatectomy can also be referred to as a sectionectomy, as two segments are resected together. A right anterior sectionectomy is resection of segments V and VIII, and a right posterior sectionectomy is resection of segments VI and VII. A right extended hepatectomy includes segment IV along with V-VIII, while a left extended hepatectomy includes segments I-IV and V.

4. Histology

The liver is composed of hepatocytes (50% by number, 80% by volume), Kupffer cells (macrophages), and endothelium. Hepatocytes are divided into three zones. Zone I cells are nearest the periportal blood supply and process incoming nutrients. These cells primarily produce protein. Zone III cells are far from arterial blood and take part in glycogenolysis and lipogenesis. Formation of urea occurs in zones II and III. Gluconeogenesis predominantly occurs in zone I.

5. Physiology

a) Hepatic Biosynthesis

Proteins created by the liver include albumin, which has a half-life of 3 weeks, prealbumin, which has a half-life of 2 days, and transferrin, which has a half-life of 10 days. Factor VII has the shortest half-life at 5 hours. The cytochrome p450 system in the liver plays a role in toxin metabolism. Phase I reactions lead to oxidation and reduction, while phase II reactions lead to conjugation. Hepatic biotransformation is dependent on the cytochrome P450 system.

b) Gluconeogenesis

During an overnight fast, 75 gm of liver glycogen is depleted rapidly through glycogenolysis and serum glucose begins to fall. The result is a decrease in insulin and an increase in glucagon, growth hormone, catecholamines, and cortisol. The net effect is stimulation of hepatic gluconeogenesis and glycogenolysis. Gluconeogenesis relies on amino acids as the main carbon source, especially glutamine and alanine. Other sources include lactate, pyruvate, propionate, and glycerol. The primary source of substrate is from proteins, where nearly 75gm of proteins are broken down every day leading to excretion of 10gm of nitrosurea products. This protein breakdown stops about a week after starvation as the body begins to shift to ketoacid use. The fuel source to the body during periods of prolonged starvation (i.e. > 2 weeks) comes from ketone bodies. These ketone bodies are generated by the oxidation of fatty acids. The primary tissues that relay upon glucose are the kidney and liver. The brain, red blood cells, and testes also require glucose.

c) Serum-Ascites Albumin Gradient

The SAAG is calculated by comparing the albumin concentration in the serum to that of the ascites fluid. If the difference between the serum and the ascites is greater than 1.1 and portal hypertension is present, it indicates the underlying etiology to likely be due to liver disease such as hepatitis, cirrhosis, liver failure, or HCC; it may alternatively be due to congestion caused by hepatic failure, heart failure, constrictive pericarditis, tricuspid insufficiency, or Budd-Chiari syndrome. A SAAG less than 1.1 with hypoalbuminemia typically indicates that nephrotic syndrome, severe malabsorption with protein loss, or malnutrition with anasarca are the cause. Other conditions that may lead to a SAAG less than 1.1 include ascites of pancreatic, bile, stomach, kidney, bladder, or ovarian origin. A diseased peritoneum can also present with a SAAG less than 1.1 with causes including infection, malignancy, and rarer conditions such as familial Mediterranean fever (FMF), vasculitis, granulomatous peritonitis, and eosinophilic peritonitis.

6. Diagnostic Imaging

The main modalities available for imaging of the liver include ultrasound, CT, MRI, and PET. Ultrasound is suitable for use for guiding needle biopsies of superficial lesions, and intraoperatively to evaluate the portal system and vascular flow. It can also be used to identify parenchymal lesions that are not immediately evident on the surface.

CT scanning can utilize arterial, portal and delayed images to better image the liver. With a resolving power of 1 cm, CT scanning has a 85% sensitivity and a 5% false positive rate for most liver masses. However, this sensitivity decreases with smaller HCC-type masses in a cirrhotic patient. In these instances, MRI has a superior sensitivity and is the preferred imaging modality. MRI is superior to CT in characterizing specific soft tissue lesions and is more sensitive for hemangioma. The biliary tree can also be imaged with MRI by way of a cholangiopancreatography scan. Both studies are invaluable for preoperative evaluation of the anatomy.

PET-CT is a highly sensitive (95%) and specific (90%) test that is useful for non-hepatocellular carcinoma masses and can change staging; the major downfall of PET-CT is the 10% false negative rate that is especially prominent with hepatocellular carcinoma. PET-CT is a sensitive method for detecting residual tumor activity and evaluating the entire body for signs of metastatic disease. The gold standard for intraoperative imaging is ultrasound, as it permits detection of small masses in relation to the surrounding vascular structures.

7. Classification of Liver Disease

a) Child-Pugh Score

The Child-Pugh score is the main method for classifying liver disease. It uses five major components: bilirubin, albumin, ascites, encephalopathy, and PT/INR time. Points are assigned for the degree of severity and broken down into three categories: A, B, and C with the latter being the most severe. The breakdown is presented below. The category and overall survival are listed in the following table. A Child score of A has a 15-20 year survival; Child class C survival has a survival of only a few years.

TABLE 1. Child-Pugh classification system.

Score	+1	+2	+3
Total bilirubin (mg/dL)	<2	2-3	>3
Serum albumin (g/L)	>35	28-35	<28
Ascites	None	Treated with medication	Refractory to medication
Encephalopathy	None	Treated with medication	Refractory to medication
PT / INR	<1.7	1.7-2.2	>2.2

TABLE 2. Child-Pugh categories and survival.

Points	Class	One Year Survival	Two Year Survival
5-6	A	~100%	85%
7-9	B	81%	57%
10+	C	45%	35%

b) MELD Score

The Model for End-Stage Liver Disease (MELD) score is used to assess the severity of chronic liver disease. The MELD score is used to help stratify patients awaiting a liver transplantation, and is predictive of short-term mortality. The MELD score is somewhat similar to the Child-Pugh score and utilizes serum bilirubin, creatinine, and PT/INR to calculate the final score. Any patient who receives regular dialysis is given a creatinine of 4.0. The formula to calculate the MELD score is below. The table below includes information about the 90 day mortality.

$$MELD = 3.78[\ln TB\ (mg/dL)] + 11.2[\ln INR] + 9.57[\ln Cr\ (mg/dL)] + 6.43$$

TABLE 3. 90 day mortality as a function of the MELD score.

<10	4%
10-19	27%
20-29	76%
30-39	83%
40+	100%

c) Liver Reserve

Evaluating the functional reserve of the liver following a planned resection is important to ensure that a sufficient volume of liver remains. The Child-Pugh score was the original method used to assess the functional status of the liver, but due to its imprecise nature, the evaluation of liver reserve has become more quantitative in nature. The clearance of galactose or indocyanine green can be used as part of the evaluation. More rigorous methods include evaluating microsomal function by way of caffeine or lidocaine clearance, or via the aminopyrine breath test. The use of SPECT and CT liver volume analysis are currently being evaluated as more sensitive quantitative methods to evaluate liver reserve.

II.B. Infectious and Inflammatory Disease

1. Liver Abscess

a) Pyogenic Abscesses

(1) *Assessment*

Bacterial abscess formation within the liver is an uncommon but potentially morbid typically secondary to instrumentation of the pancreas and biliary tree and biliary obstruction. Abscesses can also form after a liver transplant due to thrombosis of the hepatic artery. The most common organisms are bowel flora, including Escherichia coli and Klebsiella pneumoniae. Liver function tests are elevated and CT or ultrasound imaging confirms the diagnosis.

(2) *Management*

Pyogenic liver abscess is treated with broad spectrum antibiotics for 6 weeks. Ultrasound-guided percutaneous drainage can be completed in appropriately selected patients should medical management fail.

b) Amoebic Abscesses

(1) *Assessment*

Abscess formation by Entamoeba histolytica may affect up to 5% of the immigrant population in the United States. Patients are infected by a fecal-oral route and may present with fevers, night sweats, and diarrhea. Rupture can lead to peritonitis and sepsis. The diagnosis is confirmed by elevated liver function tests (especially alkaline phosphatase) and a wall-enhancing lesion on CT imaging.

(2) *Management*

Metronidazole can be used to eliminate the infection. Very large abscesses can be drained percutaneously. Open resection is used only in severe cases due to the risk of spillage into the peritoneal cavity.

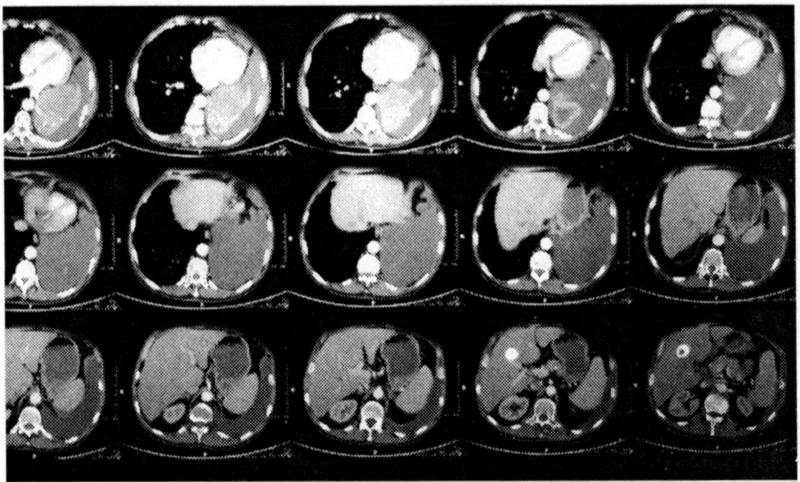

c) Hydatid Disease

Echinococcus can lead to hydatid cyst disease of the liver and lungs with parenchymal destruction and portal hypertension. Thick, fluid-filled cysts with calcification are evident on imaging studies. Pain is a common complaint from the expanding cysts. Treatment is open resection with care taken to avoid spillage.

d) Schistosomiasis

Schistosomiasis is a trematode infection of the liver that presents with a maculopapular rash and liver necrosis. Wall-thickening of the portal vein is occasionally seen on ultrasound secondary to infection, but the major change is hypertrophy of the liver with ring-enhancing lesions on CT. Treatment is with praziquantel.

2. Viral Hepatitis

a) Etiology

Viral hepatitis is an infectious process due to hepatitis A (HAV), B (HBV), C (HCV), D (HDV), E (HEV), or G (HGV). Longstanding viral hepatitis leads to symptoms of liver damage, including jaundice and dark urine, right upper quadrant (RUQ) pain, weakness and fatigue, anorexia, nausea and vomiting, low-grade fever, and general malaise. Generally, viral hepatitis presents with elevations in ALT. The increases are significant – viral hepatitis is one of three serious causes of transaminases increasing above 1,000; the other two causes are acetaminophen toxicity and septic shock leading to fulminant liver failure. Fulminant liver failure can also occur with infection by any of the hepatitis viruses except HGV. Cirrhosis is most commonly associated with chronic hepatitis, which can occur with HBV and HCV. Finally, all of the causes of viral hepatitis are due to RNA viruses except HBV, which is a DNA virus. The specific hepatitis viruses are discussed below.

b) Hepatitis A Virus

Table 4. Hepatitis A Virus

Pathophysiology	Single-stranded RNA. Spread by fecal-oral route, contaminated food.
Diagnosis	Positive for IgM and IgG to HAV in serum.
Treatment	Symptomatic management. Prophylaxis available.

c) Hepatitis B Virus

(1) *Pathophysiology*

HBV is a DNA virus in the hepadnavirus family. HBV is spread predominantly through sex, blood products, and saliva. It is found in all body fluids. HBV has a 1/10 chance of progressing to chronic hepatitis in adults, and a 90% risk in neonates. Chronic infection significantly increases the risk of hepatocellular carcinoma (HCC) due to repeated cycles of damage and healing. The risk of fulminant liver failure is approximately 1 in 100 patients, and half of all cases of fulminant hepatitis are due to HBV. HBV has a two-six month incubation period.

(2) *Diagnosis*

A number of markers for HBV infection are used to determine the infectivity and prognosis of the disease. Hepatitis B core antigen (HBcAg) is expressed in infected hepatocytes, but not detectable in the serum. HBcAg is a marker for early infection. IgM antibodies to hepatitis B core (HBcAb IgM) indicates the onset of the window period, and is the time between disappearance of hepatitis B surface antigen (HBsAg) and appearance of antibodies to HBs (HBsAb) in the serum. HBcAb IgM is detectable during the acute phase of infection, which typically occurs 1-6 months after infection. HBsAg is the antigen present on the protein coat of the virus and is a marker of active hepatitis and a carrier state. Ongoing viral replication with a high chance of infectivity is indicated by the hepatitis B "e" antigen. Both HBsAg and HBeAg are expressed between 1-6 months after initial infection. A significantly decreased risk of infection is indicated by the presence of antibodies to HBe (HBeAb), which can take several months to years and are present in the acute phase of resolution. Immunity is signified by antibodies to HBs (HBsAb). Signs of infection in the distant past are indicated by IgG antibodies to HBc (HBcAb IgG), and are detectable for the longest period of time. Essentially, if HBsAg is positive, infection is ongoing. If HBcAb IgM is present, the infection is in the window period. The presence of only HBsAb indicates immunity via vaccination.

(3) *Treatment*

Treatment of HBV is instituted with immunoglobulins to HBV (HBIG), use of alpha-interferon or lamivudine for chronic infections, and liver transplantation in the case of fulminant hepatic failure. Prophylaxis to HBV is the best way to avoid infection, and it is done with a series of three HBV IgG injections and standard precautions to body fluids should be taken. Only the hepatitis B surface antibody is present following vaccination in a hepatitis-naïve person.

d) Hepatitis C Virus

(1) *Pathophysiology*

HCV is a single-stranded RNA virus in the flavivirus family, and is spread in a manner similar to HBV. HCV is now the most common cause of viral hepatitis in the United States due to precautions against blood-borne transmission of HBV instituted earlier than HCV precautions. HCV transmission is especially common in IV drug users and in prisons. Vertical transmission is possible but minimal (5%), as is sexual transmission (5%) and via needles (5%). Like HBV, the incubation period is typically on the order of

1-6 months. About ¾ of HCV infections become chronic and there is up to a 5% risk of HCC. HCV infection can present with symptoms of hepatitis and also polyarteritis nodosa (PAN) and cryoglobulinemias. Only ¼ of patients are symptomatic.

(2) *Diagnosis*

Diagnosis is made by positive serum titers for antibodies to HCV (HCVAb). HCVAb indicates chronic infection. Repeated infections over time are possible due to poor antibody development.

(3) *Treatment*

HCV is treated with alpha-interferon and ribavirin with a 50% chance of remission. Patients who do not respond to this therapy can be given a course of amantadine or rimantadine. As with HBV, the best treatment is prevention.

e) Hepatitis D Virus

TABLE 5. Hepatitis D virus.

Pathophysiology	RNA virus. Requires HBV to be infective.
Treatment	Treat the concurrent HBV infection.

f) Hepatitis E Virus

TABLE 6. Hepatitis E virus.

Pathophysiology	RNA virus. Transmitted by fecal-oral route. Most common in Asia and Africa.
Diagnosis	No marker for diagnosis.
Treatment	Supportive therapy.

g) Other Viral Infections

CMV infections can lead to a low grade viral hepatitis that is usually asymptomatic in most patients. In susceptible individuals, fulminant liver can occur and may lead to a liver transplantation. Symptomatic infections can be treated with ganciclovir.

EBV infections can lead to a mild hepatitis in the context of mononucleosis. Similar to CMV infections, EBV can lead to a fulminant liver failure in susceptible patients. In such severe infections, the only treatment is liver transplant.

HSV can lead to hepatitis in neonates and immunocompromised patients. Treatment with acyclovir should be started if HSV is suspected due to the potential of infection progressing to end stage liver failure.

VZV can lead to Reye syndrome if inappropriately treated with aspirin during the febrile stages. Fulminant liver failure can occur and may necessitate liver transplantation.

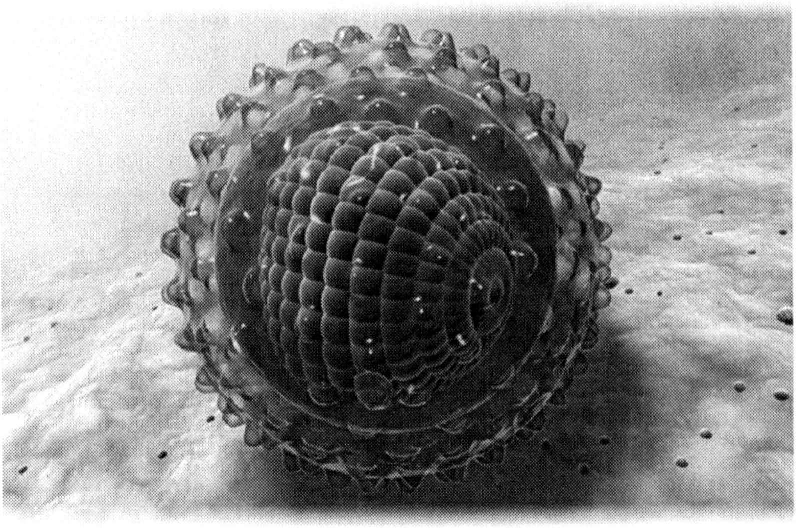

II.C. Metabolic and Degenerative Diseases

1. Cirrhosis

a) Etiology

Cirrhosis is the development of repeated liver damage leading to cycles of fibrosis, necrosis, regeneration, and eventually, HCC. Causes of cirrhosis include alcohol, viral infection, primary biliary cirrhosis (PBC), Wilson disease, alpha-1-antitrypsin deficiency, and hemochromatosis. The most common cause of cirrhosis in the United States is alcohol abuse leading to fatty liver, and eventually hepatitis and cirrhosis with continued insult.

b) Presentation

Cirrhosis presents with many of the signs discussed above for liver damage, including jaundice, nausea and vomiting, hepatomegaly, loss of appetite, angiomas, ascites, encephalopathy, palmar erythema, Dupuytren contracture, and portal hypertension. Overall, 15% of alcoholics will develop cirrhosis. There is a 10% mortality from hepatitis, and half of all cases are due to progression to cirrhosis and the other half to fibrosis.

c) Diagnosis

Diagnosis of cirrhosis is made with abnormal LFTs including an elevated AST to ALT ratio (viral disorders raise the ALT to AST ratio), elevated direct and indirect bilirubin, elevated GGT, prolonged PT, low albumin, and anemia. MELD (model for end stage liver disease) scores are the most accurate predictors for 90-daymortality in cirrhotics. It was implemented by UNOS in 2002 for liver allocation for transplantation. It is a better estimation of disease severity and allows for a more timely assessment and transplantation of the sickest patients. It consists of serum creatinine, serum bilirubin, INR, and cause of cirrhosis.

d) Treatment

Cirrhosis is treated by avoiding risk factors that can further exacerbate liver injury. Failure to do so, and continued use of alcohol, will likely lead to fulminant hepatic failure or HCC. Unlike some other hepatobiliary conditions, a high protein diet is recommended (these patients are hypermetabolic and require as much as 1.1 grams protein/kg/day to maintain nitrogen balance) with vitamin supplements to permit the liver to form the necessary proteins required for normal body function. Fluid and electrolyte management is also necessary including sodium and water restriction and cautious dieresis (over diuresing can lead to hepatorenal syndrome) Medications that can further damage the liver are avoided, including acetaminophen and isoniazid

(INH). Inflammatory changes can often be halted with the use of colchicine and glucocorticoids. Other complications of cirrhosis such as ascites should be treated as necessary. Alpha 1-antitrypsin deficiency is a defect in alpha 1-antitrypsin production leading to excess deposition of abnormal A1^{a}T protein in lung and liver. The result is COPD and cirrhosis. Treatment involves a lung and liver transplant, whenever possible.

2. Portal Hypertension

Portal hypertension is the development of elevated pressures within the portal vein from a hepatic process that raises the resistance of inflow. Since the portal vein supplies 75% of the flow to the liver but cannot generate the pressure found in the hepatic artery, the flow is shunted to collateral vessels and leads to the numerous manifestations of portal hypertension.

Specifically, dilation of the left gastric, inferior mesenteric, umbilical, and retroperitoneal veins occur. Left gastric vein dilation leads to the formation of varices by involving the venous collaterals in the esophagus. Involvement of the inferior mesenteric veins leads to an increase in pressure within the hemorrhoidal branches. The umbilical vein can lead to caput medusae, and most patients will reconstitute the entire vein within the round ligament.

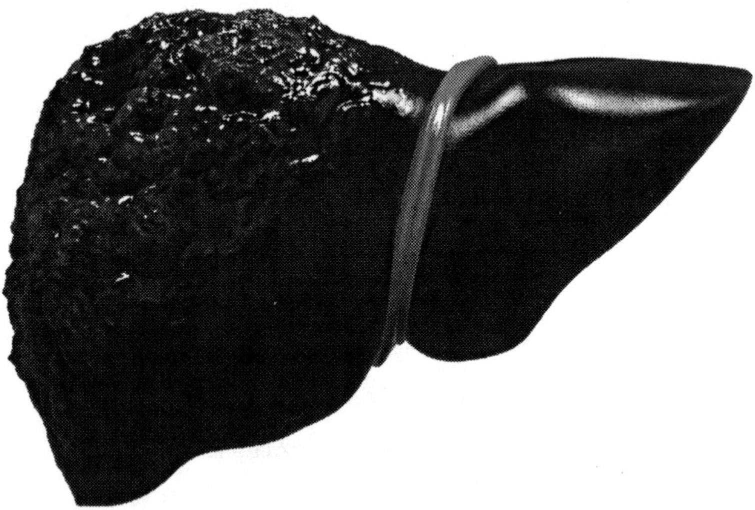

Involvement of the retroperitoneal veins leads to a bypass of nutrient flow and can exacerbate hepatic encephalopathy. The increase in pressure can also lead to splenomegaly and bleeding, which may be treated with a splenectomy.

Esophageal varices may lead to an upper gastrointestinal bleed that is difficult to control. The initial management is with beta blockers and nitrates to reduce the pressure gradient across the portal system. Octreotide and nitroglycerin can also be used. Active bleeding is treated differently: after resuscitating and stabilizing the patient, vasopressin and octreotide can be given to vasoconstrict the vessels and decrease splanchnic blood flow. Upper gastrointestinal endoscopy should be carried out to ligate the bleeding vessel. If the vessel cannot be controlled through band ligation, tamponade can be achieved with a Sengstaken-Blakemore tube placement.

TIPS may be completed in patients with severe manifestations of esophageal varices, and is quickly becoming the procedure of choice in patients with bleeding refractory to medical management. Surgical interventions include the creation of a portacaval or mesocaval shunt, an option typically reserved for Child's A or B cirrhotics who are not otherwise candidates for transplantation and have exhausted other options. Devascularization of the esophagus and stomach to reroute the venous drainage away from the splanchnic circulation can also be completed. Devascularization procedures can also be done for patients with gastric varices.

Most Child A cirrhotics with severe variceal disease that fail to respond to maximum medical management are likely to respond to TIPS. This is the procedure of choice in a patient who may eventually be a candidate for a liver transplant. Patients who are not candidates for transplant can have a splenorenal shunt created to bypass the liver and ameliorate the portal hypertension. Unstable patients who are not candidates for transplantation may fare better with a portacaval or mesocaval shunt. Child's B and C cirrhotics typically respond to a TIPS procedure.

3. Budd-Chiari Syndrome

Budd-Chiari syndrome develops with occlusion of hepatic outflow secondary to thrombosis or mechanical obstruction by cancer. This raises hepatic resistance to inflow and leads to portal hypertension. The diagnosis should be suspected in patients with an acute onset of ascites, hepatomegaly, and right upper quadrant pain. Early recognition by ultrasound, CT imaging, or angiography permits the formation of a transjugular intrahepatic portosystemic shunt (TIPS) and can forestall the development of portal hypertension and liver failure. The only treatment for more advanced disease is liver transplantation.

4. Portal Vein Thrombosis

Portal vein thrombosis may lead to portal hypertension. It is more common in children and may be due to infection of the umbilical vein. Ultrasound confirms the presence of a thrombus. Treatment is by way of a splenorenal shunt or superior mesenteric vein to left portal vein shunt.

5. Ascites

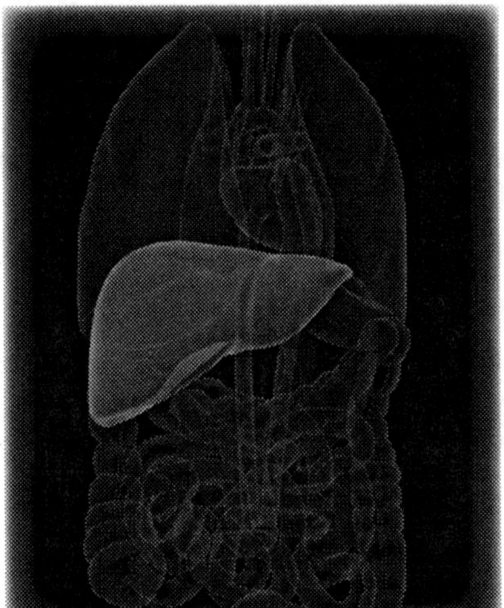

Increased resistance in the diseased liver also leads to an increase in hydrostatic pressure at the sinusoids, leading to the formation of ascites. This problem is exacerbated by sodium loading and fluid overload. Calculation of the SAAG via paracentesis can be done to evaluate the nature and potential cause of the ascites. Most patients will respond to medical management including limiting sodium intake, moderation of fluid intake, and the use of furosemide.

6. Spontaneous Bacterial Peritonitis

Spontaneous bacterial peritonitis occurs in a subset of patients with longstanding ascites, and is due to infection by enteric gram negative bacteria from the intestinal flora. Spontaneous bacterial peritonitis presents with fever and chills, rebound abdominal tenderness, and sepsis. It is diagnosed with gram stain, culture, and sensitivity following paracentesis of the ascites.

The presence of over 250 polymorphonuclear lymphocytes (PMNs) is diagnostic. Spontaneous bacterial peritonitis is treated with cefuroxime to cover the intestinal flora and electrolyte replacement for the ascites.

7. Umbilical Hernia

The increase in intraabdominal pressure from the ascites leads to the development of an umbilical hernia in a quarter of all patients. Patients with grossly symptomatic disease should be treated electively after a paracentesis is completed to drain the ascites. Drains are typically placed to continue ascites drainage while the incision heals.

8. Hepatic Encephalopathy

Encephalopathy from liver disease is commonly the result of elevated levels of ammonia leading to central nervous system (CNS) damage. The elevated amino acid content of the blood also leads to an increase in GABA levels and endogenous benzodiazepines. Hepatic encephalopathy is often heralded by signs of impaired consciousness such as drowsiness, confusion, disorientation, or coma, changes in personality, behavior, mood or judgment, changes in speech, asterixis, fetor hepaticus, and cerebral edema. Hepatic encephalopathy is worsened by acute GI bleeds, increased protein intake, and active infection. The differential diagnosis of hepatic encephalopathy includes alcohol intoxication, delirium tremens, dementia, infection, and various systemic disorders.

9. Hepatorenal Syndrome

Hepatorenal syndrome is the development of acute renal failure with worsening oliguria, azotemia, and sodium retention. It is diagnosed by very low urine sodium (<10 mEq/L). It is especially common in later stages of severe hepatic failure. There is no known treatment other than supportive therapy and palliative care. Hepatorenal syndrome is due to the inability to concentrate urine and is associated with portal hypertension. It is attributed to an alteration in blood flow to the splanchnic circulation and kidney. Type I involves a rapid increase in creatinine to over 2.5 mg/dL and a drop in creatinine clearance to less than 20 mL/min. Type I is resolved with relief of ascites and improved volume status/renal perfusion. Type II is progressive over a longer period of time and has more gradual worsening of renal function. Type II hepatorenal syndrome is typically due to ascites that is refractory to medical management. Urine sodium is typically less than 10 mEq/dL. IV albumin has been shown to improve outcomes in some studies. Type II is resolved by improved hepatic function and increased SVR. Octreotide or midodrine used individually have no beneficial effects.

10. Primary Biliary Cirrhosis

a) Etiology and Epidemiology

PBC is an autoimmune disorder that causes destruction of the intrahepatic bile ducts. It is more common in women, and is predicted by the presence of AMA and a demonstrable autoimmune response to the epithelium of the biliary tree. PBC leads to the accumulation of waste products commonly dissipated with bile secretion, namely, cholesterol, bile acids, and bilirubin.

b) Presentation

PBC presents with symptoms similar to other liver diseases, including jaundice, fatigue and weakness and pruritus. In addition, PBC presents with xanthomas from the elevated cholesterol. There is typically an additional autoimmune disorder present with PBC, such as rheumatoid arthritis (RA). Nearly ⅓ of patients are asymptomatic, and the most common initial complaint is fatigue.

c) Diagnosis and Treatment

Diagnosis of PBC is made by elevated alkaline phosphatase and GGT. AST and ALT are typically normal. There is also a positive AMA. Ultrasound is typically unremarkable. Hyperlipidemia is another feature of PBC. Treatment largely consists of surgical intervention due to the failure of medical management. Liver transplantation is necessary.

11. Fulminant Liver Failure

Fulminant liver failure presents with a rapid rise in liver function tests, jaundice, mental status changes from ammonia toxicity, and eventually multisystem organ failure if not expeditiously treated. The most common cause of liver failure is Tylenol overdose. A rise in the ALT to a peak nearly 30 times that over baseline is typically diagnostic. The rise of mental status changes indicates encephalopathy and portends a poor prognosis. Falling factor V levels, advanced coma, slowly progressive changes, and necrotic changes are also predictive of a negative outcome.

II.D. Trauma

The liver is the most common organ to be injured from penetrating or blunt trauma. Following assessment and management of the airway, breathing, and circulation, a thorough evaluation of the patient should be completed. Stable patients with suspected intraabdominal injury should undergo a CT scan. Unstable patients suspected of bleeding should go to the operating room for surgical exploration. A diagnostic peritoneal lavage (DPL) or focused abdominal sonographic test (FAST) can aid in the decision-making process.

Lacerations to the liver in a hemodynamically stable patient can often be managed conservatively. Grade I lacerations have a subcapsular hematoma affecting less than 10% of the surface area or a less than 1 cm capsular tear. Tears up to 3 cm or subcapsular hematomas affecting up to 50% of the surface area are grade II injuries. Grade III injuries have expanding hematomas or a laceration over 3 cm in depth. Grade IV lacerations involve up to 75% of a lobe or up to 3 separate segments. Grade V lacerations have significant liver disruption and injury to nearby vascular structures, and almost always require operative management. Grade VI injury is total avulsion of the liver and is not compatible with life.

II.E. Cancer

1. Cystic Disease

Noninfectious, simple cystic disease of the liver is often an incidental finding on imaging done for other reasons. In a subset of patients, cysts may become symptomatic and cause right upper quadrant or flank pain. Very large cysts may even lead to impingement upon the gastrointestinal system. The treatment of choice for symptomatic cysts is ultrasound-guided percutaneous drainage. This procedure can be repeated if unsuccessful the first time, and sclerosing agents can even be injected to facilitate closure. If the cyst reappears a third time, wide fenestration via a small laparoscopic incision can be completed.

2. Hepatic Adenoma

Hepatic adenomas are lesions commonly found in women of reproductive age who are also using oral contraceptives. The estrogen stimulation leads to the development of an adenoma. Adenomas must be differentiated from focal nodular hyperplasia (FNH), as adenomas have up to a 5% chance of harboring a focus of hepatocellular carcinoma. Larger adenomas also have a risk of rupturing and causing a potential fatal hemorrhage; early diagnosis is also important in women who may become pregnant as adenomas should be resected prior to pregnancy due to this risk of rupture.

Adenomas can be distinguished from focal nodular hyperplasia by CT and MRI imaging. Adenomas do not have a central scar like that of an FNH. Adenomas appear bright on MRI. Technetium scanning can also be done and will highlight FNH.

The optimal treatment of an adenoma less than 4 cm is stopping all oral contraceptives and monitoring the patient. If the mass does not regress or it is larger than 4 cm, surgical resection is indicated. All lesions in women who may become pregnant should also be resected, regardless of size.

3. Focal Nodular Hyperplasia

Focal nodular hyperplasia presents with a central scar evident on CT scanning. A large arterial supply is also notable. Symptomatic lesions should be resected. There is no malignant potential with FNH.

4. Hemangioma

Hemangiomas are distinguished from FNH and adenomas by their enhancement on T2 weighted MRIs. Tagged red blood cell scanning and arteriography can also be used to confirm the diagnosis. Like FNH, symptomatic lesions should be resected.

5. Hepatocellular Carcinoma

a) Etiology and Pathophysiology

Primary hepatocellular carcinoma is a highly morbid and lethal cancer that commonly occurs following chronic liver injury such as cirrhosis. Etiologies include viral hepatitis (hepatitis B carriers have 220X increased risk, alcohol consumption/cirrhosis, exogenous steroid use (3.2X increased risk), inheritable liver diseases (alpha-1 antitrypsin, hemochromatosis), cigarette smoking (2.4X increased risk), and chemical carcinogens (aflatoxin, vinyl chloride). However, up to one quarter of all patients may develop HCC spontaneously. Metastasis from the liver to the bones, brain, and lungs is common in late stage HCC. HCC composes 2% of all cancers and affects some 10,000 new persons annually. Males are more affected than females. The most common causes include chronic alcoholism, HBV, HCV, hemochromatosis, and aflatoxin poisoning. The fibrolamellar variant has the best outcome.

b) Presentation and Diagnosis

HCC presents with signs and symptoms of liver failure, including jaundice, pruritus, hepatosplenomegaly (often with hepatic nodules as in cirrhosis), bleeding diatheses, cachexia, encephalopathy, asterixis, ascites, and varices. LFTs are elevated along with AFP. Biopsy confirms the diagnosis, while imaging studies are used to determine the extent of disease and whether a surgical approach could be beneficial. The presence of a liver mass in a patient with a history of cirrhosis is hepatocellular carcinoma unless otherwise proven. Over 90% of patients will have an elevation in alpha-fetoprotein. All liver metastases must have an arterial supply and so are susceptible to chemoembolization. A liver tumor with a central, stellate scar is focal nodular hyperplasia.

c) Treatment

(1) *Preoperative Management*

Patients with significant cancer burden who cannot tolerate a straightforward liver resection either due to the volume of the tumor or because of their Child's score may undergo portal venous embolization. This procedure leads to hypertrophy of the liver in carefully selected patients and may permit interval resection of the tumor. Patients who would have less than 20% of functional liver remaining after resection are the ideal candidates.

The Milan criteria are often used to determine whether a patient is a candidate for surgical resection. Patients with a primary tumor less than 5 cm, or up to there tumors each less than 3 cm, are candidates for resection. Patients with Child's A cirrhosis and who meet Milan criteria fare equally well between a liver resection and transplant. Patients with more advanced cirrhosis who may not be candidates for surgical resection should undergo a liver transplant (see page 441).

(2) *Operative Management*

A careful study of the inflow and outflow of the liver should be made, and a thorough preoperative evaluation as discussed earlier in this chapter should be made. The anatomy of the liver should be carefully elucidated, including both the intrahepatic and extrahepatic anatomy. Involvement of the portal vein, hepatic arteries, or hepatic veins may all influence the extent of the resection. Patients that will tolerate surgery and have a sufficient volume of functional liver remaining following resection should undergo resection.

Recurrent tumors of the liver may also be amenable to repeat resection. A

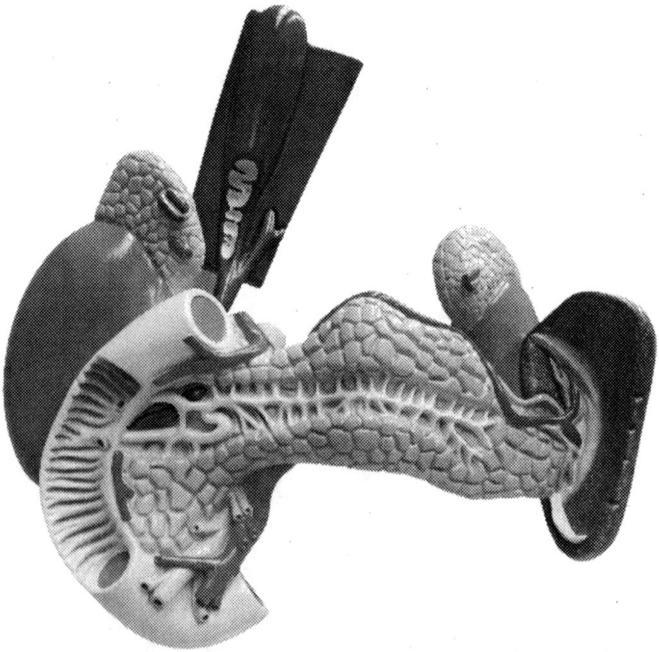

similar type of preoperative workup should take place prior to this procedure. This is also an increasing body of literature describing ablation therapies for recurrent liver cancer.

(3) Nonoperative Management

Radiofrequency ablation (RFA) is a method to eradicate or reduce the volume of a tumor while sparing the surrounding parenchyma. This is a method to precisely target the tumor itself without removing large parts of the liver along anatomic boundaries. The ideal candidate is someone who does not meet criteria for surgical resection and has no evidence of metastatic disease. RFA can also be combined with surgery in selected patients.

(4) Postoperative Management

Neoadjuvant chemotherapy is still being investigated as a potential treatment for hepatocellular carcinoma prior to surgery. Adjuvant chemotherapy is indicated in patients with metastatic cancer to the liver and involves 5-FU, floxuridine, and steroids. Adjuvant therapy has been shown to improve median survival.

d) Metastatic Colorectal Cancer

Metastatic lesions to the liver are most commonly secondary to colon cancer. Prognosis is tied to the number of lesions present. Ideal candidates for resection of liver metastases from colon cancer include those with stage I or II cancer and who originally had an R0 (margin-free) resection. Even aggressive management of more severe lesions appears to improve outcome in carefully selected patients.

III. Gallbladder and Biliary Tree

III.A. General Concepts

1. Anatomy

The biliary system is composed of the gallbladder, bile ducts, and related transport systems to deliver bile from the liver to the duodenum. The right and left hepatic ducts collect bile produced by the thousands of lobules of the liver and transport it to the common hepatic duct and then the gallbladder for bile storage. The common hepatic duct joins with the cystic duct from the gallbladder to form the common bile duct, which transports bile to the duodenum for emulsification of fats and release of waste products from the liver. The common bile duct joins the pancreatic duct to form the common duct, which empties into the duodenum at the ampulla of Vater.

The cystic artery is more commonly a branch off the right hepatic artery, but may occasionally be a branch of the left hepatic, a replaced right or left hepatic, or even the proper hepatic arteries. This artery is visualized when doing a cholecystectomy and found in the triangle of Calot.

2. Physiology

a) Bile Formation

The liver serves to regulate the concentration of toxic chemicals and byproducts within the body. It also processes ingested minerals and nutrients and converts most ingested substances into a more easily used form. The liver serves to create proteins necessary for coagulation, breaks down waste products and uses bile to carry them to the intestines, serves as a storage organ for glucose in the form of glycogen, controls the concentration of amino acids, forms urea from toxic ammonia, stores iron for use with hemoglobin, and produces a number of factors present in inflammatory and immune reactions for control of infection. Bile itself is composed of waste products, cholesterol, and bile salts and is responsible for the dark color of feces. Impaired bile secretion leads to clay-colored stools. Bile is released from the gallbladder through stimulation by CCK (cholecystokinin). Emptying of the gallbladder is inhibited by parasympathetic blockade. The gallbladder absorbs a significant amount of water and sodium through sodium diffusion created by a sodium-potassium ATPase effectively concentrating the bile. Water absorption is linked to this active sodium transport.

b) Bile Salt Metabolism

The most important bile acids are cholic acid, deoxycholic acid, and chenodeoxycholic acid. Bile acids are conjugated with either the amino acid glycine or taurine prior to secretion by the liver. Conjugation increases water solubility and thereby prevents passive reabsorption once secreted into the small intestine. Under normal circumstances, cholesterol, bile salts, and lecithin remain in aqueous solution as bile-salt-lecithin micelles. When the concentration of the bile salts or lecithin decreases, cholesterol mat precipitate out of solution forming cholesterol stones (most common in patients) The concentration of bile acids in the small intestine can thereby stay high enough to form micelles and solubilize lipids. Bile acid salts are reabsorbed in the terminal ileum. The primary bile acids are cholic acid and chenodeoxycholic acid. The secondary bile acids are deoxycholic acid and lithocholic acid formed by anaerobic bacteria in the intestine. Biliverdin is the bile pigment formed from the breakdown of hemoglobin. Urobilinogen is produced by bacteria in the intestines. It can be converted to stercobilin, which gives feces their brown color. It may be converted to urobilin, which is absorbed and secreted in urine. Conjugation of bile acids is required for absorption.

The bile salt pool is approximately 2 grams and is recycled half a dozen times a day. Cholesterol synthesis by the liver replenishes this pool. The cholesterol content in bile is entirely derived from that created by the liver. The rate of this production is inhibited by high cholesterol intake.

3. Diagnostic Imaging

a) Ultrasound

Ultrasound is the test of choice to image the gallbladder and diagnose a wide range of biliary disorders. Features on an ultrasound that are consistent with acute gallbladder disease include wall thickening, the presence of gallstones (including those that may be obstructive), free fluid around the gallbladder, and dilation of the biliary ducts (including the presence of trapped stones).

b) Nuclear Imaging

Nuclear imaging by way of a hepatic 2,6-dimethyl-iminodiacetic acid (HIDA) scan is a method to determine whether the nuclear tracer taken up by the liver makes its way into the gallbladder. Failure to fill the gallbladder indicates a blockage and is strongly suspicious for cholecystitis.

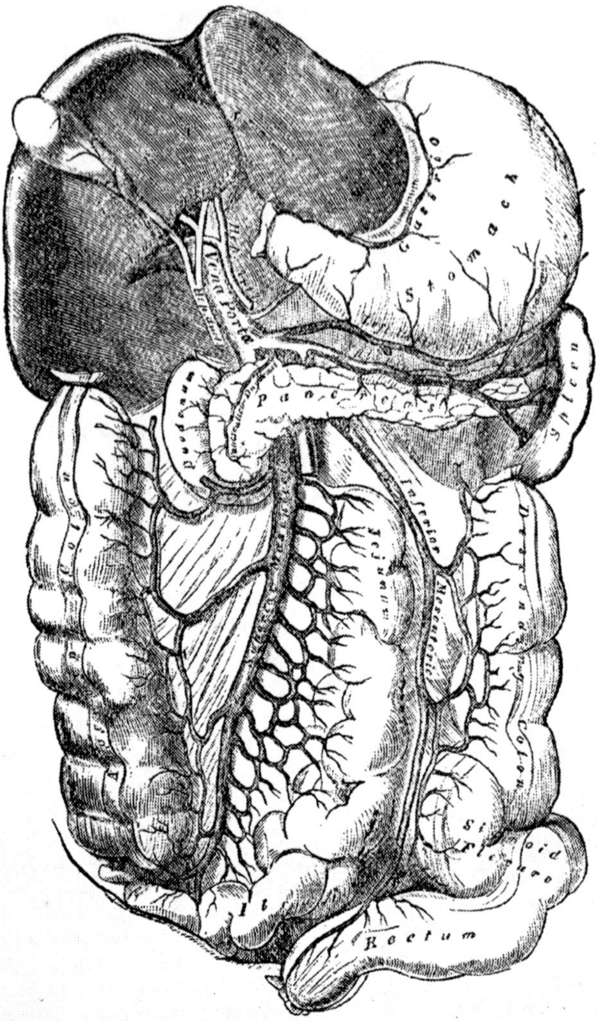

c) CT and MRI

CT imaging will find many of the same gallbladder changes as ultrasound, but has the added benefit of imaging the surrounding anatomy. This is particular valuable when dealing with neoplasms of the gallbladder and biliary system. MRI offers a similar benefit with an increased sensitivity for detecting gallstones compared to CT.

d) ERCP

Endoscopic retrograde cholangiopancreatography (ERCP) with sphincterotomy of the ampulla of Vater is a method to identify and treat stones within the common bile duct. Basket retrieval of stones is possible in most cases and can resolve the immediate presentation of choledocholithiasis. An interval cholecystectomy is still necessary due to the high likelihood of repeat obstruction. About 5% of patients will develop complications from ERCP, including pancreatitis and bleeding.

e) MRCP

Magnetic retrograde cholangiopancreatography (MRCP) is a noninvasive alternative to ERCP and is particularly useful for imaging the bile ducts. This is a sensitive method to evaluate the anatomy when dealing with soft tissue tumors such as cholangiocarcinomas.

f) Intraoperative Cholangiography

Intraoperative cholangiography (IOC) uses radioopaque contrast and fluoroscopy to detail the biliary tree. Patients found to have stones trapped within the common bile duct can subsequently undergo a common bile duct exploration

III.B. Benign Biliary Disease

1. Cholelithiasis

a) Pathophysiology

Cholelithiasis is the formation of gallstones that may lead to a cessation in bile transport. Cholesterol stones are the most common and are typically located in the gallbladder. Stones in the common bile duct tend to be pigmented stones or calcium bilirubinate stones. Pigmented stones are more common in liver disease, alcohol abuse, and hemolytic anemia. It is several times more common in women (found in 8% men, 17% women), and has a number of risk factors including patients who are in their 40's, fertile, female, overweight, currently fasting, rapid weight loss, Crohn disease, hypertriglyceridemia, a history of cystic fibrosis, a familial tendency, sickle cell disease, diabetes, or use of oral contraceptive drugs (OCDs). These risk factors generally tend to cause an increase in cholesterol content in bile, decreased secretion of bile by the liver, and lead to pooling of cholesterol-laden gallstones within the gallbladder. The sludge that is created has difficulty passing through the ducts and may become lodged within the lumen, leading to obstruction and distension of the ductal structures causing the signs and symptoms of cholelithiasis.

b) Presentation

Cholelithiasis presents with colicky, RUQ, may radiate to back or below right scapula pain that lasts several hours. The pain is severe and worsens with eating. Nausea and vomiting accompany this relentless pain, and there is some mild epigastric or RUQ tenderness to palpation but no rebound tenderness.

c) Diagnosis

Diagnosis of cholelithiasis is made by serum blood tests that demonstrate elevated alkaline phosphatase, direct bilirubin, and signs and symptoms of concomitant hepatitis and pancreatitis. As cholesterol stones tend to be radiolucent and only the minority of stones are radioopaque (pigment stones), ultrasound is the best way to detect gallstones and diagnose cholelithiasis. Stones within the common bile duct are diagnosed and treated with ERCP. Cholesterol stones make up 80% of all gallstones and are composed primarily of cholesterol. Pigment stones are found about 20% of the time and are made of calcium and bilirubin. Risk factors for pigment stones include cirrhosis, biliary tract infections, and red blood cell dyscrasias.

d) Treatment

Patients with biliary colic secondary to their gallstone burden are candidates for a cholecystectomy. Barring the presence of gallstone cancer or a particularly hostile abdomen, a laparoscopic is favored due to its shorter hospital stay and decreased pain. Patients who are poor surgical candidates, are medically unstable, or who would otherwise not realize the benefit of cholecystectomy may do better with the placement of a cholecystostomy tube.

Although there are many variations, the standard approach for a laparoscopic cholecystectomy is with the patient in the supine position. An infraumbilical incision is made and a Hasson cannula inserted to achieve pneumoperitoneum. A 30 degree laparoscopic camera is inserted and a diagnostic laparoscopy completed. An 11 mm port is established just below the xiphoid and to the right of the falciform ligament. The liver edge is retracted and the gallbladder visualized. Two 5 mm ports are established laterally to help retract the gallbladder superiorly and laterally. The triangle of Calot is identified and the critical view of safety established. The cystic artery and duct should be clearly identified, along with the inferior edge of the liver and the location of the bile duct.

The peritoneal reflection and surrounding fat are dissected away from the cystic artery and duct until both structures are clearly visualized. An angled dissector is then used to isolate each of the structures, typically starting with the cystic duct. An intraoperative cholangiogram may be performed to delineate the biliary tree and confirm the identity of the cystic duct, verify that there are no stones trapped in the common bile duct, and that there are no other accessory ducts. The cystic duct is then ligated with clips, followed by ligation of the cystic artery. Care must be taken to avoid injury to any recurrent or replaced hepatic vessels, especially a replaced right hepatic artery. The gallbladder is then dissected free from its fossa on the liver (segments 4b and 5).

The critical view of safety has been well described in the literature and is the key to preventing a common bile duct injury during dissection and ligation. Knowledge of the variations in the cystic duct and cystic artery is necessary to avoid injury to the hepatic arteries and common bile duct. Although some practitioners will complete an IOC with all cases, the specific indications include patients with jaundice, choledocholithiasis, and changes in the LFTs. An intraoperative cholangiogram performed following a laparoscopic cholecystectomy with no proximal ducts found should elicit open exploration.

Major injuries during a laparoscopic procedure include inadvertent damage to the right hepatic artery and damage to the common bile duct. Brisk bleeding that cannot be controlled laparoscopically may necessitate conversion to an open procedure via a large right subcostal incision. The Pringle maneuver in which a Penrose drain is passed through the foramen of Winslow and around the portal triad will stop inflow to the liver and permit visualization.

If a common bile duct injury occurs during a cholecystectomy, the proper treatment is returning the patient to the operating room and to permit an experienced surgeon perform a hepaticojejunostomy. Advanced gallbladder cancer is another reason to convert to an open procedure so that the appropriate liver resection can be completed.

The formation of an empyema secondary to spillage is an occasional complication of cholecystectomy. For this reason, many practitioners favor copious irrigation above and around the liver in cases that have frank spillage of bile from a ruptured gallbladder. Drain placement and antibiotic coverage will treat most cases of empyema.

The morbidity due to a laparoscopic cholecystectomy is about 3%, and the mortality about 1%. Hemorrhage, infection, disability from anesthesia, biliary tree injuries, vascular injury, and organ injury are the most common problems. The use of carbon dioxide insufflation can lead to gas embolism, which may present as a sudden decrease in end tidal CO_2. Treatment is to place the patient in the left lateral decubitus position to facilitate gas bubble absorption by the right atrium.

The presence of a cystic duct leak can be initially treated with ERCP for stenting. Otherwise, a cystic duct leak with a biloma is treated with a sphincterotomy followed by percutaneous drainage. A patient who undergoes an uncomplicated laparoscopic cholecystectomy but then develops a stricture at the left and right biliary ducts years later has cholangiocarcinoma until otherwise proven.

2. Acute Cholecystitis

a) Etiology and Pathophysiology

Cholecystitis is inflammation and infection that results following cholelithiasis and obstruction. Nearly ¾ of all presentations of cholecystitis have concurrent infection by enteric bacteria, including E. coli, Klebsiella, Enterococcus, and Bacteroides species. Other causes of cholecystitis include abscess and tumors.

b) Presentation

Charcot's triad is positive in cholecystitis, including fever, jaundice, and RUQ pain. Anorexia, nausea and vomiting are common as well. Guarding and rebound tenderness are common, and a positive Murphy's sign is often present (inspiration is suddenly arrested during palpation of the RUQ). Murphy's sign is very sensitive for cholecystitis.

c) Diagnosis and Treatment

Diagnosis of cholecystitis is best made with a HIDA scan. Elevated PMNs and positive ultrasound findings increase the clinical suspicion of cholecystitis. Cholecystitis is treated with antibiotic administration, pain control with meperidine, and cholecystectomy (preferred therapy unless high risk patient). Complications of cholecystitis include the formation of hydrops, gangrene/perforation, abscesses and fistulas, gallstone ileus, and pancreatitis.

One variant of cholecystitis is with acalculus cholecystitis, which occurs in about 10% of all cases. In this situation, there is increased morbidity and mortality. Risk factors for acalculus cholecystitis include increased age, systemic disorders such as diabetes, infections such as HIV, surgery, labor of pregnancy, gallbladder torsion, and vasculitis. Another variant of cholecystitis is emphysematous cholecystitis caused by Clostridium infection leading to gangrene and perforation. Immediate antibiotic treatment and surgery is required.

In severe cholecystitis, a cholecystoduodenal fistula may form and occasionally lead to gallstone ileus when a large gallstone causes obstruction within the small bowel. Gallstone ileus presents with nausea, vomiting, signs of a bowel obstruction, and pneumobilia on imaging. Surgical management includes removal of the gallstone via an enterostomy, cholecystectomy, and repair of the fistula.

Biliary dyskinesia occasionally occurs due to a dysfunction of the sphincter of Oddi. Treatment is by way of a sphincterotomy to relieve the high pressure within the biliary system.

Mirizzi syndrome occurs rarely and is secondary to a large gallstone within the gallbladder that causes an external obstruction upon the hepatic duct. Mirizzi syndrome presents with jaundice and is commonly secondary to chronic cholecystitis. Treatment is via cholecystectomy.

3. Choledocholithiasis

Approximately 8-16% of patients with cholelithiasis will be found to have stones in the common bile duct. Development or diagnosis of choledocholithiasis following laparoscopic cholecystectomy requires an ERCP to attempt stone removal. The success rate of this procedure is 90% with 1% mortality. A sphincterotomy is routinely done as part of this procedure. Stones larger than 1.5cm or the presence of multiple stones may require a take back to the operating room for a choledocholithotomy with choledochoduodenostomy. A contraindication to ERCP is the presence of duodenal diverticula. ESWL is a possible alternative procedure. The development of shock following ERCP may be due to a retroduodenal perforation.

4. Cholangitis

a) Etiology and Pathophysiology

Ascending cholangitis is due to obstruction of the common bile duct leading to obstruction of the biliary tree. This is a life threatening disease that requires prompt recognition and treatment. The obstruction of the biliary tract can lead to biliary stasis, bacterial overgrowth, suppuration, and subsequent biliary sepsis under pressure. Other causes include tumors, benign post procedure strictures, foreign bodies, and parasitic infections that lead to the blockade of the biliary tree.

b) Presentation

Cholangitis presents with Charcot's triad, including fever, RUQ pain, and jaundice (seen in 50-70% of the cases). Reynold's pentad may also develop, which includes the tripartite Charcot's triad in addition to altered mental status and shock. Reynold's pentad is an indicator of poor outcome.

c) Diagnosis and Treatment

Diagnosis of choledocholithiasis is made by laboratory test that show leukocytosis, hyperbilirubinemia and elevated liver function tests. Initial imaging should include ultrasound looking for the presence of ductal dilatation and gallstones along with thickening of the bile duct walls, liver abscess, gas in biliary tree to be strongly suggestive. It is treated with IV fluids and vasopressors to maintain BP, antibiotics to cover enteric flora to prevent cholecystitis, use of ERCP to remove the biliary tree blockade, and surgery to permit the resumption of bile flow. Ascending cholangitis is an emergency.

5. Gallstone Pancreatitis

a) Assessment

Gallstone pancreatitis is the development of pancreatitis due to an obstructing gallstone. This gallstone is typically located in the distal common bile duct, which shares its passageway with the main pancreatic duct. About 5% of patients with cholelithiasis present with gallstone pancreatitis. An intraoperative cholangiogram that indicates no emptying into the duodenum when performed for gallstone pancreatitis can be checked by giving glucagon to the patient.

b) Management

Therapy involves supportive care until amylase and lipase return to normal. An ERCP with sphincterotomy and stone retrieval is typically indicated in patients who do not spontaneously pass the stone and return to their baseline quickly. The presence of choledocholithiasis on gallbladder ultrasound necessitates an ERCP prior to operative intervention. A patient who has had resolution of gallstone pancreatitis should be treated with a laparoscopic cholecystectomy with a cholangiogram within the same hospitalization. The risk of recurrent disease is as high as 50% within a month without cholecystectomy.

6. Biliary Stricture

The most common causes of biliary stricture formation include trauma during a laparoscopic cholecystectomy and an inflammatory process such as Crohn disease or pancreatitis. Damage to the arteries that supply the common bile duct can also occur with extended dissection near the portal triad.

Direct repair of any bile duct injuries is also thought to increase the likelihood of future stricture development due to scarring. Stent placement is favored as the treatment for biliary stricture.

7. Primary Sclerosing Cholangitis

a) Pathophysiology

Primary sclerosing cholangitis is an inflammatory narrowing of the bile ducts that affects men ages 20-50. PSC is common in patients with ulcerative colitis, and presents as chronic, progressive inflammation and scarring of the bile ducts. It is thought that PSC is due to a hypersensitivity reaction.

b) Diagnosis and Treatment

Diagnosis of PSC is made by ultrasound (US), ERCP, and PTC. ERCP and biopsy are necessary to rule out malignancy. PSC presents with elevated alkaline phosphatase, GGT, bilirubin, and symptoms of cholestasis and liver disease. Treatment is through surgical intervention to decompress the biliary tree via a transhepatic stent placement. Worsening disease may need to be treated by way of a liver transplant.

III.C. Malignant Biliary Disease

1. Gallbladder Polyps

Polyps of the gallbladder affect about 5% of all patients and are secondary to cholesterol accumulation. Most polyps are benign; however the presence of sessile polyps increases the risk of malignancy and should be treated with a cholecystectomy. Patients with polyps over 1 cm should also be treated with removal of the gallbladder to avoid the risk of cancer.

2. Gallbladder Cancer

a) Etiology and Epidemiology

Gallbladder cancer is a rare and often fatal disease with a dismal 5 year survival. Only 1 in 100 patients who undergo a cholecystectomy are found to have gallbladder cancer. Larger gallstones are associated with an increase in risk of cancer due to chronic inflammation.

b) Pathophysiology

The majority of gallbladder cancers are adenocarcinomas that fall into the papillary, nodular, or tubular types. Papillary gallbladder adenocarcinoma has the best prognosis. Involvement of Calot's lymph node near the gallbladder occurs early via lymphatic spread and subsequent disease can lead to painless jaundice from biliary obstruction. Gallbladder cancer is associated with mutations in p53 and K-ras.

Prognosis is characterized by the depth of tumor invasion, the number of nodes affected, and the presence of metastatic disease (i.e. TNM system). Depth of tumor invasion is particularly important as the gallbladder wall is composed of only a mucosa and serosa – and the serosa is not present at the gallbladder fossa. Stage I cancers are in-situ and go no further than the perimuscular layer. Stage II cancers have penetrated the serosa and/or the liver. Stage III is locally advanced cancer, and stage IV cancers are metastatic.

c) Presentation and Diagnosis

Gallbladder cancer is often an incidental finding on imaging studies completed for other reasons. Occasionally, cancer will present with cholelithiasis or cholecystitis. Ascites and jaundice are also sometimes evident. Although not as specific as once believed, a porcelain gallbladder on imaging studies is also highly suspicious for underlying malignancy. The diagnosis of cholelithiasis or cholecystitis is confirmed by ultrasound, while CT or MRI will be more specific. Asymmetrical wall thickening and evidence of invasion are specific signs seen on CT or MRI.

d) Treatment

Most stage I tumors are diagnosed after the gallbladder is already removed for symptomatic disease. As a result, most patients will undergo a laparoscopic cholecystectomy. However, if the diagnosis is made a priori, a diagnostic laparoscopy is completed first to evaluate for metastatic or unresectable disease. If stage I cancer is confirmed, a simple cholecystectomy will suffice and is likely to lead to a cure. Stage II cancer should ideally be treated by way of a radical cholecystectomy, which includes resection of at least a 2 cm margin of the liver, but more commonly a sectionectomy with segments 4b and 5. Lymphadenectomy is also completed due to the potential of lymphatic spread. 5 year survival in these patients approaches 100%.

Stage III and IV cancer should be treated surgically if there is a chance for near R0 resection as there is evidence for improved survival. A sectionectomy is commonly completed for stage III cancers, but most authors favor an extended right hepatectomy. An extended right hepatectomy is also the procedure of choice for stage IV cancer. Reconstruction of the biliary tree via a Roux-en-Y hepaticojejunostomy is often completed due to the involvement of the common bile duct. Skeletonization of the portal triad is done if there is no direct involvement of the common bile duct.

3. Cholangiocarcinoma

a) Etiology and Epidemiology

Cholangiocarcinoma can arise anywhere along the biliary tree (see separate discussion in pediatric surgery chapter on page 513). Cholangiocarcinoma affects about 1 in 100,000 patients and is among the rarest of the hepatobiliary tumors. The risk of cancer goes up in patients with inflammatory diseases, biliary infections, and exposure to carcinogens. At the time of diagnosis, many tumors are locally advanced and with a poor outlook.

b) Pathophysiology

Cholangiocarcinomas are commonly adenocarcinomas. The papillary subtype has a superior prognosis. Anatomy guides surgery: tumors within the liver may only be treatable with liver transplant; tumors along the portal triad may be treated with excision and hepaticojejunostomy; tumors within the pancreas may require a pancreaticoduodenectomy.

c) Presentation and Diagnosis

Extrahepatic cholangiocarcinoma typically presents with painless jaundice, but occasionally leads to cholangitis in about a quarter of patients. Intrahepatic cholangiocarcinoma is often asymptomatic, but alkaline phosphatase tends to be elevated. Ultrasound, CT scanning, MRCP, and MRI confirm the diagnosis and are useful for anatomic guidance.

d) Treatment

Prior to surgery, patients with severe symptoms may benefit from an ERCP-guided stent placement. Routine placement is not recommended due to the risk of infection. As discussed above, patients with disease restricted to the head of the pancreas benefit from a pancreaticoduodenectomy. In the rare case that the disease is restricted to a portion of the common bile duct that can be resected, primary resection with formation of a hepaticojejunostomy can be completed. Proximal tumors (i.e. Klatskin tumor) can be treated with an extended hepatectomy in carefully selected patients. Despite maximum medical and surgical management, five year survival rates are dismal and hover at about 10-30%.

Adjuvant therapy is still being explored as an option.

IV. Pancreas

IV.A. General Concepts

1. Anatomy

The pancreas occupies a retroperitoneal position in the abdomen located dorsal to the stomach and extends between the right and left upper quadrants. The widest part of the pancreas is known as the head, and is located within the first section of the intestines. In its entirety, it extends from the duodenal c-shaped loop (second portion of the duodenum) to a more cephalad position in the hilum of the spleen. The left side tapers and travels somewhat superiorly and is known as the body of the pancreas. The pancreas is composed of exocrine tissue that secretes digestive enzymes into the small intestine and endocrine tissue that secretes hormones into the bloodstream.

The blood supply to the head of the pancreas is from the superior and inferior branches emanating from the gastroduodenal artery and superior mesenteric artery, respectively. The head of the pancreas is intimately associated with the second portion of the duodenum and anterior and posterior pancreaticoduodenal vessels supply both structures (originating from the superior and inferior pancreaticoduodenal vessels off gastroduodenal and superior mesenteric arteries). In the event of a transection of the pancreatic neck, a distal pancreatectomy should be done. The dorsal pancreatic artery is a branch of the splenic artery, and supplies (along with the transverse pancreatic artery off the left gastroepiploic artery) the body and tail of the pancreas along with a bit of the head. Posterior arcades of the left gastroepiploic artery anastomose with dorsal and transverse pancreatic arteries to provide additional blood supply.

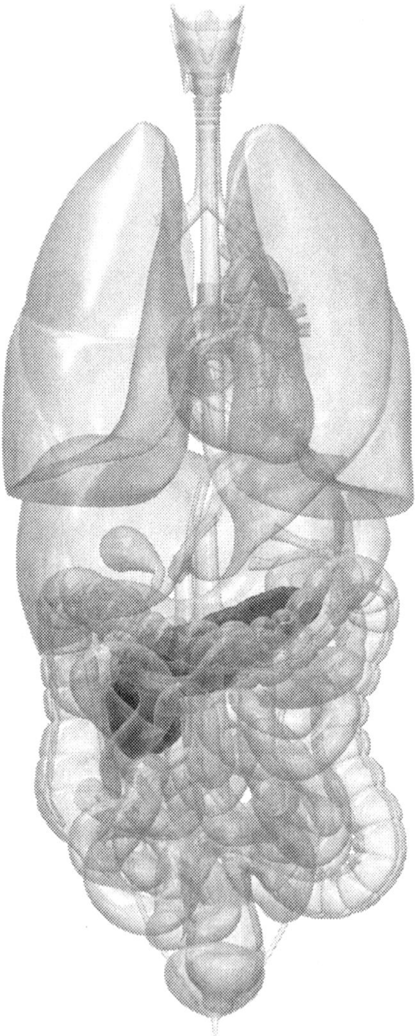

Venous drainage of the pancreas parallels the arterial supply and lies superficial terminates in the portal vein which arises posterior to the neck of the pancreas at the confluence of the superior mesenteric and splenic veins. As a result, splenic vein occlusion leading to gastric varices is possible with pancreatic cancer. Gastric varices occur due to retrograde venous drainage from flow diversion into the short gastric and left gastroepiploic veins.

2. Physiology

The exocrine pancreas serves a distinct function from the endocrine pancreas, even though the two tissues are juxtaposed within the same organ. The exocrine pancreas releases a number of enzymes into the pancreatic duct in an inactive form. These digestive enzymes are activated by the acidic environment within the duodenum and break down carbohydrates, proteins, and fats. The exocrine pancreas also secretes bicarbonate to neutralize the hydrochloric acid produced by the parietal cells of the stomach. Nearly 3L of bicarbonate and enzyme-rich fluid are produced every day by the pancreas, and the release of these compounds is facilitated by cholecystokinin (CCK), secretin, and bile salts.

The endocrine pancreas secretes insulin and glucagon to regulate the titer of sugar within the bloodstream, and also somatostatin to control the function of the intestines and modulate the concentration of insulin and glucagon. The amount of bicarbonate secretion from the pancreas is inversely related to the amount of chloride secretion.

IV.B. Benign Pancreatic Disease

1. Pancreas Divisum

Fusion failure between the minor (Santorini) and major (Wirsung) pancreatic ducts leads to pancreatic divisum. Pancreatitis is common from the insufficient drainage. ERCP is difficult to complete due to the small size of the duct. Treatment is via stent placement into the minor papilla.

2. Annular Pancreas

An annular pancreas wraps around the entire duodenum and is due to failure of normal clockwise rotation of the ventral pancreas during ontogeny. The eventual presentation is a partial small bowel obstruction, peptic ulcer disease, and chronic pancreatitis. Treatment involves a duodenojejunostomy; resection of the pancreas is not indicated.

3. Pancreatic Fisulta

The formation of a pancreatic fistula typically results between the pancreas and transverse colon. Greater than 200 ml / day output is classified as a high output fistula. Treatment involves conversion to TPN, use of somatostatin, and time to permit spontaneous closure. Failure of a high output fistula to close requires a roux-en-Y diversion to the fistula. A distal pancreatectomy can also be performed if the fistula is located in the body or tail.

4. Acute Pancreatitis

a) Etiology

Acute pancreatitis is the result of direct damage from prematurely activated pancreatic enzymes digesting the parenchyma of the organ. 80-90% of patients with chemical pancreatitis will experience only mild symptoms with self limiting course and recover fully with supportive care. Severe disease can lead to systemic inflammatory response syndrome (SIRS) and subsequently progress to severe septic shock, multi-organ system failure, and adult respiratory distress syndrome (ARDS).

b) Pathophysiology

Causes of acute pancreatitis include perforation of a alcoholism, peptic ulcer, neoplastic disorders, cholelithiasis, end stage renal disease (ESRD), endoscopic retrograde cholangiopancreatography (ERCP), malnutrition leading to anorexia, direct trauma to the pancreas, certain infections, use of drugs that lead to toxic byproducts, burn injuries, surgery, and scorpion bites. The most common causes are alcohol abuse and gallstones. Metabolic conditions that predispose to pancreatitis include severe hypertriglyceridemia, and hypercalcemia. Medications that can lead to pancreatitis include oral hypoglycemic agents, thiazide diuretics, furosemide, pentamidine, TMP-SMX, and DDI.

Acute pancreatitis is divided into one of six major classes depending on the severity of the inflammation. Mild acute pancreatitis presents with rapid onset of symptoms and self-limiting pancreatic dysfunction. Severe acute pancreatitis leads to systemic manifestations of disease and involves disruption of the pancreas. Acute fluid collections may occur with acute pancreatitis and are reactionary to the ongoing pancreatic dysfunction. Pseudocyst formation with fluid enclosed by a reactionary fibrotic process may develop in acute pancreatitis. Pancreatic necrosis is a more serious manifestation of acute pancreatitis secondary to premature release of active digestive enzymes from the pancreas. Infection in the setting of acute pancreatitis may manifest as abscess formation at the pancreas.

c) Presentation

Acute pancreatitis presents as severe epigastric pain that radiates to the back. The pain worsens after consumption of food and may improve if the patient leans forward. Nausea and vomiting are common, as is fever, tachypnea (to avoid deep breaths that may lead to further irritation of the already inflamed pancreas), a positive Cullen sign, and a positive Turner sign. Cullen sign is the presence of a bluish hue to the umbilicus due to hemorrhaging within the peritoneum – it is most commonly found in necrotizing pancreatitis. Turner sign is a bluish discoloration in the flanks due to hemoglobin deposition and decomposition in the soft tissue. Abdominal exam typically reveals tenderness and involuntary guarding, but no rebound tenderness. Metabolic derangements in pancreatitis include a decrease in calcium, magnesium, and hematocrit. An increase in WBC, BUN/Cr, bilirubin, LFTs, and glucose can occur.

d) Diagnosis

Acute pancreatitis is diagnosed primarily by blood tests that indicate elevations in amylase and lipase. Neither of these two enzymes are 100% specific to the pancreas, and they may be elevated in a number of other conditions. Perforation of the gastrointestinal system may lead to elevations in amylase; this enzyme is also found in the salivary glands, small intestine, reproductive organs such as the testes and ovaries, and in striated muscle. Renal disease and hypertriglyceridemia also lead to elevations in amylase. Lipase is found throughout the gastrointestinal system and the liver. Notwithstanding, very high elevations in both amylase and lipase are often pathognomonic for acute pancreatitis. Overall, the most specific test for pancreatitis is lipase levels, while the most sensitive test is amylase titers. The presence of acute pancreatitis with hyponatremia may be due to significant hypertriglyceridemia.

e) Diagnostic Imaging Tests

The diagnosis of acute pancreatitis can be confirmed through various imaging tests. As acute pancreatitis progresses, various anatomical changes can occur including the development of a pseudocyst, abscess, phlegmon, splenic vein thrombosis, and clear evidence of pancreatic necrosis. These changes are detectable on a CT scan. The earliest changes that can be detected are the development of a phlegmon, which is typically obvious within a couple of days. Pancreatic necrosis and pseudocyst formation are typically apparent within a couple of weeks. Abscess formation is clear within a month or two. Plain films are also of some value in diagnosis. Chest X-rays (CXR) are taken

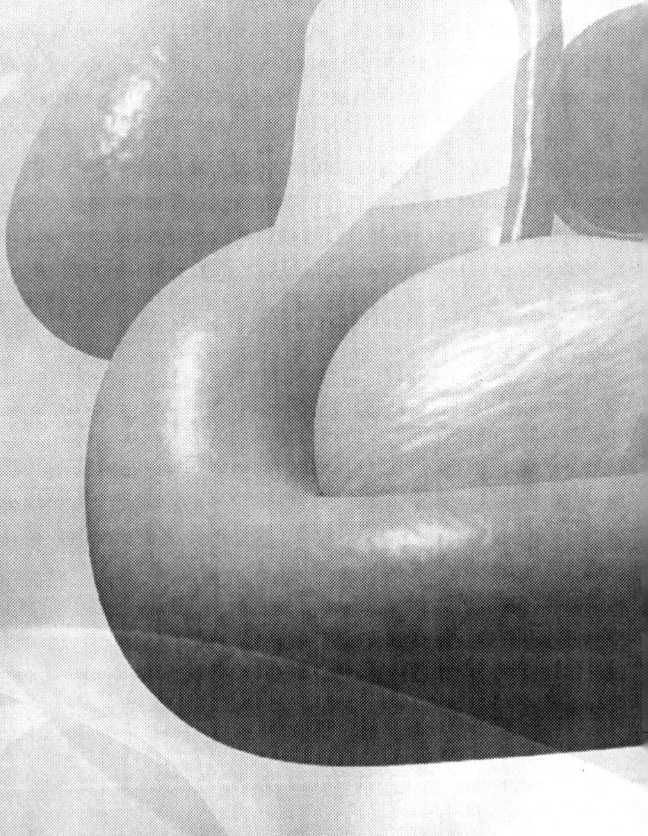

to determine pancreatitis-induced pleural effusions or elevations in part of the diaphragm. Abdominal X-rays (AXR) are taken to detect calcification within the pancreas, which is actually a better predictor of chronic pancreatitis instead of acute pancreatitis. Ultrasound is used to identify gallstones as the causative agent of pancreatitis, and once identified; they may be removed with ERCP. Amylase has a sensitivity of 90%.

f) Treatment

Treatment of acute pancreatitis is to treat reversible causes such as alcoholism and gallstones (treat with ERCP). Complications of acute pancreatitis such as pseudocyst or abscess formation may be drained with CT-guided aspiration. Most cases are self-limited, and so the standard of care is to provide supportive therapy, IV fluids, pain control with meperidine or fentanyl, and bowel rest. A nasogastric tube is used to decompress the GI system. Morphine is historically not used with pancreatitis due to the risk of sphincter of Oddi spasms, but this has not been borne out in clinical practice. Surgical debridement is used in with infected pancreatic necrosis. Gastric varices may be treated with splenectomy to avoid splenic vein thrombosis.

Prolonged bowel rest may be required to minimize the extent of inflammation and damage. Total parenteral nutrition (TPN) may be necessary in this case. Extended periods of nil per os (NPO) status may be beneficial in patients with severe systemic manifestations of pancreatitis and evidence of ongoing injury (i.e. severe acute pancreatitis). Patients with less severe disease may benefit from placement of a post-pancreatic feeding tube (i.e. jejunostomy tube) so that enteral nutrition can be implemented.

g) Prognosis

The prognosis of acute pancreatitis is gauged by Ranson criteria. Mortality depends on the number of risk factors present. The risk factors are divided into those present on admission and those that develop after two days. Risk factors that increase the risk of mortality and may present on admission include age over 55, elevations in blood sugar over 200, elevated white blood cell (WBC) counts over 16,000, elevated aspartate transaminase (AST) over 250, and elevated lactate dehydrogenase (LDH) over 350. Risk factors present after two days include a decrease of more than 10% in the hematocrit (HCT), increase in BUN over 5, calcium less than 8, PO2 less than 60 mmHg, a base deficit greater than 4, and a fluid deficit of more than 6 L. The risk of mortality is low if less than two risk factors are present. Two through four risk factors carries a 1/6 risk of death. Five or 6 risk factors increase the mortality to 2/5, and more than 6 risk factors have a mortality that approaches 100%.

Table 7. Ranson criteria for pancreatitis.

Criteria on Admission	Criteria Within 48 Hours	Mortality
Age over 55	Hct decrease over 10%	Less than 2 criteria: 1% mortality
WBC over 16,000	BUN increase over 5	2-4 criteria: 16% mortality
Blood glucose over 200	Serum calcium less than 8	5-6 criteria: 40% mortality
AST over 250	PO2 less than 60mmHg	More than 6 criteria: Nearly 100%
LDH over 350	Base deficit greater than 4	
	Fluid deficit more than 6L	

5. Pancreatic Necrosis

a) Assessment

The development of pancreatic necrosis may occur following the onset of acute pancreatitis, sustained chronic pancreatitis, infection, or trauma. Early signs on imaging tests may include gas within the pancreas on CT scan, sometimes referred to as a "soap bubble" sign. CT scan is the gold standard for imaging. Failure to diagnose and treat early may lead to sepsis and ARDS with abdominal findings on physical exam. Amylase tends to be elevated in the early stage of disease, along with an elevation in WBC.

b) Management

For necrotizing pancreatitis, prophylactic antibiotics are not used. Sterile necrosis does not require debridement or drainage. Only evidence of gas or frank abscess needs drainage. Necrosectomy and drainage should happen only 4 weeks after diagnosis and only in symptomatic patients; routine necrosectomy is no longer recommended. Enteral nutrition is preferred. Patients that are not stable for an operation can be treated with a CT-guided drain placement with broad spectrum antibiotics such as imipenem or fluoroquinolones.

About half of all patients with necrotizing pancreatitis will develop an acute infection of the necrosed segment, leading to severe sepsis and death if not immediately corrected. Diagnosis is confirmed by ultrasound or CT-guided aspiration of the potentially infected segment or strong CT evidence of an infection. Treatment involves completion of a necrosectomy, wide drainage, and long term antibiotics. In patients with very severe disease, repeat surgical interventions may be necessary and open packing can be instituted. Despite aggressive surgical management, mortality still hovers near 25%.

6. Pancreatic Pseudocyst

About 1 in 10 patients with pancreatitis will develop a walled off fluid collection known as a pseudocyst. Pseudocysts have the risk of becoming infected. Patients with symptomatic disease should undergo percutaneous drainage. Very large pseudocysts may be drained on an individual basis. Recurrence following percutaneous drainage remains high, and selected patients may undergo a cystgastrostomy or cystduodenostomy to facilitate drainage.

7. Hemorrhagic Pancreatitis

Hemorrhagic pancreatitis, also known as Flitz syndrome, is a severe complication of acute pancreatitis with a dramatic increase in morbidity and mortality. Severe acute pancreatitis can lead to bleeding due to erosion of proximal vascular structures leading to uncontrolled bleeding. Patients with active bleeding should be managed with an emergent celiotomy following aggressive resuscitation and ventilatory support. Antibiotics are also necessary. In one series of 68 patients found to have hemorrhagic pancreatitis, 16 made it to the operating room and only 6 survived after surgery.

8. Chronic Pancreatitis

a) Etiology and Pathophysiology

Repeated episodes of acute pancreatitis can lead to chronic injury and scarring to the pancreas, thereby inducing the development of chronic pancreatitis. The most common cause of chronic pancreatitis is continued abuse of alcohol. Approximately ¾ of patients with chronic pancreatitis have their disease from alcohol abuse, the remainder tend to be generally idiopathic in nature. Presentation of chronic pancreatitis in younger patients may be a result of cystic fibrosis. Other causes include genetic defects (i.e. PRSS1), inflammatory disorders (i.e. Sjögren syndrome, primary biliary cirrhosis), recurrent acute pancreatitis, and obstruction of the pancreatic duct. About 1 in 10,000 patients are affected with chronic pancreatitis.

b) Presentation

Chronic pancreatitis presents with signs and symptoms similar to acute pancreatitis, including epigastric pain that radiates to the back, and diarrhea with steatorrhea. Malabsorptive disorders are typically present including vitamin deficiencies, elevated blood sugars and polyuria due to damage to the endocrine pancreas leading to diabetes and chronic liver disease.

c) Diagnosis

Diagnosis of chronic pancreatitis is made by history and blood tests that indicate normal amylase and lipase levels but decreased pancreatic enzyme levels such as trypsin deficiencies. Calcifications are seen on abdominal plain films, which strongly raise the clinical suspicion for this disorder. Finally, the secretin stimulation test is used to stimulate bicarbonate production by the pancreas. The pancreatic duct is typically dilated, and calcification with atrophy of the pancreas is a common finding in late disease.

d) Treatment

Treatment for chronic pancreatitis is primarily supportive with modification of risk factors and avoidance of exacerbating activities. Replacement of pancreatic enzymes is often required in addition to dietary changes such as decreased fat intake, vitamin supplements, and use of spontaneously absorbed medium-chain fatty acids. Diabetes induced by chronic pancreatitis should be controlled carefully due to the decrease in both insulin and glucagon. An ERCP should be done to assess the biliary tree and pancreatic duct. If no dilation is found, a pancreaticoduodenectomy, distal pancreatectomy, or Beger procedure can be completed. A dilated pancreatic duct over 7 mm should be treated with either a Puestow or Frey procedure.

Patients with longstanding chronic pancreatitis who have had numerous complications but do not have a dilated pancreatic duct may do better with resection of the entire pancreas via a pancreaticoduodenectomy (Whipple procedure). This resection also includes cholecystectomy, antrectomy, and distal common duct resection, though there are variants that spare the pylorus. This procedure is favored over simple distal pancreatectomy whenever a complex mass or a suspicion of pancreatic cancer exists. A radical distal pancreatectomy removes the vast majority of the pancreas and spleen and retains only the segment that abuts the duodenum.

The Beger procedure is pancreatic head resection, distal pancreaticojejunostomy via a Roux-en-Y, and sparing of the duodenum. The outcome is similar to a radical distal pancreatectomy or Whipple procedure.

The Puestow procedure is creation of a longitudinal pancreaticojejunostomy with the pancreatic duct. The Frey procedure adds a pancreatic head resection to the Puestow and is associated with a higher rate of pain amelioration compared to Puestow alone.

9. Pancreatic Trauma

Patients with pancreatic transection injuries sustained in the course of a trauma should be treated with distal pancreatectomy with splenic preservation. If the patient is not stable or has other major injuries, splenectomy should also be done.

IV.C. Malignant Pancreatic Disease

1. Pancreatic Adenocarcinoma

a) Etiology and Pathophysiology

Pancreatic cancer is an aggressive, often fatal cancer that has an annual incidence of about 1 in 10,000 people. Elderly patients, those with inflammatory gastrointestinal disorders or chronic pancreatitis, and smokers are at increased risk of developing disease.

Defects in BRCA2, DPC4, p53, and p16 have all been implicated as strong risk factors for carcinogenesis in the pancreas. Of these, DPC4 is the most specific risk factor for pancreatic cancer. More advanced disease metastasizes to the liver. A point mutation in K-ras is attributed as the underlying cause for most pancreatic adenocarcinomas.

Over half of all tumors are primarily located in the head or neck of the pancreas, a quarter are in the body or tail, and the remainder affect the entire pancreas. Adenocarcinoma is the most common type of pancreas cancer.

b) Presentation and Diagnosis

Few patients with pancreatic cancer present with obvious symptoms. Anorexia, painless jaundice, pain, and diabetes are some of the potential hallmarks of disease, but many of these become evident only after the onset of locally advanced (i.e. stage III) disease. Diabetes and acute pancreatitis may be earlier indicators of pancreatic cancer, but this is still under investigation. CA 19-9 in conjunction with CT and ERCP can improve the specificity and sensitivity of diagnosis to nearly 100%. CA 19-9 is also used as an indicator for tumor recurrence and is followed similar to how PSA levels may be followed for prostate cancer. CT imaging is the noninvasive test of choice as it provides information about the tumor location and the surrounding anatomy. ERCP has the added benefit of potentially providing a tissue diagnosis, but biopsy-proven cancer is not necessary prior to proceeding to the operating room.

Several criteria are used to assess patients as potential candidates for operative intervention. Cancer that invades the superior mesenteric vein (SMV) or portal vein in the context of pancreatic head cancer indicates a potentially unresectable cancer. However, involvement of the SMV with pancreatic tail cancer is only a relative contraindication. Involvement of major arteries or nearby organs is typically an indication to proceed with palliative management. Endoscopic ultrasound (EUS) may assist with the staging of pancreatic cancer.

The TNM classification is used for pancreatic cancer. Unlike most other cancers, even patients with stage IA cancer have only a 20% 5 year survival. Significant 5 year survival for stage III or IV cancer is virtually unheard of.

c) Treatment of Resectable Cancer

For cancer located in the head of the pancreas without extensive metastasis, a Whipple procedure is the surgery of choice. A Whipple procedure consists of an antrectomy, cholecystectomy, choledochectomy, pancreaticoduodenectomy, proximal jejunectomy, excision of all regional lymph nodes, followed by reconstruction via a gastrojejunostomy, pancreaticojejunostomy, and choledochojejunostomy. Mortality following a Whipple surgery is about 5-10%. A fully resected tumor still requires 5-FU and radiation. A pylorus-preserving procedure can be done in selected patients and recent research indicates no difference in survival between the procedures. Modifying the procedure to include a total pancreatectomy and splenectomy has also shown no difference in survival.

The operation begins with an examination of all structures to ensure that the cancer is resectable. The Kocher maneuver is performed to evaluate the retropancreatic space and to ensure that the pancreas can be separated from the underlying portal vein, SMV, IVC, and aorta. The uncinate process is examined in relation to the SMA. The distal stomach and pylorus are mobilized and the anchoring ligaments (hepatogastric and hepatoduodenal) examined, along with the portal triad. The base of the transverse mesocolon is examined to ensure that the root of the mesentery is intact without deformities, and that the blood supply is intact without evidence of invasive cancer. The lesser sac is explored to examine the anterior pancreas. Resection proceeds with transection of the common hepatic duct and clearing of the local nodes along the celiac axis. The stomach is then transected at the body and antrum and a truncal vagotomy performed. The neck of the pancreas is then transected just left of the portal vein. Reconstruction then occurs by way of gastrojejunostomy, pancreaticojejunostomy, and choledochojejunostomy.

d) Treatment of Unresectable Cancer

The criteria for unresectable pancreatic cancer include the presence of distal metastasis (i.e. liver, pelvis, ligament of Treitz), regional metastasis to celiac nodes or lymph nodes posterior to the common bile duct, and locally invasive tumor into the portal vein or superior mesenteric vein. The presence of unresectable pancreatic cancer in the setting of worsening pain may be treated with a double pancreatic bypass and injection of the splanchnic bed with ethanol. Chemoradiation with 5-FU is typically used as a palliative measure. Treatment is centered on reducing the clinically-significant symptoms, including jaundice, gastric obstruction, and pain. A cholecystojejunostomy or choledochojejunostomy can both be done for palliation in patients who are developing painless jaundice or more serious manifestations of biliary obstruction. Gastrojejunostomy can be done for bowel obstruction. Pain can be treated through destruction of the celiac plexus with ethanol.

2. Pancreatic Lymphoma

Primary lymphoma of the pancreas, such as from NHL, is rare. When present, a CT-guided biopsy is typically used for diagnosis. Staging with bone marrow biopsy and pan-CT scan is necessary. Patients with clinical symptoms, including anorexia, jaundice, and abdominal pain, may need biliary decompression via percutaneous transhepatic catheterization. Localized disease can be successfully treated with local resection. Chemotherapy with doxorubicin has been shown to be successful for more advanced disease.

V. Spleen

V.A. General Concepts

1. Anatomy

The spleen is a 200 g organ that abuts the stomach and pancreas in the left upper quadrant of the abdomen. The vascular supply to this organ arises from the splenic artery, a major branch of the celiac artery. The splenic artery divides into 3-5 branches that become end arteries within the spleen. The left gastroepiploic artery gives off the short gastric arteries, which also supply the spleen. The splenic artery travels outside the pancreas, while the splenic vein penetrates the parenchyma of the pancreas. The splenic vein joins the inferior mesenteric vein, then coalesces with the superior mesenteric vein to form the portal vein.

Suspensory ligaments of the spleen keep this organ in its shielded position under the rib cage. The splenogastric ligament contains the short gastric

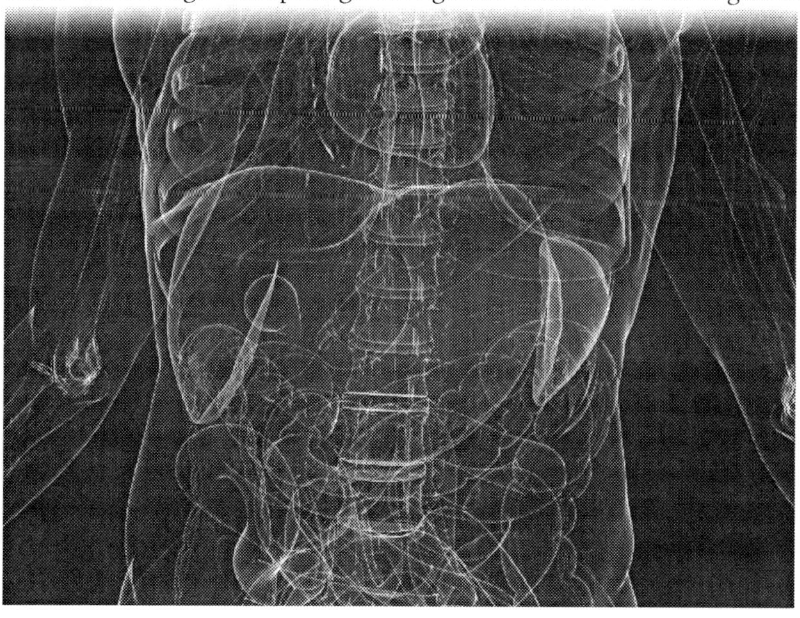

arteries; the splenorenal ligament is avascular and connects the spleen to Gerota's fascia. The splenic flexure of the colon is tented to the spleen via the splenocolic ligament.

2. Physiology

The spleen plays an important immunologic role in cultivating B and T cells and enhancing immunoreactivity against encapsulated organs. This predominantly occurs in the white pulp of the spleen. The red pulp plays a hematologic role and eliminates red blood cells from the circulation that have become senescent or damaged. This typically occurs within the trabeculae of the spleen. Hematopoiesis briefly occurs in the spleen during ontogeny. At any time, 5% of the blood flow in the body will travel through the spleen. The spleen also serves as a large reservoir for platelets and macrophages.

Destruction of the spleen removes the ability to combat encapsulated organs and can make an individual susceptible to specific types of infection. Overwhelming postsplenectomy sepsis (OPSS) can occur in susceptible individuals, particularly the very young or those with hyposplenism. OPSS leads to a rapid and fulminant infection by S. pneumoniae, H. influenzae, N. meningitides, S. aureus, E. coli, or P. aeruginosa. Vaccination against S. pneumoniae, H. influenzae, and N. meningitides are recommended two weeks prior to elective surgery, or as soon as possible following emergent surgery. Hyposplenism can present with a reactive leukocytosis and thrombocytosis following surgery. Hypersplenism traditionally presents with pancytopenia prior to surgery and nearly normal counts following surgery.

V.B. Metabolic and Degenerative Disease

1. Thrombotic Thrombocytopenic Purpura

Thrombotic thrombocytopenic purpura (TTP) is platelet hyperreactivity that leads to plugging of arterioles, organ damage, and fever. Treatment is with FFP, steroids, and plasmapheresis. Patients with severe disease who have failed medical management are candidates for splenectomy, and most patients who have had TTP for an extended period of time have undergone this procedure.

2. Immune Thrombocytopenic Purpura

Immune thrombocytopenia purpura (ITP) is the development of an IgG antibody against platelets that leads to their destruction within the spleen. Symptomatic disease that leads to plummeting platelet counts and subsequent spontaneous bleeding is an indication for splenectomy. There is a nearly 10% chance of death per year in patients with platelet counts near 10,000. Alternatives to surgery include steroids and intravenous IgG (IVIG).

3. Hemolytic Disorders

a) Autoimmune Hemolytic Anemia

Hemolytic anemia secondary to autoantibodies against red blood cells (i.e. spectrin) presents with anemia and jaundice. A direct Coombs test is positive and the disease may be instigated by an allergic reaction to hydralazine, quinidine, or penicillin. Involvement of the spleen typically involves IgG, which is positive on a warm antibody test and a potential indication for splenectomy. Involvement of IgM leads to destruction of RBCs within the liver, and splenectomy in these patients is not beneficial.

Felty syndrome is an autoimmune neutropenia secondary to IgG antibodies against neutrophils. Felty syndrome also presents with splenomegaly and rheumatoid arthritis. The treatment for these patients is also splenectomy and helps to avoid the febrile neutropenic complications that can occur.

b) Hereditary Spherocytosis

Decreased deformability of the red blood cells occurs in hereditary spherocytosis and leads to a higher than normal rate of destruction of RBCs. Symptomatic disease presents with anemia, jaundice, pigmented cholelithiasis, and splenomegaly. The treatment for these patients is splenectomy – a partial splenectomy may be sufficient in selected patients.

c) Sickle Cell Anemia

Most patients with sickle cell anemia develop splenomegaly in their formative years from the enhanced RBC destruction, but ultimately develop a fibrosed spleen from repeated cycles of ischemic necrosis. Occasional surgical resection of the spleen may be necessary in young patients with gross symptomatic hypersplenism.

d) Thalassemia

Symptomatic thalassemia major may lead to splenomegaly from increased destruction of red blood cells. Similar to hereditary spherocytosis, this disease may be treated with splenomegaly and may lead to symptomatic improvement.

4. Splenic Vein Thrombosis

Thrombosis of the splenic vein is typically secondary to acute pancreatitis affecting the splenic vein as it passes through the parenchyma of the distal pancreas. Gastric varices may occur from the outflow limitation and may be the only presenting sign. The treatment for symptomatic patients is splenectomy.

V.C. Trauma

Many cases of trauma to the spleen may be managed conservatively. Grade I injuries to the spleen involve lacerations less than 1 cm deep with hematoma involving less than 10% of the surface. Grade II lacerations are up to 3 cm deep and may involve hematoma of less than half of the splenic surface. Grade III lacerations are over 3 cm deep and may have significant hematoma formation. These injuries may need vascular interventional embolization of the affected arteries in order to stabilize the injury.

Grade IV injuries involve major splenic branches, while grade V injuries result in splenic avulsion or total disruption. Most patients with grade IV injuries who are stable will benefit from conservative management and embolization of the affected regions. All unstable patients and those with grade V injuries should be managed in the operating room via splenorraphy, partial splenectomy, or total splenectomy. The most common cause of splenic injury is from blunt trauma. Children with splenic injuries require surgical exploration if significant blood products are required for resuscitation. They may be observed if hemodynamically stable.

V.D. Cancer

1. Leukemia

Advanced chronic lymphocytic leukemia (CLL) can lead to splenomegaly from hypersplenism. CLL in particular can lead to enormous increases in spleen size to the point that it impinges on nearby structures. Radiotherapy can be used to decrease the mass of the spleen, and may be helpful as a pre-operative procedure to make resection easier. Surgery can reduce the effects of the anemia and can quell the effects of the leukemia.

Chronic myelogenous leukemia (CML) also leads to some splenomegaly, and is secondary to the Philadelphia chromosome (t 9,22). Splenectomy in patients who are in the acute phase of CML may have symptomatic relief from splenectomy.

2. Lymphoma

Non-Hodgkin lymphoma presents as a diffuse lymphadenopathy that responds to chemotherapy. Some patients will have disease that involves the spleen and may benefit from splenectomy to help ameliorate their anemia.

Hodgkin lymphoma is occasionally an indication to complete a diagnostic laparoscopy and evaluate the spleen as the nidus of the disease. A diagnostic laparoscopy can change staging and removal of the spleen in affected individuals does not appear to change survival except in patients with stage I or early stage II disease where the lymphoma is still restricted to the spleen. Chemotherapy has been shown to have an improved outcome in patients with more advanced disease.

3. Myelodysplastic Syndrome

Myelodysplastic syndrome can lead to excessive splenomegaly secondary to hypersplenism. Symptomatic disease leads to anemia and sequelae of splenic impingement upon nearby intraabdominal structures; this syndrome typically responds to splenectomy.

ENDOCRINE

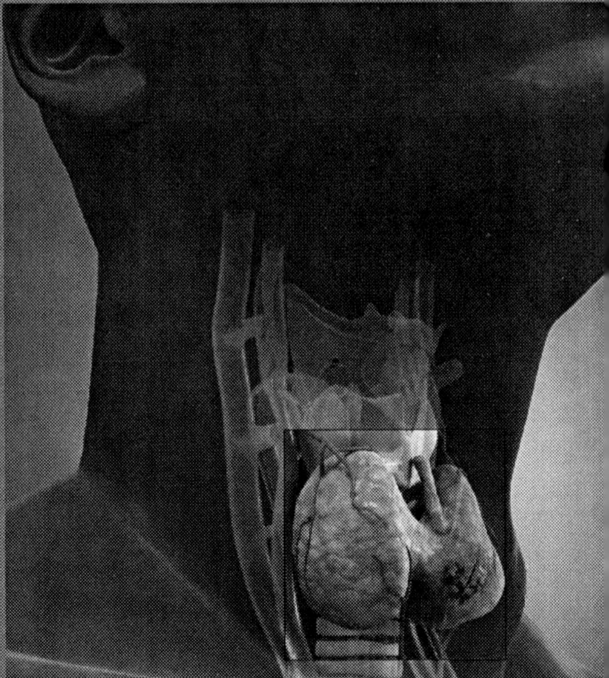

I would like to see the day when somebody would be appointed surgeon somewhere who had no hands, for the operative part is the least part of the work.

Harvey Cushing
Father of Neurosurgery (1869-1939)

SURGISPHERE

ENDOCRINE SURGERY

Sapan S. Desai, M.D., Ph.D. and Randall Scheri, M.D.

I. Breast

I.A. General Concepts

1. Introduction

Surgical evaluation for clinically-significant breast disease is a significant proportion of clinic visits. Breast cancer is the second most common cause of death in women, with nearly a million cases a year throughout the world and 50,000 deaths annually in the US. A multimodal approach toward early diagnosis and decisive treatment is necessary. The selected topics that follow are the most common pathologies and procedures seen in general surgery practice.

2. Anatomy

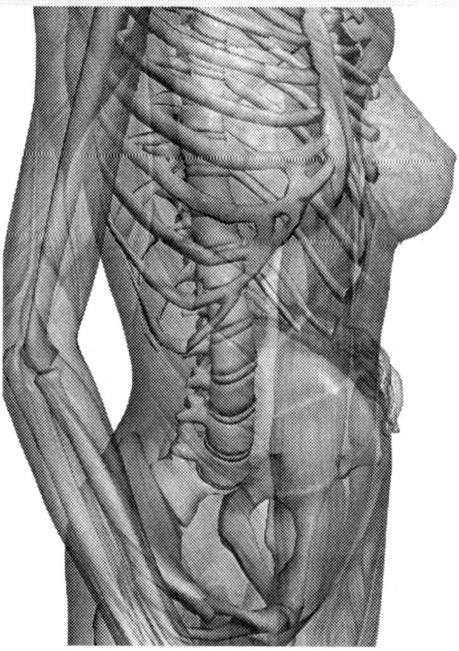

The female breast spans the region between the midline and midaxillary line and extends as a tail into the axilla. The posterior extent is the pectoralis major. Perforating vessels through the pectoralis major supply blood to the breast; these vessels are branches of the internal thoracic and lateral thoracic arteries.

The majority of the lymphatic drainage from the breast is to the axillary lymph nodes. A small portion drains into the internal mammary lymph nodes. The axillary lymph nodes are located within the axillary space, bounded laterally by the latissimus dorsi, inferomedially by the serratus anterior, and superiorly by the axillary vein. The posterior wall of the axilla is the teres major and latissimus dorsi; the anterior wall is the pectoralis major.

Surgeons frequently divide the axillary nodes into three levels: level I lymph nodes are lateral to the pectoralis minor; level II lymph nodes are posterior to the pectoralis minor; level III lymph nodes are medial to the pectoralis minor and are not resected in a modified radical mastectomy. Lymph nodes located between the pectoralis minor and pectoralis major are sometimes known as Rotter's nodes.

Within this space lie a number of critical nerves and vessels. The long thoracic nerve travels closely along the chest wall and innervates the serratus anterior. Damage to this nerve can lead to winged scapula. The thoracodorsal nerve starts posterior to the axillary vessels and crosses the floor of the axilla to reach the latissimus dorsi. Damage to this nerve leads to difficulty while doing pull ups. Damage to the intercostobrachial nerve is common and usually intentional. Resection of this nerve presents with loss of sensation to the proximal medial portion of the arm and occasionally to the upper lateral thorax.

3. Physiology

A variety of hormones interact during gestation and puberty to form the mature breast. Development of the lactiferous ducts is stimulated by estrogen and growth hormone. Both estrogen and progesterone are required to continue normal breast development through puberty. Prolactin and oxytocin are released at various stages of pregnancy to stimulate development of milk production. Lactation occurs at the conclusion of pregnancy with the fall of estrogen and progesterone levels.

4. Diagnostic Imaging and Tests

a) Mammogram

Mammograms visualize the majority of breast cancers in women over 35 years of age. In women over the age of 40, annual mammograms can decrease mortality through early detection of breast cancer by over 20%.

Earlier screening is recommended in any woman with findings suspicious for breast cancer, or risk factors for the development of early breast cancer. Digital mammography is particularly suitable for younger women with dense breasts. Mammograms should be continued in any patient in whom it would change management if cancer was detected, regardless of age.

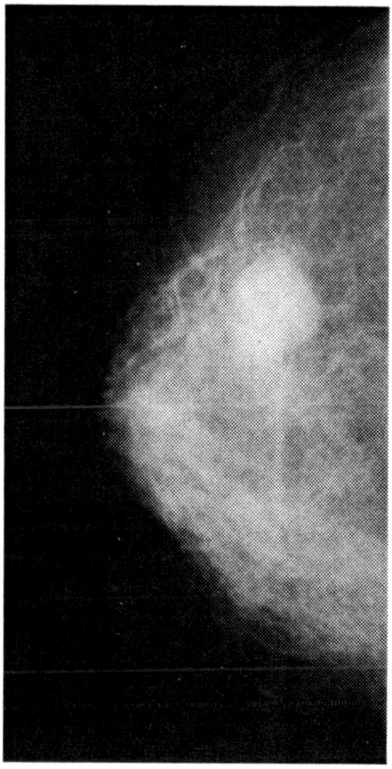

The classification of breast lesions is done by the breast imaging reporting and data system (BI-RADS), a standardized schema that ranks the suspicion of a particular lesion from 1 through 5. Category 4 or 5 lesions require biopsy or excision due to their high suspicion for cancer. Category 5 lesions have a high suspicion for invasive breast cancer.

TABLE 1. BI-RADS classification of breast lesions.

BI-RADS	Finding	Decision-Making
1	No suspicious findings	Continue annual mammograms
2	Benign lesion	Continue annual mammograms
3	Potentially benign lesion	Close follow up (i.e. repeat study in 3-6 months)
4	Suspicious lesion	Biopsy
5	Malignant lesion	Biopsy and resection

b) Ultrasound

Breast ultrasound is an invaluable tool in the office and operating room to differentiate various types of lesions and to assist with guided aspirations and biopsies. Ultrasound is able to differentiate fluid-filled cysts from solid masses, detects calcification, and assists with surgical planning by better characterizing the lesion. Used in conjunction with fine needle aspiration

(FNA) or core biopsy, ultrasound permits collection of samples in an office setting. Ultrasound provides more accurate information about the dimensions of a lesion compared to mammogram, and is a sensitive test for potential malignancy when used in conjunction with mammography.

c) MRI

Breast MRI is particularly useful in younger women as masses that may otherwise be hidden by the dense breast tissue can more easily be elucidated. MRI is also more sensitive in the detection of invasive lobular carcinoma and more precisely delineating invasive cancers. MRI is also a highly sensitive test for detecting multicentric disease, which may change clinical decision-making by leading to mastectomy instead of a simple lumpectomy. MRI is a good test for monitoring the response of a tumor to neoadjuvant and adjuvant therapy, and also for evaluating the breast in women at high risk for breast cancer.

d) PET-CT

PET scanning is a useful for prognostic purposes. Uptake of 18-F fluorodeoxyglucose (FDG) is an indicator of enhanced metabolic activity potentially found in tumor cells, and a focus of activity elsewhere in the body may indicate metastatic disease.

e) FNA

In conjunction with ultrasound, FNA provides a reliable method for aspirating a cyst. Cystic masses that resolve after aspiration should have a repeat ultrasound in six weeks to confirm that there is no recurrence. Recurrent cysts should be surgically excised. Aspiration of an orange, yellow, or green fluid is likely normal if the mass resolves. Bloody output should be followed by wire-localized surgical excision. Unilateral cysts are more worrisome than bilateral cysts as the underlying cause may be intraductal papilloma leading to obstruction of the ducts.

f) Core Biopsy

Core biopsy uses a special needle to obtain a tissue sample with intact cytoarchitecture. Core biopsy is a more sensitive and specific test for sampling masses suspicious for breast cancer compared to FNA. There are several benefits of core biopsy including excellent sensitivity and specificity and the ability to obtain tumor markers including ER, PR, and HER-2.

g) Excisional Biopsy

Excisional biopsies can be completed with wire-localization or with ultrasound / mammogram guidance. Due to the highly three dimensional nature of the breast and the need to maximize cosmesis, wire-localized excisional biopsies have gained favor as a means of minimizing trauma and precisely locating the suspicious lesion. Wire-localization is particularly beneficial in small lesions that are not easily palpated. Excisional biopsy permits full removal of the suspicious lesion and a potential cure in the appropriate setting.

I.B. Benign Breast Disease

1. Mastodynia

Breast pain is a common complaint among females presenting for clinical evaluation, but it is rarely the initial presenting sign of cancer. Cyclical breast pain in particular may be attributable to hormonal changes leading to secondary changes in the breast cytoarchitecture. Noncyclical breast pain is more concerning, but the primary causes are likely to be fibroadenomas and benign cystic disease. All patients presenting with breast pain should be evaluated; women over 35 should receive a mammogram, while those under 35 can be evaluated with either a digital mammogram or MRI. Continuing breast pain can be treated with antigonadotropins such as danazol. Surgery is not indicated if a specific cause of the breast pain is not elucidated.

Trauma to the breast may lead to a palpable cord and pain in a condition known as Mondor disease. Relief from pain is the standard management after malignant causes have been ruled out; surgical resection is not indicated in this self-limited and spontaneously resolving disease. Trauma to the breast may also lead to focal fat necrosis, which presents as a firm, nontender mass on exam. Biopsy is necessary to rule out a potential malignancy as fat necrosis appears similar to malignant lesions on diagnostic imaging studies.

2. Mastitis

Mastitis is most likely to occur in postpartum women who are breast feeding and is secondary to *S. aureus* infection. Signs of infection include fever, swelling, and abscess formation. Antibiotics are the first line of treatment with aspiration of any potential abscess. Recurrent mastitis in nonlactating women that is unresponsive to antibiotics and needle aspiration may require open incision and drainage, particularly for lesions located in the periphery of the breast tissue.

3. Fibroadenomas

Fibroadenomas are rubbery, mobile lesions especially common in women of childbearing age. Fibroadenomas are particularly sensitive to estrogen. Fibroadenomas appear as a homogenous mass on ultrasound without surrounding calcification. Core biopsy should be performed to confirm the diagnosis. Surgical excision should be reserved for fibroadenomas that are large, increase in size or are symptomatic.

4. Intraductal Papilloma

Intraductal papillomas are associated with a bloody nipple discharge and are typically less than 1 cm in size. Papilloma is rarely associated with invasive breast cancer. However, peripheral papillomas in particular should be fully resected due to the risk of transformation to invasive disease. All symptomatic central lesions should be excised via a circumareolar incision. Lesions deeper than 2-3 cm may require a ductogram with needle localization.

5. Pseudoangiomatous Hyperplasia

Pseudoangiomatous hyperplasia (PASH) is a benign, enlarging breast mass that has extensive empty spaces flocked by stromal cells on histology. Endothelial markers are negative (unlike angiosarcoma, which has markers for VEGF). Simple observation is typically all that is needed.

I.C. Malignant Breast Disease

1. Paget Disease

Paget disease is a small constituent of breast cancer involving the nipple. Eczematous nipple changes with erythema and discharge is a common presentation. Paget disease is associated with underlying invasive ductal carcinoma. Localized disease can be treated with breast conservation surgery. However, diffuse disease requires a mastectomy.

2. Phyllodes Tumor

Phyllodes tumor are fibroepithelial breast tumors with a wide range of biological behaviors. The majority of these tumors is benign and behaves similar to fibroadenomas but tend to recur after local excision; however there is a small proportion that does metastasize distantly.

Wide local excision with 1 cm margins is sufficient treatment for localized tumors. Phyllodes tumors behave like sarcomas in that they spread hematogenously instead of via the lymphatics. As a result, axillary node dissection and sentinel lymph node biopsy (SLNB) are not required. Very large tumors may require a mastectomy. Malignant tumors are usually unresponsive to chemotherapy. Distant spread to the lungs and liver can occur with malignant phyllodes tumor.

3. Inflammatory Breast Cancer

Inflammatory breast cancer typically presents with an erythematous, enlarged, indurated breast with edematous skin characterized by a peau d'orange appearance. Inflammatory breast cancer can be mistaken for mastitis, but lack fever, elevated white blood cell count and do not respond to antibiotics. A punch biopsy should be done on all patients with suspected inflammatory breast cancer to evaluate for dermal lymphatic plugging by tumor emboli. Therapy includes neoadjuvant chemotherapy followed by radiotherapy and a modified radical mastectomy.

4. Lobular Carcinoma In Situ

Lobular carcinoma in situ (LCIS) is a major risk factor for the eventual development of breast cancer. Diffuse disease with hyperplasia and atypia characterize advanced forms of this disease. Patients with LCIS have a 1% chance per year of developing invasive ductal or lobular carcinoma, which may occur in either breast. Women with LCIS have the option of watchful monitoring with mammograms and MRI, medical management with tamoxifen, or prophylactic bilateral mastectomy.

Tamoxifen reduces the risk of invasive ductal carcinoma by 49%. Prophylactic bilateral mastectomy is potentially curative. Women with additional risk factors for breast cancer may opt for bilateral mastectomy at a younger age to their higher relative risk of developing invasive breast cancer.

5. Ductal Carcinoma In Situ

a) Assessment

Ductal carcinoma in situ (DCIS) is an intraductal cancer with a high risk of progressing to invasive carcinoma. DCIS may take the form of localized disease amenable to breast conservation therapy, multicentric disease, or isolated Paget disease of the nipple. The most common presentation of DCIS is an asymptomatic finding of microcalcification on a screening mammogram. Nearly half of all such findings on mammography are likely to be DCIS.

b) Management

Local disease can be treated with breast conservation therapy (i.e. lumpectomy and radiation) or mastectomy. Multicentric disease, large tumors, or patients with contraindications to radiotherapy may require mastectomy. Locally recurrent disease manifest with invasive ductal carcinoma following breast conservation therapy occurs in about 1 in 10 patients after a decade; this is 50% higher compared to mastectomy. However, there is no overall difference in survival between breast conservation therapy and modified radical mastectomy. Radiation with lumpectomy is required as it reduces local recurrence by 50%. Tamoxifen decreases the incidence of contralateral breast cancer by 38% and reduces the progression of DCIS to invasive cancer by over 50%. Microinvasive or multicentric disease should have a sentinel lymph node biopsy (SLNB) for staging and prognosis.

6. Invasive Breast Cancer

a) Pathophysiology

Invasive breast cancer most commonly takes the form of ductal carcinoma or lobular carcinoma. Ductal carcinoma is divided into lobular, medullary, and tubular subtypes based on their histological appearance. Tubular ductal carcinoma has the best prognosis.

b) Risk Factors

Risk factors for development breast cancer include early menarche, late menopause, nulliparity, obesity, alcohol abuse, hormone replacement therapy (but not oral contraceptives), positive family history for cancer, radiation exposure, and LCIS. There was a controversial lack of association between smoking and breast cancer in the past, but recent studies have confirmed a link between the two.

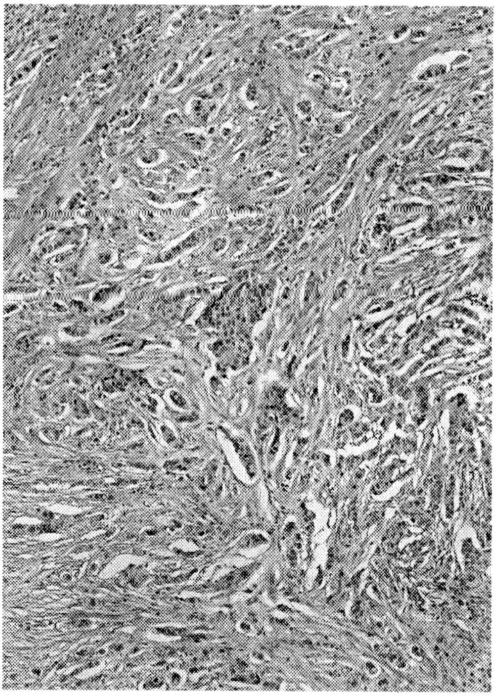

The GAIL breast cancer model quantifies several of these risk factors and comes up with a risk assessment score for the future development of breast cancer. This model takes into account present age, age at onset of menarche, total prior breast biopsies, first-degree relatives with breast cancer, and atypical ductal hyperplasia on a diagnostic biopsy to determine the overall risk of developing breast cancer. Patients that have a risk that exceeds 1.6% are started on tamoxifen and can achieve a 50% risk reduction.

c) Presentation

Breast cancer most commonly presents on routine screening mammogram or as an asymptomatic, firm, fixed mass. Occasionally, it may present with pain, unilateral bloody nipple discharge, retraction of the skin, nipple ulceration, and erythema. Advanced disease that has metastasized may present with bone pain, pleural effusion, and hepatomegaly.

Breast cancer in men presents similar to cancer in women. However, since the index of suspicion is lower in men, they are more likely to present with advanced disease and a poorer prognosis. Management is the same as it is for women. Klinefelter disease is a major risk factor for male breast cancer.

d) Evaluation

Breast cancer evaluation includes a determination of hormone status, which fundamentally guides medical management. ER+ and PR+ tumors are highly responsive to endocrine therapy with tamoxifen and portends a favorable outcome compared to triple negative (ER, PR, and HER-2) tumors. HER-2 positive tumors are responsive to herceptin, a monoclonal antibody against the HER-2/neu growth factor receptor.

e) Staging

The American Joint Committee on Cancer (AJCC) system is used to stage breast cancer, which is based on the TNM status of the tumor.

TABLE 2. TNM classification of breast cancer.

T Status	Criteria
T0	No tumor
Tis	In situ tumor
T1	Tumor size < 2 cm
T2	Tumor size between 2-5 cm
T3	Tumor size > 5 cm
T4	Tumor that involves skin or chest wall, or inflammatory cancer
N Status	Criteria
N0	Lymph nodes negative for cancer
N1	Metastatic disease to 1-3 axillary nodes or microscopic disease to internal mammary nodes
N2	Metastatic disease to 4-9 axillary nodes or internal mammary nodes
N3	Disease that affects 10+ axillary nodes, infraclavicular nodes, supraclavicular nodes, or multiple intramammary and axillary nodes
M status	Criteria
M0	No metastasis
M1	Distant metastasis

TABLE 3. Breast cancer staging.

Stage	TNM Status	Optimal Intervention
Stage I	T1N0M0	Breast conservation therapy with SLNB
Stage II	T1-3, N0-1, M0	Breast conservation therapy with SLNB (if N0) or modified radical mastectomy with axillary node dissection (if N+)
Stage III	T1-4, N0-3, M0	Most cases require modified radical mastectomy with axillary node dissection
Stage IV	TXNXM1	Neoadjuvant therapy, surgical resection, adjuvant therapy

TABLE 4. Medical treatment.

Drug	Indications	Mechanism of Action	Complications	Notes
Tamoxifen	ER+ PR+ breast cancer, DCIS	Selective estrogen receptor modulator (SERM)	DVT / PE, endometrial cancer, retroperitoneal fibrosis	STAR trial compared tamoxifen with raloxifene; tamoxifen is best for breast cancer, raloxifene for osteoporosis. 50% annual risk reduction in recurrence
Raloxifene	Osteoporosis and invasive breast cancer in postmenopausal women with osteoporosis	SERM	Lower risk of DVT / PE than tamoxifen	See above
Anastrozole (Arimidex)	ER+ breast cancer and metastatic disease	Aromatase inhibitor that blocks estrogen synthase	Osteoporosis with fracture risk; give with statins or bisphosphonates (the latter is associated with mandibular osteonecrosis)	ATAC trial indicates improved outcome in postmenopausal women with ER+ breast cancer compared to tamoxifen. Benefits in ER- disease and 40% reduction in recurrent disease.
Trastuzumab (Herceptin)	HER-2/neu+ breast cancer	Monoclonal antibody to HER-2/neu receptor that suppresses cell cycle and angiogenesis	Cardiac toxicity requires echocardiography/MUGA scanning prior to use	HER-2/neu influences CDK-2
Doxorubicin (Adriamycin), cyclophosphamide (Cytoxan), and taxol (Paclitaxel)	Multimodal chemotherapy regimen for breast cancer	DNA intercalation; DNA crosslinking with disruption of mitosis; inhibition of mitosis	Neutropenia, cardiac toxicity; hemorrhagic cystitis, transitional cell carcinoma of bladder; arthralgia	Regimen typically consists of eight regimens over 5 months; variable schedules and combinations are common

f) Surgical Treatment

(1) *Breast Conservation Therapy*

Breast conservation therapy is indicated for all focal, clearly delineated tumors that are amenable to radiation treatment. Breast conservation therapy may be particularly effective following neoadjuvant chemoradiation to reduce the tumor burden. Absolute contraindications to wide local excision include multicentric disease, positive margins after multiple attempts at resection, and diffuse disease. Patients with connective tissue disease, multifocal disease in the same area, and women who may have a potentially poor cosmetic outcome from breast conservation therapy may not be ideal candidates for this approach.

Recurrent disease following breast conservation therapy with radiation therapy have long term survival on par with mastectomy if R0 (margin-negative) resection is completed and postoperative radiation is used.

(2) *Modified Radical Mastectomy*

A modified radical mastectomy is resection of all breast tissue and level 1 and 2 lymph nodes of the axilla. The borders of the resection include the clavicle and axillary vein on the superior extent, the sternum medially, latissimus dorsi laterally, and the inframammary fold inferiorly. The posterior margin is the pectoralis major.

Modified radical mastectomy is the standard approach for breast cancer with metastases to the axillary lymph nodes that is resectable but otherwise not amenable to breast conservation surgery. Women early in pregnancy require a modified radical mastectomy as they will be unable to tolerate radiation.

Mastectomy followed by immediate reconstruction can be completed with a variety of approaches. Tissue expanders with subsequent implant placement are the most frequently chosen path, but require a follow up procedure to place the permanent implant. A transverse rectus abdominis myocutaneous (TRAM) flap can be used to fill the space formerly occupied by breast tissue but requires a reasonably healthy patient who can tolerate the extended operation. The TRAM can be performed as either a pedicle or free flap.

Latissimus dorsi flaps can also be used, but are relatively contraindicated in very active patients.

The use of flaps and immediate reconstruction may be a poor option in women who will require postoperative radiation therapy due to destruction of the flap. These women may be better candidates for delayed reconstruction.

(3) *Axillary Lymph Node Dissection*

In the past all patients with breast cancer required axillary lymph node dissection (ALND) to stage the axilla and for local control. Sentinel lymph node biopsy (SLNB) was developed as an alternative to stage the axilla and avoid the comorbidities associated with full ALND. This approach is highly accurate and is indicated for patients with biopsy proven breast cancer with clinically negative nodes. Contraindications to SLNB are pregnancy (due to the exposure to the radioisotope and isosulfan blue dye), inflammatory breast cancer and extensive previous axillary surgery.

A SLNB begins with injection of a radioactive nucleotide tracer near the tumor site. This is followed by injection of a lymphazurin blue dye in the operating room into a nearby region in the breast. The goal is to identify the lymph nodes that are draining the tumor. Nodes that are either blue or "hot" (radioactive) are resected and sent to pathology for evaluation. Positive lymph nodes imply spread of tumor to the axillary nodes and require a full axillary node dissection. Negative nodes are highly sensitive for localized disease only and prevent the risk of complications associated with completing an axillary node dissection in all patients. If no lymph nodes are identified at all, an axillary node dissection is necessary.

g) Breast Cancer Genetics

BRCA-1 is associated with breast cancer, ovarian cancer, colon cancer, and prostate cancer in men. BRCA-1 accounts for 40% of familial breast cancer and is due to a defect in a tumor suppressor gene on chromosome 17. BRCA-1 has a higher association with ovarian cancer than BRCA-2.

BRCA-2 is associated with breast cancer, ovarian cancer, and male breast cancer. BRCA-2 is due to a defect in a tumor suppressor gene on chromosome 13. BRCA-1 or 2 mutations lead to a 30% increase in risk of contralateral cancer. A bilateral salpingo-oopherectomy reduces the risk of breast cancer incidence in these patients. Prophylactic mastectomy specimens are often found with premalignant lesions. Nearly 85% of women with BRCA-1 or 2 mutations are likely to develop breast cancer by the age of 70.

II. Pituitary

II.A. General Concepts

1. Anatomy

a) Hypothalamus

The pituitary is situated below the hypothalamus and is suspended by the hypophyseal stalk. The hypothalamus receives input from the external environment and the internal environment. In addition it receives negative feedback from hormones such as glucocorticoids, estrogen, testosterone, and thyroid hormone. Thus, the hypothalamus integrates sensory and hormonal inputs and provides coordinated responses. These responses include responses to the anterior and posterior pituitary, among many other areas.

b) Anterior and Posterior Pituitary

The pituitary is divided into two parts, the anterior (adenohypophysis) and posterior (neurohypophysis) sections. The posterior portion is directly innervated from the hypothalamus and releases oxytocin and vasopressin. The anterior portion is controlled by the releasing factors of the hypothalamus. Each anterior pituitary hormone has its own unique hypothalamic releasing factor (hormone). The main releasing hormones are: thyrotropin-releasing hormone, corticotropin-releasing hormone, luteinizing hormone-releasing hormone, growth hormone-releasing hormone, prolactin-releasing peptide, gonadotropin-releasing hormone.

2. Physiology

a) Antidiuretic Hormone

Antidiuretic hormone (ADH) is synthesized in the hypothalamus and released by the posterior pituitary as a response to hypotension or increased osmolarity. The response to hypotension is mediated by a decrease in left atrial filling pressure, leading to activation of baroreceptors. ADH increases permeability of the collecting duct, leading to reabsorption of free water and an increase in intravascular volume. However, an increase in osmolality is the more potent stimulus for ADH secretion.

II.B. Metabolic Disorders

1. Hyperprolactinemia

Table 5. Hyperprolactinemia.

Etiology	Prolactinomas and dopamine inhibition.
Presentation	Amenorrhea, gynecomastia and galactorrhea, bitemporal hemianopsia.
Diagnosis	Exclusion of other conditions and excluding medication-induced hyperprolactinemia. Prolactin greater than 100 ng / mL.
Treatment	Reversing elevated levels of prolactin. Disease refractory to medical management requires surgical excision or radiation therapy.

2. Hypopituitarism

Table 6. Hypopituitarism.

Etiology	Lesions may be the result of trauma or damage from tumor overgrowth. Infarction of a pituitary tumor, infection by TB and syphilis, along with sarcoid and various autoimmune disorders.
Presentation	Inability to lactate in pregnant women; amenorrhea, infertility, decreased sexual desire, impotence, loss of sexually-mature hair patterns, insulin-sensitivity, growth failure in children, symptoms of hypothyroidism, symptoms of aortic insufficiency.
Diagnosis	Insulin-challenge test to see if growth hormone increases, measuring the titers of cortisol, LH, FSH, and either estrogen or testosterone, and thyroid hormones.
Treatment	Replacement of the lost hormones, especially cortisol. Reversal of any underlying etiology should be undertaken immediately.

3. Diabetes Insipidus

a) Etiology and Pathophysiology

Diabetes insipidus (DI) may be due to either decreased production of antidiuretic hormone (ADH) by the posterior pituitary or hypothalamus, or decreased renal response to ADH. Central DI occurs with decreased hormone production and is secondary to trauma (the most common cause), tumor, vascular disease, medications, and hypophysectomy. Nephrogenic DI is due to a lack of renal response and may be due to electrolyte imbalances, sickle cell anemia, sarcoid, or medications such as lithium and colchicine.

b) Presentation and Diagnosis

Central DI presents with concomitant loss of anterior pituitary hormones. The result is the inability to concentrate urine and loss of salt excretion with excess diluted urine secretion and increased water intake from hypernatremia. Diagnosis of DI is made by comparing urine to plasma osmolarity, but a careful history often yields clues to the correct diagnosis. Nephrogenic DI is the diagnosis if there is no change in osmolarity following administration of ADH.

c) Treatment

Central DI is treated with ADH replacement along with any other missing pituitary hormones. Either vasopressin or desmopressin (DDAVP) may be used as synthetic analogues. Increased ADH secretion can be induced by chlorpropamide, clofibrate, and carbamazepine. Nephrogenic DI is best treated with hydrochlorothiazide (HCTZ), amiloride, or chlorthalidone.

4. Secretion of Inappropriate Antidiuretic Hormone

a) Etiology and Pathophysiology

Secretion of inappropriate antidiuretic hormone (SIADH) may occur with ectopic ADH secretion (the result of endocrine activity by tumors such as oat cell carcinomas of the lung, pancreatic tumors, infections such as TB or pneumonia), CNS trauma, and by various medications (chlorpropamide, clofibrate, various chemotherapeutic agents, and carbamazepine).

b) Presentation and Diagnosis

SIADH presents with dilutional hyponatremia with hypernatriuria. In severe cases, central edema may lead to CNS symptoms. Concentrated urine is formed in SIADH with sodium concentration over 20 mEq / L. The renin-angiotensin system (RAS) is also suppressed. Normal renal, adrenal, and thyroid function is necessary before making this diagnosis.

c) Treatment

SIADH is treated with fluid restriction to minimize the dilutional hyponatremia, the use of furosemide or demeclocycline to cause a water diuresis, and saline infusion as indicated in when sodium concentration falls below 110 mEq/L (rarely used to avoid central pontine myelinolysis [CPM]). The rate of correction should not exceed 0.5 mEq/L/hr for the first 24 hours. Cerebropontine myelinolysis can lead to seizure, coma, and death.

II.C. Cancer

1. Pituitary Adenoma

a) Assessment

Tumors of the pituitary comprise some 10% of all intracranial tumors. The majority is benign and slow growing, but over time, may manifest as impingements on the optic nerve (leading to bitemporal hemianopsia) and various endocrinologic effects. The anterior pituitary is the only portion that develops primary tumors, including adenomas and craniopharyngiomas. Craniopharyngiomas develop from the remnants of Rathke's pouch and occur primarily in children; they are typically suprasellar, solid calcified tumors. Adenomas may have abnormal formation of various hormones with expected side effects. Microadenomas are found in a significant number of women, but tend to be asymptomatic. Pituitary tumors present with headache, compression of the optic chiasm, and the endocrinologic effects of the adenoma. Diagnosis is by plain films, CT, and MRI. Hormone studies identify the nature of the endocrinologic excess. The sudden onset of acne, hirsutism, hypertension, amenorrhea, and hypertension may be attributed to a pituitary adenoma.

b) Management

Pituitary tumors are treated by medical management to decrease hormone production, radiation therapy, or surgical excision.

TABLE 7. Pituitary tumors.

Etiology	Adenomas, craniopharyngiomas,
Presentation	Headache, compression of the optic chiasm, and endocrinologic effects.
Treatment	Decrease hormone production, radiation therapy, or surgical excision.

III. Thyroid

III.A. General Concepts

1. Anatomy

a) Embryology

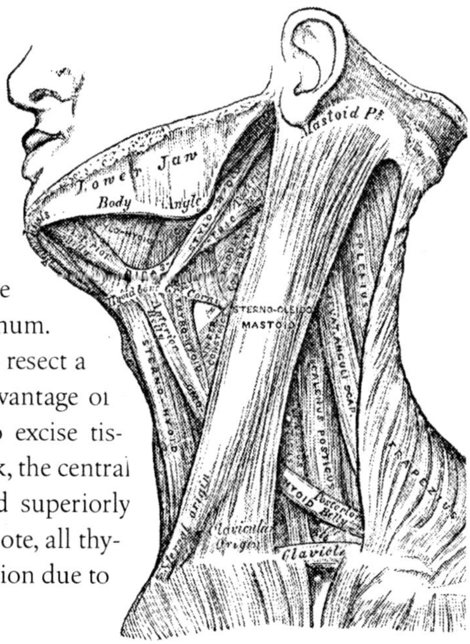

The thyroid gland develops at the base of the tongue at the foramen cecum and descends into its space near the cricoid cartilage via the thyroglossal duct. It is for this reason that thyroid tissue can be located anywhere between the base of the tongue and the sternum. The Sistrunk procedure, used to resect a thyroglossal duct cyst, takes advantage of these anatomic relationships to excise tissue along the midline of the neck, the central portion of the hyoid bone, and superiorly into the base of the tongue. Of note, all thyroglossal duct cysts require excision due to their potential for infection.

Endocrine Surgery

b) Surgical Anatomy

(1) *Anatomic Relationships*

The thyroid gland is inferior to the thyroid cartilage and extends between the fourth and sixth tracheal rings. The infrahyoid muscles, including the sternothyroid, sternohyoid, thyrohyoid, and omohyoid lie anterior to the thyroid; the posterior layers include the cricoid and thyroid cartilages and the posterior suspensory ligament of Berry. The superior laryngeal nerve is located superior and medial to the thyroid. The recurrent laryngeal nerve is

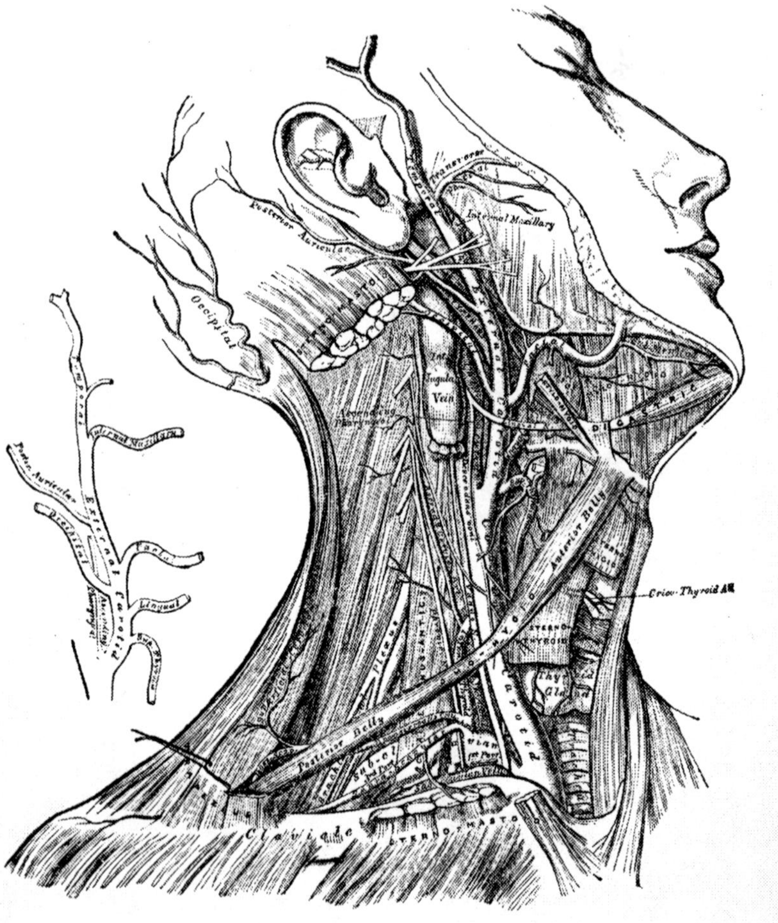

found in the tracheoesophageal (TE) groove and is located near the inferior thyroid artery.

The parathyroid glands are located on the posterolateral aspect of the thyroid gland. Variation in location may occur in up to 20% of individuals, and ectopic glands may be located in the thyrothymic ligament, tracheoesophageal groove, and carotid sheath. Ectopic thyroid tissue found in the lateral neck is not normal thyroid tissue and frequently represents a thyroid cancer. Disruption of various nerves related to the thyroid gland is discussed in the Head and Neck Surgery chapter on page 63.

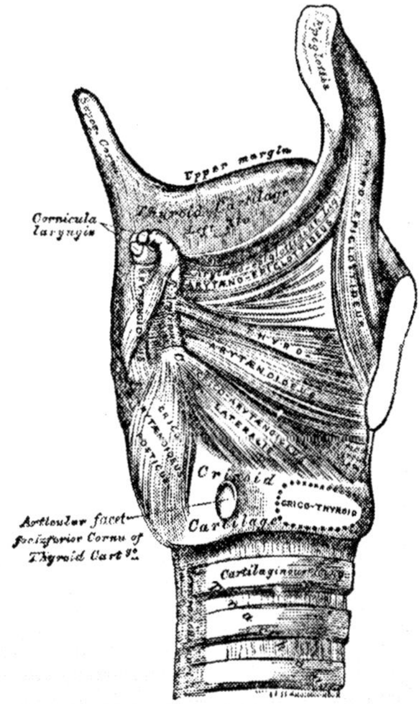

(2) *Vascular Supply*

The blood supply is via the superior thyroid artery (a branch of the external carotid artery), and the inferior thyroid artery (a branch of the thyrocervical trunk). A branch directly from the arch of the aorta supplies the thyroid in about 10% of patients and is known as the thyroid ima. Venous drainage is by three paired veins, the superior, middle and inferior thyroid veins. These drain into the left brachiocephalic vein. The lymphatic drainage is into the deep cervical nodes and the pretracheal nodes.

2. Physiology

a) Thyroid Hormones

The thyroid produces thyroxine (T4), triiodothyronine (T3), and calcitonin. The majority of T4 is converted into T3 peripherally via a deiodinase enzyme; T3 is ten times more active than T4. The majority of hormone is bound by albumin and thyroxine-binding globulin. Production is regulated by thyroid-stimulating hormone (TSH), produced by the anterior pituitary, in turn regulated by thyrotropin-releasing hormone (TRH) via the hypothalamus. Follicular cells of the thyroid are involved in iodine uptake.

b) Calcitonin

Calcitonin is produced by parafollicular C cells of the thyroid. Calcitonin opposes parathyroid hormone (PTH) and leads to increased calcium resorption by bone. Loss of calcitonin via a total thyroidectomy does not significantly affect calcium homeostasis.

c) Iodine

Iodine is required for thyroid hormone production; a lack of iodine in the diet (and incidentally, the rise to fame for the Mayo brothers in Rochester, MN) leads to goiter due to accumulation of thyroglobulin.

3. Diagnostic Studies

a) Ultrasound

Ultrasound is used to differentiate between cystic and solid nodules, but does not necessarily imply that the nodule is benign. A high-frequency probe at about 10 MHz is used. Ultrasound in conjunction with fine needle aspiration is the initial diagnostic test of choice to assess all neck masses.

b) Technetium Scanning

Radioisotope scanning permits a physiologic analysis of the thyroid and is used to identify hyperfunctioning and hypofunctioning areas (either of which may be indicative of malignancy). Technetium pertechnetate has a rapid absorption profile. I^{123} has a lower radiation dose and can be used to identify ectopic thyroid tissue. I^{131} has a longer half-life and is suitable for identifying thyroid cancer and metastatic disease.

c) CT and MRI

CT and MRI are reserved for metastatic thyroid cancer or for substernal disease. Non-contrast CT imaging is preferred in patients suspected of having thyroid cancer as the iodinated contrast may lead to saturation of iodine receptors in the thyroid and thereby delay the function of radioactive iodine.

d) Fine Needle Aspiration

Fine needle aspiration (FNA) is the initial diagnostic modality for the work-up of all neck masses. In conjunction with ultrasound, the sensitivity and specificity approaches 90%. FNA that indicates follicular cells may be either follicular adenoma or follicular thyroid cancer, and up to 1 in 5 cases may end up being a malignancy. As a result, most practitioners will continue with a diagnostic thyroid lobectomy. The finding of macrophages and colloid indicates benign disease.

III.B. Metabolic Disorders

1. Hypothyroidism

a) Epidemiology

Hypothyroidism affects 2% of the United States population and is secondary to a lack of iodide (an international concern). Thyroid disease is up to 8 times more common in women. The incidence increases with age, but there is little mortality attached to this disorder. Hypothyroidism as a congenital condition is known as cretinism.

b) Etiology and Pathophysiology

Hypothyroidism is commonly due to congenital disease, autoimmune disease, inflammation leading to transient symptoms, medications leading to thyroid toxicity, prior injury from correction of hyperthyroidism, postpartum hypothyroidism, and a variety of central causes leading to decreased hormone production. Low production of TH leads to decreased BMR, myxedematous infiltration of tissue leading to decreased cardiac function, pericardial effusions, decreased CO, decreased GI transit with achlorhydria, delayed puberty, infertility, and worsening of the lipid profile.

c) Presentation and Diagnosis

Hypothyroidism sometimes presents with asymptomatic goiter (especially in Hashimoto thyroiditis) that may lead to local impingement. Weight gain commonly occurs with concomitant lethargy and decreased energy. Cold intolerance and constipation are commonly present. Dry coarse hair is typically seen along with myxedema. Diagnosis is made by examination and a full thyroid panel to identify deficiencies. TSH is typically elevated but T4 and T3 are decreased.

d) Treatment

Hypothyroidism is treated by supportive therapy and by hormone replacement using levothyroxine. Goiter resection may be necessary in patients with symptomatic disease.

2. Hashimoto Thyroiditis

a) Assessment

Hashimoto thyroiditis is an autoimmune disease that leads to lymphocytic fibrosis with painless goiter formation, primarily in women of childbearing age. Hashimoto disease will eventually degenerate into hypothyroidism in 5% of patients per year; however, a similar number of patients may experience a transient thyrotoxicosis during this period. Hashimoto thyroiditis (which eventually leads to primary hypothyroidism) is also associated with thyroid lymphoma, which presents as an enlarging, painful mass. FNA is the first step in diagnosis; the majority of lymphomas tend to be B-cell in nature. Multimodal treatment with CHOP and radiation is the best treatment; surgery is a less preferred option.

b) Management

Most cases of primary (i.e. intrinsic thyroid dysfunction), secondary (i.e. pituitary gland damage), and tertiary (i.e. hypothalamus dysfunction) hypothyroidism can be treated with supplementation of thyroid hormone. Surgery is restricted only in the setting of symptomatic goiter formation that is refractory to medical management.

3. Subacute Thyroiditis

a) Assessment

Subacute thyroiditis is sometimes referred to as de Quervain thyroiditis, which commonly follows viral illness in young women and is thought to be of viral origin. A painful enlarged gland is initially hyperthyroid but progress to a hypothyroid state. At resolution, a euthyroid state is common.

b) Management

Treatment of subacute thyroiditis involves pain control with NSAIDs, corticosteroids to decrease the inflammatory reaction, and occasionally beta-blockers for hyperthyroidism. Surgery is typically not required or necessary.

4. Hyperthyroidism

a) Etiology

Hyperthyroidism leads to excessive amounts of triiodothyronine (T3) and / or thyroxine (T4) leading to thyrotoxicosis. Common causes include Graves disease, toxic multinodular goiter (also known as Plummer disease), toxic adenomas, and subacute thyroiditis. Less common types of thyrotoxicosis emanate from iodide-induced disease, amiodarone toxicity, excess beta-human chorionic gonadotropin (B-hCG), factitious disease, pituitary adenomas that produce an excess of thyroid stimulating hormone (TSH), metastatic cancer from the thyroid, and struma ovarii. Graves disease is a diffuse goiter leading to exophthalmos, pretibial myxedema, palpitations, and goiter. It is more common in females and is associated with autoantibody formation that stimulates thyroid function.

b) Pathophysiology

Thyrotoxicosis exerts its effects systemically through excess production of T3 and T4. Basal metabolic rate (BMR) increases significantly leading to increased cardiovascular work and heat production. This increase leads to the symptoms of sweating, heat intolerance, and palpitations. Anxiety often occurs as a sympathetic response. Tremor and tachycardia are also common due to activation of the sympathetic nervous system (SNS). Graves disease is the most common cause, and is due to thyroid stimulating antibodies that bind to thyroid thyrotropin receptors leading to the synthesis of excessive thyroid hormone. The result of this antibody is thyroid hormone synthesis and thyroid hypertrophy. Subacute thyroiditis, a cause of thyrotoxicosis in about 20% of patients, is discussed separately below. Plummer disease occurs in a subset of patients, and is the development of a toxic multinodular goiter.

c) Presentation and Diagnosis

Hyperthyroidism presents with anxiety, anorexia, heat intolerance, diaphoresis, tremor, hyperactivity, palpitations, and oligomenorrhea. HTN may occur. On physical exam, the thyroid may be diffusely enlarged and firm as in Graves disease. Graves disease itself may present with the triad of proptosis, exophthalmos, and pretibial myxedema. Signs of thyrotoxicosis include tachycardia, atrial fibrillation, HTN, smooth skin, diaphoresis, lid lag, tremor, and hyperkinesis. Diagnosis involves a full thyroid panel, including TSH, T3 (measured by T3 resin uptake) and T4 (measured by the free T4 index). Imaging involves the use of a nuclear thyroid scintigraphy with iodine 123 or technetium-99m. Graves disease will have elevated uptake with those isotopes.

d) Medical Treatment

The majority of cases of hyperthyroidism can be treated medically. Hyperthyroidism involves the use of beta-blockers to reduce the activity of the sympathetic nervous system. Iodine, in the form of potassium iodide, can be given as a temporary measure to block the release of TH. The mainstay of treatment involves anti-thyroid drugs such as PTU or methimazole and radioactive I^{131}. The most common complication of radioactive iodine ablation of the thyroid is hypothyroidism.

e) Surgical Treatment

Surgical management of hyperthyroidism is less common than in the past due to the increased efficacy of medical management. However, specific indications where surgery may be warranted is patients with poorly managed disease, especially children; pregnant patients; patients with severe external manifestations of disease such as goiters; and patients who develop hyperthyroidism secondary to amiodarone toxicity. Surgery for Graves disease leads to nearly immediate resolution of Graves disease. Total thyroidectomy is the preferred option given the difficulty of managing the fluctuations in thyroid hormone levels associated with Graves disease. Hyperthyroidism in pregnancy that is refractory to medical management should be treated with surgery in the 2nd trimester.

5. Thyroid Storm

a) Assessment

The most significant complication of thyroidectomy for hyperthyroidism is thyroid storm, which can be mitigated with preoperative therapy with methimazole or PTU, propranolol to moderate heart rate, SSKI, and careful manipulation of the thyroid gland during surgery. Thyroid storm presents with tachycardia, hyperthermia, hypertension, followed by systemic decompensation leading to hypotension and death. Thyrotoxicosis occurs when autonomous thyroid hormone production occurs, and may be the result of longstanding multinodular thyroid disease, Graves disease, or exogenous iodine loading (Jod-Basedow effect).

b) Management

Treatment of thyroid storm involves supportive treatment, glucose, antithyroid agents, and beta-blockers. Dexamethasone is sometimes given to block further release of TH. After medical control of hyperthyroidism is obtained definitive therapy with I^{131} of thyroidectomy is performed.

6. Toxic Adenoma

a) Assessment

Toxic adenomas present as a single, palpable mass thyroid mass in a hyperthyroid patient. The first step in diagnosis is fine needle aspiration. A radioactive iodine scan demonstrates a hot nodule. In the setting of elevated thyroid hormones and suppressed TSH, the diagnosis is more likely to be a single toxic adenoma. In the absence of abnormal endocrine activity, the diagnosis is more likely to be a thyroid cancer.

b) Management

Single nodules tend to be amenable to radioactive iodine therapy. Failure of this often leads to a thyroid lobectomy.

III.C. Cancer

1. Papillary Thyroid Carcinoma

a) Etiology

Papillary thyroid carcinoma (PTC) comprises 70% of all thyroid cancers. Radiation exposure, female gender, and age under 40 years are all associated with PTC. Papillary carcinoma is highly amenable to treatment and has a low morbidity and mortality due to its slow growing nature. The most common causative factor is with prior radiation exposure to the neck.

b) Pathophysiology

PTC is a well-differentiated cancer with a 10-year survival of nearly 95%. FNA is diagnostic for this type of cancer; the presence of papillary thyroid tissue elsewhere in the neck is virtually diagnostic for PTC. Specific variants of PTC such as tall cell, columnar, and insular carcinomas are very rare and have a poorer prognosis. The AMES and AGES scoring criteria utilize age, metastasis (or grade), extent, and size are predictive of overall mortality. Age under 40 (or 50 for women), lack of metastatic disease, focal tumors, and masses less than 4 cm in size are predictors for a positive outlook. Psammoma bodies are present on histologic analysis.

c) Presentation and Diagnosis

The initial presenting sign of PTC may be a palpable thyroid mass. The initial diagnostic study is a fine needle aspiration in conjunction with ultrasound.

d) Treatment

Lesions under 1 cm in size can be treated with a lobectomy and isthmectomy. Tumors larger than 2 cm require a total thyroidectomy. Intermediate tumors are typically treated with a total thyroidectomy to permit future use of radioactive iodine therapy, but this procedure risks bilateral recurrent laryngeal nerve (RLN) damage. All patients with suspicious disease should receive an ultrasound of the neck followed by biopsy of all suspicious nodes and masses. A modified neck dissection and central lymph node dissection is necessary in all patients with confirmed cancer and spread to lymph nodes. Otherwise, a total thyroidectomy is sufficient with node-negative disease. Radiotherapy with I^{131} typically follows surgery.

Unfavorable prognosis for PTC include age over 50 for women, or 40 for men, lymphatic invasion (but no lymphocytic thyroiditis), and tall cell variant. Thyroidectomy for a substernal thyroid should be done with a collar incision. If the thyroid extends substernally, a sternotomy may be necessary.

2. Follicular Thyroid Carcinoma

a) Etiology and Pathophysiology

Follicular thyroid cancer (FTC) affects between 10-20% of all patients with thyroid cancer. It is more common in women, like papillary thyroid cancer; FTC is also more common in patients with deficient iodine intake. FTC is highly differentiated and is similar to the normal thyroid parenchyma. It has been postulated that a long-standing goiter or prior radiation exposure may predispose certain individuals to developing FTC. Mutations in ras and dysfunction in various cytokines may lead to FTC as well. Spread is hematogenous, with the most common sites being to the bone, lung, and liver. Hürthle cell carcinoma is a variant of follicular carcinoma; this type contains oxyphilic cells, is more common in the elderly, is not responsive to RAI, and has a worse prognosis compared to FTC.

b) Presentation and Diagnosis

Nodal presentation of FTC is very uncommon. However, like PTC, a painless thyroid mass is often the first presenting sign. FTC requires a tissue diagnosis; FNA is insufficient to make a formal diagnosis as cytoarchitecture must be preserved to see follicular cells invading nearby vessels and structures. Frozen sections taken intraoperatively have a low sensitivity for diagnosis.

c) Treatment

The most appropriate treatment for FTC is completing a lobectomy with isthmectomy for lesions smaller than 1 cm, and a total thyroidectomy for larger masses. If a lobectomy is completed for other reasons and the pathology yields follicular carcinoma, a total thyroidectomy is typically indicated, especially for higher risk patients. Unlike PTC, node dissection is not necessary since this cancer spreads hematogenously. Survival is comparable with PTC for the first 10 years, and then drops off. This is especially the case for poorly differentiated tumors like Hürthle cell cancer. Radiotherapy with I131 typically follows surgery.

3. Medullary Thyroid Carcinoma

a) Etiology and Pathophysiology

Medullary thyroid cancer (MTC) comprises 5% of all thyroid cancers. Medullary thyroid carcinoma (MTC) arises from derangements in the parafollicular C cells that produce calcitonin. MTC is associated with MEN 2A and MEN 2B, but the majority of patients have spontaneous disease. Unilateral disease arises spontaneously, while bilateral disease is more common in those with a familial heritage. Derangements in the ret oncogene have been identified in some cases of familial MTC.

b) Presentation and Diagnosis

Like PTC and FTC, a single thyroid nodule is the most common presentation of MTC. The combination of a mass and elevated calcitonin level is virtually diagnostic, but an FNA is required for formal diagnosis.

c) Treatment

Due to the significantly higher morbidity and mortality associated with MTC, a total thyroidectomy is completed in all cases. Most patients will also have a resection of all central nodes with a conversion to a modified radical neck dissection in the presence of lymph nodes confirmed to contain cancer by FNA. Of note, a single nodule is typically present with spontaneous disease, while masses throughout the thyroid are associated with MEN 2.

d) Modified Radical Neck Dissection

The superior border for a modified radical neck dissection is the inferior border of the mandible; the lateral border is the anterior border of the trapezius; the medial border is the sternohyoid and digastric muscles; the inferior border is the clavicle. Major nervous structures include the hypoglossal nerve, sympathetic chain, and spinal accessory nerve. Damage to the superior laryngeal nerve may occur as part of a routine thyroidectomy and presents with loss of high-pitched tones. Damage to the recurrent laryngeal nerve leads to paralysis of the vocal cords and requires cord medialization to protect the airway.

4. Anaplastic Thyroid Carcinoma

a) Assessment

Anaplastic thyroid cancer (ATC) comprises less than 5% of all thyroid tumors and typically has a dismal prognosis. It presents as an enlarging, painful neck mass that impinges on other structures of the neck. Early spread and rapid progression occurs in ATC leading to a variety of systemic symptoms. It is related to C-myc, H-ras, and other oncogenes, and may be the end result of a longstanding papillary or follicular thyroid cancer. Like other thyroid cancers, diagnosis proceeds with an FNA.

b) Management

Treatment involves resection for all tumors that do not show evidence of gross invasion of surrounding structures, but most tumors are metastatic and unresectable at diagnosis. While chemoradiation does not alter the natural course of this cancer, it is used for palliation therapy. The prognosis is grim for most patients.

IV. Parathyroid

IV.A. General Concepts

1. Anatomy

a) Anatomical Relationships

The parathyroid glands are located in the posterolateral quadrants of the thyroid gland, proximal to the superior thyroid artery for the superior two glands within 1 cm of the junction of the recurrent laryngeal nerve and inferior thyroid artery. The inferior glands are found inferior to the thyroid and within the thyrothymic ligament. Parathyroid chief cells produce parathyroid hormone (PTH).

The parathyroid is derived from the neural crest and endoderm. The superior glands come from the fourth branchial pouch, while the inferior glands descend from the third branchial pouch. The inferior parathyroid glands may occasionally descend with the thymus into the mediastinum. Failure to cure primary hyperparathyroidism in the first operation may require a reoperation to find the missing gland. The entire extent of the parathyroid tissue may lie anywhere between the pharynx superiorly, the anterior mediastinum inferiorly, and the esophagus posteriorly. However, reoperation is associated with up to a 10% risk of damage to the recurrent laryngeal nerve.

b) Vascular Supply

Both the superior and inferior parathyroid glands are supplied by the inferior thyroid artery. The superior parathyroid glands are occasionally supplied by the superior thyroid artery.

2. Physiology

a) Calcium and Phosphate Homeostasis

Parathyroid hormone (PTH) maintains calcium levels between 9-10.5 mg/dL by controlling its absorption by the duodenum and jejunum, absorption via modification of renal sodium transporters, and resorption in the bone via osteoclasts. PTH functions via a cAMP-mediated mechanism. The absorption of calcium via the GI tract is primarily controlled by vitamin D. Hypocalcemia is the chief stimulus for PTH and vitamin D production. Phosphate excretion and bicarbonate excretion are stimulated by PTH. Hyperparathyroidism may therefore lead to hyperchloremic, hypophosphatemic, metabolic acidosis.

b) Hypercalcemia

(1) *Pathophysiology*

Hypercalcemia is the most common presentation of primary hyperthyroidism; when detected in the general population and outpatients, the most common cause is primary hyperthyroidism. However, hypercalcemia in hospitalized patients is more likely to be due to a malignancy. Serum phosphate concentrations are reduced with hypercalcemia. However, a small subset of patients with cancer will have hypercalcemia and hyperphosphatemia; this is thought to be from bone resorption due to tumor-induced osteoclast activity.

(2) *Presentation*

Hypercalcemia presents with CNS changes (psychiatric overtones), nausea and abdominal pain (groans), bradycardia and shortened QT intervals with wide T waves, nephrolithiasis (stones), and bone pain (bones). Excess vitamin A and D, milk-alkali syndrome, and thiazide diuretics can also lead to hypercalcemia.

(3) *Treatment*

Most patients present with asymptomatic disease, and patients requiring aggressive medical or surgical management are uncommon. Hospitalization is mandated for patients with altered mental status or arrhythmia secondary to severe hypercalcemia. Hydration with normal saline to maintain a high urine output in conjunction with furosemide is typically sufficient. Calcitonin can be given exogenously in patients with severe symptoms, along with bisphosphonates, oral phosphates, and glucocorticoids. Surgery should be undertaken as soon as calcium levels normalize.

c) Familial Hypocalciuric Hypercalcemia

This is a genetic disorder that leads to mild, asymptomatic hypercalcemia with relatively normal PTH levels and is due to a defect in the calcium sensor. Surgical resection is contraindicated as it will not repair the root cause of this disease.

d) Hypocalcemia

(1) *Pathophysiology*

Hypocalcemia is sometimes manifested following a total thyroidectomy that leads to disruption of the blood supply or accidental resection of the parathyroid glands. The incidence is approximately 5% but most patients will resolve spontaneously as long as at least a single functional gland remains. If left uncorrected, hypocalcemia leads to osteomalacia in adults and rickets in the pediatric population. Magnesium deficiency also leads to hypocalcemia via inhibition of PTH release and action.

(2) *Presentation*

The key signs of hypocalcemia include tetany (i.e. Tinel sign or Chvostek sign), circumoral paresthesia, numbness and tingling, and peaked T waves with tachycardia. Patients who have undergone a parathyroidectomy or thyroidectomy will reach their lowest calcium level approximately 2-3 days after surgery; continuing symptoms require calcium and vitamin D supplements.

(3) *Treatment*

Most patients can be treated with oral calcium and vitamin D supplements. Severe symptoms should be treated with intravenous calcium gluconate and oral supplementation using calcium carbonate. Calcium chloride requires a central line for infusion.

IV.B. Metabolic Disorders

1. Hypoparathyroidism

a) Etiology and Pathophysiology

Hypoparathyroidism is the development of decreased PTH leading to a decrease in calcium homeostasis. Primary hypoparathyroidism is the result of parathyroidectomy, destruction of the glands in radiation therapy or accidental excision in thyroidectomy, autoimmune syndromes, various congenital causes, and defects in the calcium-sensing receptor.

Secondary disease is due to low PTH levels due to hypercalcemia caused by another etiology. Decreases in PTH lead to bone resorption, increased phosphate excretion, and poor absorption of calcium in the diet. Hypocalcemia is the result.

b) Presentation and Diagnosis

Hypoparathyroidism presents with symptoms of hypocalcemia. Seizures, personality and mood changes, paresthesias, hoarseness, muscle cramps, and irritability are the result. Positive physical exam signs such as Chvostek sign (facial twitching as a result of facial nerve stimulation) and Trousseau sign (carpal spasm due to blood pressure cuff on arm), and choreoathetosis may occur. Paraplegia, Parkinsonism, dystonia, and other motor defects may also occur due to metastatic calcifications in the basal ganglia. PTH titers are decreased in primary disease with hypocalcemia; secondary hypoparathyroidism may present with low PTH and elevated calcium, pseudohypoparathyroidism presents with elevations in PTH due to hormone insensitivity.

c) Treatment

Treatment of primary disease involves calcium and vitamin D supplements. The primary goal is to avoid hypocalcemia and bone resorption.

2. Pseudohypoparathyroidism

a) Assessment

Pseudohypoparathyroidism is typically due to genetic defects that lead to hypocalcemia, hyperphosphatemia, increased PTH, and insensitivity to PTH. PHP typically presents early especially with hypocalcemia. It is an exceedingly rare disorder. Patients present with a complex known as Albright hereditary osteodystrophy (AHO), which includes short stature, rounded facies, shortened metacarpals and metatarsals, obesity, dental hypoplasia, and metastatic calcifications. Diagnosis is made by confirmation of hypocalcemia, PTH assays, assessing PTH responsiveness (or lack thereof), and conducting other endocrine function tests. Basal ganglia calcification may also be present on CT.

b) Management

Treatment of PHP involves IV calcium, vitamin D, calcitriol, and careful management of calcium and phosphate homeostasis. Calcium chloride is the preferred agent.

3. Primary Hyperparathyroidism

a) Etiology and Pathophysiology

Primary hyperparathyroidism is due to increased production of PTH, typically from a hormone-secreting adenoma but sometimes from carcinoma. Although many cases of primary disease are mildly symptomatic, there are nearly 100,000 new cases per year in the United States. It is more common in women in their postmenopausal years. Adenoma development may be due to irregularities in the PRAD 1 / Cyclin D oncogene.

b) Presentation and Diagnosis

Primary hyperparathyroidism typically leads to a single gland hyperplasia primarily affecting chief cells. Multigland disease may occur in 1/10 of all cases. Identification of the affected gland can be done by a visual survey of all four glands during surgery, or via a gamma probe isolation technique using 99m technetium sestamibi scintigraphy. High resolution ultrasound localization has a similar sensitivity to ^{99}technetium sestamibi scintigraphy. Intraoperative measurement of PTH levels can also be used to confirm that the affected gland has been removed; this may mitigate the need to explore the opposite side of the neck and thereby reduce morbidity. While a mass in the neck may indicate parathyroid cancer, the most common cause of an anterior neck mass is a nodule in the thyroid. Elevated calcium to phosphate ratios of 30:1 or more are typically diagnostic. Twenty four hour urine collection studies are necessary to rule out FHH.

c) Treatment

The primary treatment for primary hyperparathyroidism is removal of the affected gland(s). Due to early detection of disease, few patients now present with nephrolithiasis and osteitis fibrosa cystica with pathologic fractures; however, decisive surgical treatment is necessary to forestall the progression of the disease. Natural history studies that have been done on primary hyperparathyroidism suggest that nearly 50% will require surgery within 10 years, and that waiting until the development of advanced disease to treat the hyperparathyroidism will yield less benefit compared to early intervention.

Specific indications for surgical excision include elevations in serum calcium, impairment of renal function or nephrolithiasis, a history of symptomatic hypercalcemic episodes, and symptomatic osteoporosis. Based off the 2002 NIH consensus statement on asymptomatic patients with hyperparathyroidism, surgery is indicated in patients with an elevated serum calcium that is 1.0 mg/dL above the upper limit of normal, a 24 hour urinary calcium secretion over 400 mg, a reduction in creatinine clearance of over 30%, T scores more than 2.5 standard deviations below normal on a bone scan, and patients younger than 50 years of age.

Pregnant females with hyperparathyroidism should have surgery in the second trimester. The majority of tumors are cured by excision; if there is incomplete treatment, care must be taken to identify any aberrant glands through ultrasound and sestamibi scans. The most common site of ectopic glands are those higher in the pharynx due to failure to descend (i.e. near the base of the tongue), along the carotid sheath, near the thymus, or elsewhere within the mediastinum. A sternotomy should not be done during initial surgery. Blind thyroid lobectomy is not recommended due to the rare occurrence of intra-thyroid parathyroid glands. Four gland hyperplasia is managed by subtotal 3 ½ gland resection as the incidence of permanent hypoparathyroidism is unacceptably high with four gland resection.

4. Secondary Hyperparathyroidism

a) Assessment

Secondary hyperparathyroidism is due to a defect in calcium homeostasis, often secondary to renal disease. It is commonly found in patients receiving dialysis leading to metastatic calcification, osteitis fibrosa cystica, bone erosions (leading to a ground-glass appearance in the skull), hyperphosphatemia, and normal calcium. Bone pain with fractures, peptic ulcer disease, and metastatic calcification are all presenting signs. The inability to hydrolyze vitamin D into the active form by poor functioning of 1-alpha-hydroxylase leads to an elevation in PTH to maintain serum calcium levels.

b) Management

The goal of therapy is to normalize serum calcium levels through moderation of aluminum intake (which exacerbates the osteoporosis), correcting hyperphosphatemia, and providing oral calcium and vitamin supplementation. Surgery is the next step for any patient who remains symptomatic and refractory to medical management, especially for patients who are candidates for renal transplant. A subtotal parathyroidectomy should be completed.

5. Tertiary Hyperparathyroidism

a) Assessment

Long term activation of the parathyroid gland, as in patients with calcium maintenance problems from end stage renal disease, may lead to production of PTH that is no longer responsive to the calcium sensor; this is termed tertiary hyperparathyroidism. Continued hypercalcemia one year after a renal transplant confirms the diagnosis.

b) Management

Tertiary hyperparathyroidism is treated with parathyroidectomy with removal of all affected glands. A subtotal parathyroidectomy should be completed.

IV.C. Cancer

1. Parathyroid Carcinoma

a) Assessment

Parathyroid cancer is typically evident in the setting of hyperparathyroidism with fibrotic and inflammatory changes and possible invasion into nearby structures. The long term prognosis of parathyroid cancer tends to be poor unless there is satisfactory wide excision of the tumor with negative margins. Parathyroid cancer affects about 1 in 100 patients who present with hyperparathyroidism. With parathyroid cancer, PTH, alkaline phosphatase, and hypercalcemia are evident.

b) Management

Treatment of parathyroid cancer requires a parathyroidectomy with ipsilateral thyroid lobectomy and lymph node dissection. Chemoradiation is not necessary. Recurrent disease is best treated with resection using wide margins.

V. Endocrine Pancreas

V.A. General Concepts

1. Anatomy

a) Embryology

The ventral bud forms the uncinate process and a portion of the head, while the dorsal bud becomes the remainder of the pancreas. Their fusion is required to avoid pancreas divisum or annular pancreas; fusion forms the duct of Wirsung, also known as the main pancreatic duct. The duct of Santorini, or the accessory pancreatic duct, arises from the dorsal bud.

b) Anatomic Relationships

The pancreas is a retroperitoneal organ located posterior to the pylorus and anterior to the gastric wall. The head of the body is nestled within the 2nd and 3rd portion of the duodenum. The head becomes the neck at the gastroduodenal artery and is proximal to the superior mesenteric artery. The body continues as the enclosure to the splenic artery and vein. The tail of the spleen is near the spleen, while the left adrenal gland is proximal to the juncture of the body and tail. The Kocher maneuver is used to mobilize the pancreas and duodenum.

c) Vascular Supply

The blood supply to the pancreas comes from branches of the celiac artery and superior mesenteric artery (SMA). Collateral branches of the gastroduodenal artery (GDA) become the superior anterior and superior posterior pancreaticoduodenal artery, while branches of the SMA become the inferior anterior and inferior posterior pancreaticoduodenal artery. As the pancreas shares its blood supply with the duodenum, resection of the head of the pancreas also requires a duodenectomy. The venous drainage of the pancreas is eventually into the portal vein.

2. Physiology

a) Insulin

Normal insulin formation leads to the production of C peptide; hence, exogenous abuse of insulin will have low C peptide levels while an insulinoma will have high C peptide levels. Insulin leads to glucose absorption throughout the body except in the brain and liver. Insulin is secreted by beta cells of the pancreas.

b) Glucagon

Glucagon is secreted by alpha cells of the pancreas and leads to glycogenolysis. Glucagon balances the effects of insulin. Glucagon leads to glucose release and provides energy during times of physiologic stress. Glucose uptake in the intestines is an active process and requires a sodium gradient. Glucose metabolism in early sepsis is retarded due to decreased utilization. The intermediary between lactate and glucose is pyruvate. A hormone present in early septic shock is glucagon.

c) Somatostatin

Somatostatin is a gastrointestinal inhibitory hormone that shuts down GI activity. It is released by delta cells within the pancreas. Octreotide is the synthetic form of somatostatin.

V.B. Cancer

1. General Evaluation

If a pancreatic neoplasm is suspected, the workup begins with a pancreas-protocol triple-phase CT scan with thin cuts. The purpose is to identify any suspicious masses, evaluate the burden of disease, and for surgical planning. Following a CT, endoscopic ultrasound (EUS) is completed for anatomy and to potentially obtain a tissue diagnosis; given how sensitive this study is for insulinomas and glucagonomas, it may even be used as the initial diagnostic study. An ERCP may be completed if there is suspicion for a cholangiocarcinoma. If additional imaging is necessary, MRI may help confirm unclear CT findings. A thorough biochemical evaluation is completed including titers of all hormones, cancer markers, and end products. Finally, nuclear medicine imaging through an octreotide scan can be completed to identify pancreatic neoplasms.

In particularly difficult diagnostic cases when a neoplasm is strongly suspected but not evident on imaging studies, sampling of the portal venous supply can be done to help identify the location of the tumor. Finally, intraoperative ultrasound has a sensitivity and specificity that exceeds EUS and may be used to find small masses.

2. Gastrinoma

a) Assessment

Gastrinomas present with an elevation of gastrin leading to GERD, abdominal pain, diarrhea, and ulcer formation within the stomach and duodenum.

Serum gastrin levels over 1,000 pg/mL are diagnostic for gastrinoma; levels between 200 and 1,000 pg/mL requires a secretin stimulation test. This test must be done off PPIs or H_2 blockers.

b) Management

Unresectable disease may be managed using PPIs but may still require a gastrectomy for refractory disease. The majority of gastrinomas are found within the gastrinoma triangle, the bounds of which are the neck of the pancreas, porta hepatis, and third portion of the duodenum. All attempts to fully resect the gastrinoma should be made as this can be potentially curative.

3. Insulinoma

a) Assessment

Insulinoma presents with hypoglycemia during fasting with glucose levels below 50 mg/dL that requires intake of carbohydrates. Catecholamine release is triggered from the hypoglycemia and leads to sympathetic overdrive, while CNS changes occur from the decrease in substrate to the brain. The diagnosis of an insulinoma relies on documenting the presence of insulin despite a continued decline in glucose below normal and an insulin-to-glucose ratio over 0.4. C peptide is also elevated, indicating that surreptious use of insulin is not the case. Detailed imaging of the pancreas is necessary as insulinomas can occur anywhere within the pancreas. About 1 in 10 insulinomas are malignant.

b) Management

Enucleation, even with a laparoscopic approach, can be used to excise focal masses. A distal pancreatectomy can be completed for tumors within the body and tail. A pancreaticoduodenectomy is done for deep tumors within the head. If the tumor cannot be found despite the use of intraoperative ultrasound, sampling of various arteries and veins supplying or leaving the pancreas is done using calcium as the stimulant. A specific excision can be done in this case; failing this, a pancreaticoduodenectomy must be completed. Octreotide and diazoxide can be used for malignant, unresectable tumors.

4. Glucagonoma

a) Assessment

Glucagonoma presents with necrolytic migratory erythema, diabetes, anorexia, anemia, and angular stomatitis. Diagnosis is made clinically in the context of an elevated glucagon level during fasting. Most tumors are located within the body and tail of the pancreas.

b) Management

Octreotide is the standard therapy for all tumors that cannot be surgically resected. Most patients will present with metastatic disease, and a diligent search and resection must be completed for the best chance of a cure.

5. VIPoma

a) Assessment

VIPoma presents with watery diarrhea, hypokalemia, and achlorhydria with acidosis (WHDA syndrome). Elevated levels of VIP must be documented. Most tumors are located within the body or tail or the pancreas.

b) Management

The best treatment of patients with VIPoma is surgical resection, typically a distal pancreatectomy. A search for metastatic disease should be done, especially at the liver where ablation is curative. Octreotide can be used for unresectable tumors.

6. Somatostatinoma

a) Assessment

Somatostatinomas are a rare pancreatic neoplasm and tends to present with near complete shutdown of the gastrointestinal system. This includes cholelithiasis, achlorhydria, steatorrhea from lack of pancreatic enzymes, and diabetes. An elevated somatostatin level in the context of these clinical findings is diagnostic. Most tumors are located within the head of the pancreas.

b) Management

The best treatment for a somatostatinoma is resection and debulking of the tumor. Most tumors are found within the head of the pancreas and tend to metastasize to the liver.

VI. Adrenal Glands

VI.A. General Concepts

1. Anatomy

a) Embryology

The adrenal medulla is derived from the neural crest while the cortex arises from the mesoderm. The adrenal cortex matures into the zona glomerulosa, zona fasciculata, and zona reticularis. Remnants of the neural crest may remain as the organ of Zuckerkandl at the bifurcation of the aorta.

b) Surgical Anatomy

The adrenal glands are composed of the cortex and medulla and are located at the superior pole of the kidney. The right adrenal gland is proximal to the inferior vena cava, while the left adrenal gland is proximal to the tail of the pancreas. The zona glomerulosa is the outermost layer of the adrenal cortex and produces mineralocorticoids. The zona fasciculata is the middle layer of the cortex and produces glucocorticoids. The innermost layer of the cortex is the zona reticularis and produces androgens.

2. Physiology

a) Glucocorticoids

Cortisol production occurs in the zona glomerulosa and is regulated by the hypothalamic-pituitary-adrenal axis. The hypothalamus produces CRH, which stimulates ACTH production by the pituitary gland. This stimulates cortisol release by the adrenal gland. Cortisol is a steroid hormone that binds to intracellular receptors, which is then transported across the nuclear membrane to bind to promotors of transcription. Cortisol helps maintain volume homeostasis, regulate the immune system, modulate glucose control, and maintain blood pressure. The metabolite of cortisol is 17-hydroxycorticosteroids and can be measured in the urine as part of the work up of a suspicious adrenal mass.

b) Mineralocorticoids

Aldosterone is the primary mineralocorticoid produced by the zona fasciculata and is the end point of the renal-angiotensin-aldosterone axis. Aldosterone leads to sodium retention by the kidney and thereby increases intravascular volume; aldosterone also leads to vasoconstriction.

c) Androgens

DHEA production occurs within the zona reticulata and is regulated by ACTH.

d) Catecholamines

The adrenal medulla produces epinephrine through the function of PNMT, which converts norepinephrine into epinephrine. Catecholamines play an important role in maintaining the cardiovascular system and function through both alpha and beta receptors. The metabolites of catecholamines include metanephrines and VMA, which are excreted in the urine.

VI.B. Metabolic Disorders

1. Hypercortisolism

a) Etiology and Pathophysiology

Cushing syndrome, or hypercortisolism, is the excess production of cortisol or intake of exogenous steroids. Cushing syndrome is typically secondary to increased secretion of ACTH by the pituitary gland (known as Cushing disease). In about 1 in 10 patients, the production of ACTH may be by an ectopic source such as a non-small cell lung cancer. ACTH-dependent hypercortisolism leads to bilateral gland hyperplasia. Primary adrenal hypercortisolism is due to single gland disease with nodular hyperplasia. Females are more affected than males.

b) Presentation

Cushing syndrome presents with the typical signs of moon facies, buffalo hump, fat pads in the head and neck, truncal obesity, striae, proximal muscle weakness, bruising, hirsutism, HTN, DM, and symptoms related to other etiologies. Subclinical disease may also be found as part of a CT scan completed for other reasons, leading to the diagnosis of an adrenal mass termed an "incidentaloma."

c) Diagnosis

The first step in the diagnosis of Cushing syndrome is a low-dose dexamethasone suppression test; patients with the disease will not suppress. Urine collections for free cortisol are also used. A high-dose dexamethasone suppression test distinguishes between pituitary tumors (suppresses), and ectopic ACTH production from tumors (no suppression). Anatomic imaging is required to assist with surgical planning. A CT scan or MRI of the abdomen is sensitive for adrenal masses, while an MRI with contrast is sensitive for the detection of pituitary tumors.

d) Treatment

Cushing disease (i.e. pituitary derangement) may require radioablation or transphenoidal resection. Cushing syndrome (i.e. adrenal derangement) may require adrenalectomy with glucocorticoid replacement or medical ablation with ketoconazole, mitotane, metyrapone, aminoglutethimide, and etomidate. Tertiary disease (i.e. ectopic production of hormone) should be treated with surgical excision whenever possible.

2. Pseudo-Cushing Syndrome

a) Assessment and Management

Pseudo-Cushing syndrome is a transient excess in cortisol due to increased release of corticotrophin-releasing hormone (CRH). This disorder is commonly due to excess alcohol consumption. Pseudo-Cushing syndrome presents like Cushing syndrome with spontaneous resolution within a matter of weeks or months after avoiding alcohol.

3. Hyperaldosteronism

a) Etiology and Pathophysiology

Excess secretion of aldosterone leads to a derangement of normal sodium and potassium balance with subsequent hypernatremia and hypokalemia with increased volume retention. The end result is a suppression of the RAA axis. Hyperaldosteronism is also known as Conn syndrome.

b) Presentation

Primary hyperaldosteronism may be the underlying diagnosis in up to 10% of patients with essential hypertension. The most common presentation is a single adrenal adenoma. Idiopathic bilateral adrenal hyperplasia is a cause of hyperaldosteronism while adrenocortical cancer is a rare cause. Secondary hyperaldosteronism is due to increased renin, which in turn leads to higher levels of aldosterone through the RAA axis.

c) Diagnosis

The combination of hypertension with hypokalemia and decreased renin levels is strongly suggestive of hyperaldosteronism. A renin to aldosterone ratio over 30 is virtually diagnostic. A CT scan is necessary for anatomic imaging and to determine whether disease affects a single gland or is bilateral in nature. Adrenal vein sampling can be used to identify the affected gland; this test is the gold standard in diagnosis but is limited by its technical challenges.

d) Treatment

All functional adenomas should be removed whenever possible. Unilateral disease is often treated with an adrenalectomy and a laparoscopic approach can be used if cancer is not suspected. Prior to surgery, potassium stores must be repleted. Adrenal hyperplasia is treated medically.

4. Hypoaldosteronism

a) Etiology and Pathophysiology

Hypoaldosteronism is due to decreased renin production in CRF, leading to defects in potassium handling and subsequent hyperkalemia. Aldosterone is required for proper sodium-potassium exchange by the principal cells of the cortical collecting tubule; defects in aldosterone lead to excess potassium retention. Hyporeninemic hypoaldosteronism is also known as RTA type IV.

b) Presentation and Diagnosis

Hypoaldosteronism may lead to arrhythmia from the excessively high potassium levels. Mild acidosis may also be present, along with HTN. Other than these manifestations, hypoaldosteronism is typically subclinical, but presenting signs may include fever, nausea, and vomiting. CRF with hyperkalemia confirms the diagnosis.

c) Treatment

Loop and thiazide diuretics are used to correct the hyperkalemia in hypoaldosteronism. Sodium bicarbonate corrects acidosis, while fludrocortisone serves as an analogue to aldosterone. Resins that bind to potassium are used to remove potassium from the body on an emergent basis.

5. Congenital Adrenal Hyperplasia

a) 21-Hydroxylase Deficiency

Congenital adrenal hyperplasia is a spectrum of enzyme deficiencies that lead to abnormalities in genitalia, salt wasting syndromes, and abnormal virilization. The most common disorder is 21-hydroxylase deficiency (17-hydroxyprogesterone elevation). In females this disorder presents with ambiguous genitalia due to virilization from androgens. Males present with normal genitalia but can develop hypotension, hyponatremia, hyperkalemia, and shock.

b) 11-Beta-Hydroxylase Deficiency

11-beta-hydroxylase deficiency (11-deoxycortisol elevation) presents with masculinization in females and precocious puberty in males due to elevation in aldosterone and androgens. Hypertension and hypernatremia are common.

c) 3-Beta-Hydroxysteroid Dehydrogenase Deficiency

3-beta-hydroxysteroid dehydrogenase deficiency (DHEA elevation) presents with clitoromegaly in females and hypospadia with gynecomastia in males. Adrenal insufficiency with glucocorticoid and mineralocorticoid deficiency is common.

6. Primary Adrenal Insufficiency

a) Etiology and Pathophysiology

Adrenal insufficiency is the acute development of nausea, vomiting, abdominal pain, shock, and subsequent death due to adrenal failure. This leads to the inability to produce cortisol, aldosterone, and various androgens. Prompt diagnosis is essential to avoid death. It may occur in patients who are withdrawn from steroid therapy, as a consequence of septic shock, in patients who use medications including ketoconazole, phenytoin, rifampin, and mitotane, Waterhouse-Friderichsen syndrome (adrenal hemorrhage due to meningococcal-induced sepsis), cancer, and infection such as tuberculosis.

b) Presentation and Diagnosis

Addison disease is primary adrenal insufficiency and leads to a decrease in cortisol production with a concomitant rise in ACTH. This leads to ACTH-induced hyperpigmentation, while the hypocortisolism leads to weakness, fatigue, hyponatremia, hyperkalemia, and hypotension. Abdominal pain is common. Diagnosis is made by an abnormal ACTH test that leads to little change in cortisol. Electrolyte abnormalities in adrenal insufficiency include hyperkalemia and hyponatremia. EKG is often done to rule out cardiac manifestations of hyperkalemia. Adrenal insufficiency is diagnosed when the corticotrophin response is less than a 20 mcg/dL increase.

c) Treatment

Other than malignant invasion of the adrenal gland leading to adrenal insufficiency, the primary therapy is nonsurgical and includes exogenous steroid administration. Fluid and electrolyte correction are also necessary. Hypotension is reversed with dopamine or norepinephrine. The glucocorticoid of choice is dexamethasone. Fludrocortisone is a drug sometimes used to correct aldosterone defects.

d) Perioperative Management

Patients with significant adrenal insufficiency should be given 100 mg cortisol 1 hour prior to surgery, followed by a taper of 25 mg Q6H for 2 days, then 25 mg Q12H for 1 day with resumption of the outpatient regimen.

e) Adrenal Crisis

Abrupt cessation of adrenal function may lead to hypotension, cardiovascular collapse, and shock. Common causes include trauma, poor cardiac function secondary to a major cardiac event, and acute thromboembolic events that compromise the adrenal glands. Urgent treatment is required and includes intravenous steroids, cardiovascular support with saline, and monitoring in an ICU environment.

7. Secondary Adrenal Insufficiency

a) Assessment

ACTH deficiency may present with adrenal insufficiency and is commonly the result of long-term steroid administration that blunts the release of ACTH by the pituitary. It may also present with adrenalectomy completed for Cushing disease. The presentation is similar to Addison disease. Other causes include Sheehan syndrome (infarction of the pituitary during childbirth), and other syndromes that lead to compromise of the pituitary or hypothalamus.

b) Management

Secondary adrenal insufficiency is a nonsurgical problem and is treated with steroid administration followed by a gradual taper.

VI.C. Cancer

1. Adrenocortical Carcinoma

a) Etiology and Pathophysiology

Adrenocortical cancer comprises less than 1% of all clinically significant adrenal masses, and tends to occur in perimenopausal females. P53 mutations tend to be ubiquitous. The majority of these tumors is malignant and is metastatic at the time of diagnosis.

b) Presentation

Adrenocortical cancer typically presents with symptoms of enhanced adrenal hormone production. A constellation of symptoms consistent with more than one type of adrenal dysfunction is specific for adrenocortical cancer. Asymptomatic masses are less common.

c) Diagnosis

A full biochemical evaluation and a series of imaging tests are done to confirm the diagnosis. CT scans of the chest, abdomen, and pelvis are necessary to establish the burden of disease and also for surgical planning. Masses over 6 cm, especially those with evidence of local or regional spread, are more likely to be carcinoma than adenoma. Stage I cancers have a less than 50% 5-year survival, and this drops precipitously as staging advances. Most adrenocortical tumors are over 6 cm in size, are irregular in shape, typically produce cortisol or androgens / estrogens, are active about 66% of the time, and typically present with Cushing syndrome.

d) Treatment

The most appropriate treatment for an adrenal carcinoma is surgical resection of the entire tumor with wide margins. All resectable metastatic masses should also be removed. Despite aggressive surgical management, over half of all patients will have recurrent disease. Mitotane, cisplatin, doxorubicin, and 5-FU have all been used with varying degrees of success as chemotherapy.

2. Pheochromocytoma

a) Etiology and Pathophysiology

Norepinephrine- and epinephrine-secreting tumors of the adrenal medulla typically arise from the neuroectoderm and comprise about 0.5% of all cases of essential hypertension. About 1 in 10 tumors are bilateral, extraadrenal, multicentric, malignant, part of the MEN syndrome, or present in children. The majority of extraadrenal tumors are located at the organ of Zuckerkandl, located at the bifurcation of the aorta and another source of neuroectoderm. These sites tend to produce norepinephrine. Pheochromocytoma may be secondary to MEN 2, NF-1, or von Hippel-Lindau syndromes. Both familial disorders tend to have bilateral disease. MEN syndrome is discussed separately below. Defects in the succinate dehydrogenase complex are nearly universal in pheochromocytoma; defects in the RET oncogene tends to occur with MEN 2.

b) Presentation

Pheochromocytomas manifest their effects through a cyclical release of epinephrine and/or norepinephrine, leading to hypertension, headaches, palpitations, and diaphoresis. Careful preoperative evaluation and management prior to surgery is required to avoid a hypotensive crisis and sudden death. Metanephrine is elevated, along with vanillylmandelic acid and catecholamines.

c) Diagnosis

Pheochromocytoma is diagnosed by clinical symptoms and verified by the presence of metanephrines in the plasma and catecholamines in the urine. A 24 hour urine collection is the standard. The presence of chromogranin A can also help confirm the diagnosis. A clonidine suppression test can be used when the diagnosis is unclear. Calcium channel blockers should be used in lieu of beta blockers while undergoing diagnostic testing. CT and

MRI have similar sensitivity for diagnosis, but MRI is preferred for metastatic disease. An ^{131}I-metaiodobenzylguanidine (MIBG) nuclear study is very specific for pheochromocytoma and should be done for all malignant pheochromocytomas.

d) Treatment

Pheochromocytoma is optimally treated with 1 week of full alpha-blockade via phenoxybenzamine, followed by beta-blockade and fluid resuscitation, then surgical resection. Beta-blockade is optional and is typically done for reflex tachycardia from alpha-blockade; however, alpha-blockade is mandatory. A nitroprusside drip may be required intraoperatively. Unresectable disease should be treated with tumor debulking, radiotherapy, and radioablation. Vincristine, dacarbazine, and cyclophosphamide have all been used with positive effect. Five year survival for metastatic disease is less than 50%.

3. Incidentaloma

a) Etiology and Pathophysiology

The most common tumors that metastasize to the adrenal glands are breast cancer, lung cancer, and melanoma. Barring such a significant history, the diagnosis of incidentaloma is becoming more common as various imaging modalities are completed more frequently for other reasons. Subclinical disease is commonly present but recent evidence indicates that surgical resection improves long term morbidity and mortality. Of all incidental masses that are identified, about 40% will be adrenocortical adenomas, 20% metastatic tumors to the adrenal gland, 10% as pheochromocytomas, and 10% as adrenocortical cancers. The remaining 20% are benign soft tissue changes such as lipomas.

b) Presentation and Diagnosis

The initial management of any incidentally-found adrenal masses requires biochemical exclusion of all other adrenal tumors. This is followed by CT and/or MRI; the latter is preferred if metastatic disease is suspected.

c) Treatment

All functioning adrenal masses should be removed surgically, and all tumors that are not obviously malignant may be removed laparoscopically. All non-functioning masses over 3-4 cm should be removed, especially if there is the consideration of cancer.

VI.D. Multiple Endocrine Neoplasia

1. Overview

Multiple endocrine neoplasia (MEN) are inherited in an autosomal dominant fashion with mutations in either the MENIN gene for MEN I, or RET gene for MEN IIA and IIB. MEN I presents with pituitary adenoma, parathyroid hyperplasia, and pancreatic islet cell tumor. MEN IIA presents with parathyroid hyperplasia, MTC, and pheochromocytoma. MEN IIB presents with MTC pheochromocytoma, neuromas, and a marfanoid body habitus. Need to spell out abbreviations

2. MEN I

a) Pituitary Tumors

The most common type of pituitary tumor in MEN I is a prolactinoma, which often presents with bitemporal hemianopsia from impingement upon the optic chiasm. Amenorrhea, galactorrhea, and hypogonadism are other presenting signs. Most tumors can be treated with bromocriptine; however, a transsphenoidal pituitary resection can be completed if the tumor is refractory to medical management and radioablation. Less commonly, the pituitary tumor may manifest with Cushing disease.

b) Hyperparathyroidism

MEN I is transmitted as an autosomal dominant mutation, but it has a variable phenotype. The majority of patients present with hyperparathyroidism in their 30s to 40s. Only half of these patients will also have tumors that affect the pituitary and pancreas; however, it is these tumors that are most likely to lead to death.

Most patients have asymptomatic disease and are only found incidentally to have hypercalcemia. Hyperparathyroidism in MEN I affects all four glands via metachronous lesions and requires either a subtotal parathyroidectomy (preferred) or total parathyroidectomy with autoimplantation.

The initial treatment is to correct the hyperparathyroidism via surgery. This may improve the calcium levels sufficiently to mitigate symptoms from a potential gastrinoma. Continuing disease or evidence of malignant disease requires resection.

c) Pancreatic Tumors

Pancreatic tumors are variable and may be either benign or malignant, and may come in a variety of forms (i.e. insulinoma, gastrinoma, somatostatinoma, glucagonoma, VIPoma, etc.). Given the variability, the standard procedure is to completely excise the entire tumor. The most common type of pancreatic tumor is a gastrinoma (discussed earlier). Insulinoma tends to present as a multifocal disease with MEN I.

3. MEN IIA

a) Hyperparathyroidism

Clinically significant hyperparathyroidism affects about 10-25% of patients with MEN IIA, and most patients tend to be entirely asymptomatic. Due to the need for thyroidectomy with the MTC, most patients will undergo a total parathyroidectomy with autoimplantation.

b) Medullary Thyroid Carcinoma

Medullary thyroid carcinoma presents in nearly all patients with MEN IIA. About 20% of patients with MTC will eventually be diagnosed with MEN IIA. The initial presenting sign is a growing neck mass leading to impingement upon nearby structures. Calcitonin is elevated and may lead to diarrhea, but other hormones may also be produced. Screening is completed by genetic evaluation. Calcitonin levels are followed for recurrent disease. Surgery may be necessary for recurrent disease and can lead to cure.

c) Pheochromocytoma

Half of all patients with MEN IIA will develop a pheochromocytoma, and the majority of these will affect both adrenal glands. Most patients will present with episodic hypertension leading to headache, anxiety, and palpitations. The diagnostic workup has already been discussed. Briefly, surgical resection after full alpha-blockade and beta-blockade preoperatively is necessary.

4. MEN IIB

Pheochromocytoma is part of the presentation of MEN IIB, along with medullary thyroid cancer. Neuromas may occur on various mucosal membranes. A marfanoid habitus is typically present, including kyphosis and pectus excavatum. Gangliomas may lead to Hirschsprung disease.

5. Treatment for MEN

As MEN subtypes present with several distinct tumors, a careful search for other tumors should take place, and the patient should be closely followed. Treatment of hyperparathyroidism is completed with subtotal parathyroidectomy. Pancreatic tumors are ameliorated with medical and surgical therapy. Pituitary tumors are treated with transsphenoidal resection for refractory or enlarging tumors. Medullary thyroid cancer is treated with total thyroidectomy with central node dissection and is treated first in MEN IIA and IIB; chemoradiation is not indicated. Pheochromocytoma is treated with adrenalectomy.

Endocrine Surgery

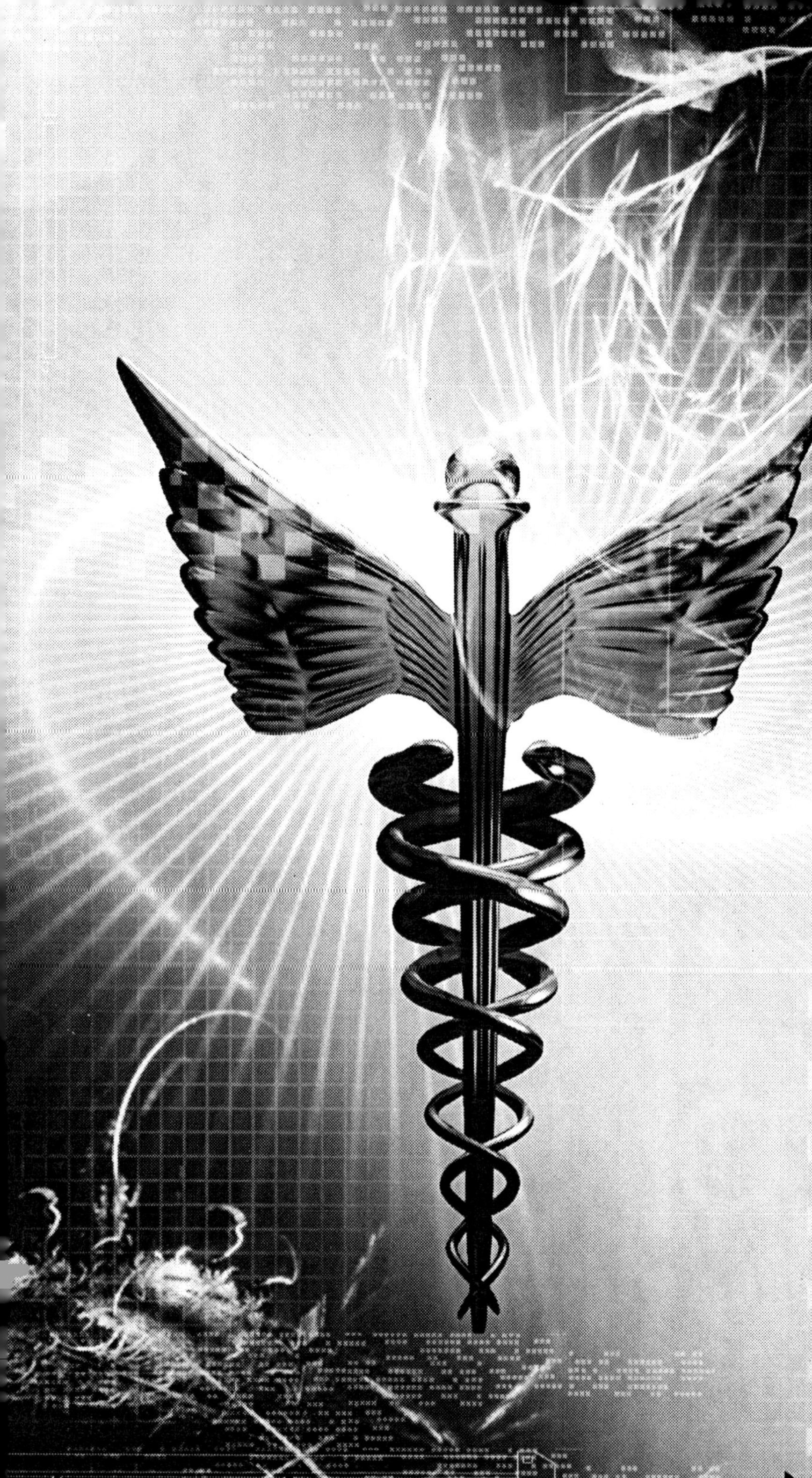

SURGICAL ONCOLOGY

Issam Koleilat, M.D. and Prateek Gupta, M.D.

I. Epidemiology

I.A. Introduction

The first half of the chapter focuses on fundamental concepts in surgical oncology, while the latter half is a review of major clinical oncologic principles. Detailed discussions on various tumors can be found in their respective sections, organized by body system.

I.B. Top 10 Causes of Death

1. Heart disease (29%)
2. Cancer (23%)
3. CVA (7%)
4. COPD
5. Accidents
6. Diabetes
7. Influenza and pneumonia
8. Alzheimer disease
9. Nephritis, nephrotic syndrome, nephrosis
10. Sepsis

I.C. Cancer Statistics

1. Top 3 Cancers by Incidence

- Prostate / Breast Cancer
- Lung Cancer
- Colorectal Cancer

2. Top 3 Cancers by Death

- Lung Cancer
- Prostate / Breast Cancer
- Colorectal Cancer

II. Tumor Biology

II.A. G-Proteins

G-proteins are cellular transmembrane receptors embedded within the plasma membrane that activate signal transduction pathways when stimulated by extracellular molecules. G-proteins are made up of alpha, beta, and gamma subunits. Gs proteins stimulate cAMP and PKA formation, Gi proteins inhibit cAMP and PKA formation, and Gq proteins stimulate IP_3 and DAG formation to increase Ca^{2+} and PKC, respectively. Gs proteins are activated by B1, B2, D1, D5, H2, and V2 receptors. Gi proteins are activated by A2, M2, M4, D2, D4 receptors. Gq proteins are activated by A1, M1, M3, M5, D3, H1, and V1 receptors.

II.B. Receptor Subtypes

1. Adrenergic

- A1 – Vasoconstriction
- A2 – Decrease SNS activity
- B1 – Increase SNS activity
- B2 – Bronchodilation, vasodilation

2. Muscarinic

- M1 – Cortex and hippocampus
- M2 – Decrease heart rate
- M3 – Increase exocrine gland and GI activity
- M4 – Neostriatum
- M5 – Substantia nigra

3. Dopaminergic

- D1 – Renal vasodilation
- D2 – Caudate, putamen, nucleus accumbens, olfactory tubercle, septum, hypothalamus, cortex
- D3 – Limbic structures (cognitive, emotional)
- D4 – Limbic structures (cognitive, emotional)
- D5 – Hippocampus, hypothalamus (pain, affective)

4. Histamine

- H1 – Bronchoconstriction, mucus production in respiratory tract, pruritus
- H2 – Increase GI activity

5. Vasopressin

- V1 – Vasoconstriction (target for antidiuretic hormone)
- V2 – Increased water reabsorption by the kidney (target for antidiuretic hormone)

II.C. Growth Factors

1. Epidermal Growth Factor

EGF is released by macrophages, skin, and neurons. It functions via the tyrosine kinase receptor and leads to elevations in calcium, glycolysis, and protein synthesis leading to cell proliferation. Derangements contribute to tumorigenesis.

2. Erythropoietin

EPO is released by mesangial cells of the kidney and induces erythrocytosis in bone marrow. Overexpression leads to polycythemia vera. EPO functions via EpoR receptors in RBC precursors.

3. Platelet-Derived Growth Factor

PDGF is released by platelets, macrophages, and neurons. Its primary function is regulation of cell growth, migration, angiogenesis, and embryonic signaling. It exerts its effects via the tyrosine kinase receptor. Major pathologies associated with derangements in PDGF include atherosclerosis, fibrosis, and malignancy.

4. Transforming Growth Factor α

TGF-α is released by macrophages, skin, and neurons. Its major function is in epithelial development, neuronal proliferation, and stem cell development via the tyrosine kinase receptor. Pathology related to TGF-α leads to cancer.

5. Transforming Growth Factor β

TGF-β is released by a variety of sources and functions chiefly as a modular of inflammation. It also leads to tissue regeneration, differentiation, and embryonal signaling primarily through the serine, threonine kinase receptors. Complications associated with TGF-β include renal fibrosis following damage, diabetes (treated by ACE-inhibitors), and tumorigenesis.

6. Types of Signaling

Autocrine reactions lead to activation of the cell that secretes the cytokine or other signaling molecule. Paracrine reactions lead to regional activation of signaling pathways. Endocrine reactions involve hormone secretion into the blood and subsequent remote stimulation of signaling pathways throughout the body.

II.D. Cancer Genetics

1. APC

Familial adenomatous polyposis (FAP) is associated with the APC gene on chromosome 5q21 and is an autosomal dominant defect (loss of function mutation). Besides colorectal cancer, other associated tumors include duodenal and gastric cancers, desmoids, papillary thyroid cancer, and osteomas. Gross polyposis occurs throughout the colon, and the overall number of simultaneous events leads to the increase in risk of cancer. Clinically-significant disease is typically present in most people in their 30s. Prophylactic total abdominal colectomy treats the primary manifestations of disease, but most people will eventually die from a secondary manifestation elsewhere. Mutations in APC are also associated with Gardner's syndrome which manifests with colon polyps and dental osseous abnormalities. This is discussed in more detail on page page 262.

2. BRCA-1 and BRCA-2

BRCA-1 and BRCA-2 are associated with breast cancer. BRCA-1 mutations are found on 17q21; BRCA-2 mutations on 13q12. While both increase the risk of breast, ovarian, and prostate cancer, BRCA-2 also leads to an increase in risk for various gastrointestinal and hepatobiliary tumors. BRCA-1 and 2 are discussed in more detail on page 348.

3. c-kit

C-kit mutations are associated with gastrointestinal stromal tumor development. The most appropriate therapy is Gleevec, or imatinib, a tyrosine kinase receptor antibody. C-kit normally functions as a receptor for certain growth factors. This is discussed in more detail on page 216.

4. MLH and MSH

MLH1, MSH2, and MSH6 are associated with HNPCC (Hereditary nonpolyposis colon cancer) and are found on chromosomes 2 and 3. Mutations of these genes are associated with colorectal cancer, bladder and renal cell cancer, and various gastrointestinal malignancies. This autosomal dominant defect disrupts DNA mismatch repair genes and accelerates tumorigenesis with clinically-significant disease present in just a couple of years after the mutation. The typical adenoma to cancer sequence in sporadic colon cancer typically takes up to a decade. Early detection is necessary so that a prophylactic total abdominal colectomy can be completed. This is discussed in more detail on page 253.

5. P16

P16 is one of the proteins involved in cell cycle regulation and is associated with malignant melanoma and pancreatic cancer. Mutations are found on chromosome 9p21.

6. P53

The most commonly mutated gene in most cancers is p53. Also heavily involved in cell cycle regulation and apoptosis, p53 is associated with Li-Fraumeni syndrome and has a mutation in chromosome 17p13. Li-Fraumeni syndrome is associated with a diverse group of cancers throughout the body. Any patient who develops a cancer before the age of 45 is suspected of having this autosomal dominant mutation. Radiation exposure is major risk factor for the development of this defect.

7. Rb

Rb is a mutation on 13q14 associated with retinoblastoma. Normally, Rb is involved in cell cycle regulation. Other tumors associated with Rb mutations include sarcomas and melanomas. Hereditary tumors present in infants and typically with bilateral ocular disease. Sporadic forms present early in childhood and are unilateral. An epigenetic phenomenon with hypermethylation of the retinoblastoma promoter element is also associated with carcinogenesis. Other tumors may have genetic instability induced by hypomethylation.

8. SMAD and DPC

These proteins are part of a superfamily of proteins that modulate the downstream effects of TGF-B signaling, resulting in inhibition of cellular growth. Defects in SMAD and DPC occur on chromosome 18q21 and are associated with juvenile polyposis coli and pancreatic cancer. This is discussed in more detail on page 334.

9. VHL

Von Hippel-Lindau is associated with a VHL mutation on 3p25 and leads to renal cell cancer, pheochromocytoma, and CNS hemangioblastomas. This autosomal dominant mutation leads to a defect in a tumor suppressor gene leading to unopposed angiogenesis.

10. WT

Wilms tumor is due to a mutation on 11p13 that leads to mental retardation, renal agenesis, and profound defects in the genitourinary system including Wilms tumor of the kidney.

II.E. Tumor Markers

1. CEA

Carcinoembryonic antigen (CEA) is a glycoprotein marker for colorectal cancer. Like all other cancer markers, it is neither very sensitive nor specific for cancer and there are numerous false positives and false negatives. Smoking, COPD, and IBD can all falsely elevate CEA levels. Like most other tumor markers, CEA is used to indirectly assess the tumor burden; it is expected to decrease following a surgical resection, and a subsequent increase is thought to indicate recurrent disease.

2. AFP and Beta-HCG

Alpha-fetoprotein (AFP) is a polypeptide formed by the liver and various gastrointestinal organs. It is an indirect maker for hepatocellular carcinoma and nonseminomatous testicular cancer (especially yolk sac tumors). Beta-HCG (human chorionic gonadotropin) is secreted by the placenta during pregnancy and is more likely to be elevated in choriocarcinoma. Like other tests, it is used in combination with multiple studies to arrive at a diagnosis and prognosis.

3. CA 19-9

CA 19-9 is a glycoprotein found in the pancreas and biliary system. It can also be positive for colorectal cancer, but its utility in making this diagnosis is very limited. This is discussed in more detail on page 253.

4. CA 125

CA 125 is an indirect glycoprotein marker for cervical and endometrial tumors. This is discussed in more detail on page 602.

II.F. Cell Processes

1. Apoptosis

Apoptosis is programmed cell death and is a part of normal development. Apoptosis occurs in response to cell damage, infection, stress, or DNA damage. Morphologic features include rounding of the cell, karyolysis (dissolution of the nucleus), pyknosis (condensation and degradation of chromatin), karyorrhexis (rupture of the nucleus and extrusion of the degraded chromatin), blebbing of plasma membrane, and the formation of apoptotic bodies that eventually undergo phagocytosis. Mediators of apoptosis include PARP-1 (poly-ADP ribose polymerase-1), caspases, and fas-associated death domain (FADD).

2. Necrosis

Cell necrosis is unprogrammed, disordered cell death and occurs due to direct injury to cells. Damage to nearby cells occurs due to release of toxic byproducts, such as lysosomal enzymes.

II.G. Transformation

1. Metaplasia

Replacement of one cell type by another as part of an adaptive response is termed metaplasia. This is not defined as a tumor or carcinoma in-situ. An example of metaplasia is Barrett esophagus in GERD in which columnar cells from the stomach replace the squamous cell layer in the esophagus. Metaplasia can be reversed.

2. Dysplasia

Dysplasia is the loss of cell polarity with hyperplastic changes leading to carcinoma in-situ. This is a pre-cancerous change. Changes in cellular size from one to another occur with an increased nucleus to cytoplasm (N:C) ratio. Numerous mitotic spindles are present. Dysplasia occurs due to underlying accumulated genetic mutations.

3. Anaplasia

Anaplasia is the loss of apical/basolateral cell polarity with cells able to survive without being anchored to a basement membrane. There is significant variability in cell size, regression to immature-looking cells, increased N:C ratio, multiple, odd-looking mitotic spindles, and multiple genetic abnormalities and mutations. Anaplasia is the lack of visible cellular differentiation, whereas dysplasia is the lack of normal cellular arrangement.

4. Angiogenesis

Initially cancerous cells receive nutrients by simple diffusion. Beyond a certain diameter, this no longer remains feasible for the tumor. VEGF (Vascular Endothelial Growth Factor), FGF (Fibroblast Growth Factor), and PDGF lead to angiogenesis and expression of these factors is required by tumor cells in order for additional growth to occur. Inhibition of angiogenesis by IFN-A, or synthetic agents such as bevacizumab, leads to inhibition of tumor cell growth.

5. Invasion and Metastasis

Tumors become invasive and start to seed metastatic foci when adherence to the basement membrane via E-cadherins and other members of the extracellular matrix fails. E-cadherin binds to catenins, which in turn bind to the cell cytoskeleton via actin filaments. Metastatic potential is amplified by disruption in integrins, expression of proteases, and disruption of protease inhibitors.

II.H. Carcinogens

A variety of carcinogens have been implicated in the development of cancer. While the damage has typically been done at the time of diagnosis, early recognition in a patient with a relevant past medical history is important to permit expeditious surgical and medical measures. Radiation is a major risk factor for a variety of tumors, particularly skin and soft tissue cancers.

There are two stages for carcinogenesis. Initiation occurs following exposure to a specific stimulus and leads to a permanent change in the genome. Promotion leads to repeated exposure to adverse events causing more mutations. Growth eventually becomes unregulated and a tumor forms.

TABLE 11. Carcinogens.

Skin and soft tissue cancers	Arsenic and coal tars
Nasopharyngeal cancer	Epstein-Barr virus (EBV)
Lung cancer	Asbestos, heavy metals, radon gas, toxins in cigarettes
Hepatocellular cancer	Aflatoxin, vinyl chloride, azathioprine, and hepatitis B and C
Leukemia	Benzene, cyclophosphamide, human T-cell leukemia virus (HTLV)

III. Skin Cancer

III.A. Desmoid Tumor

Desmoid tumors arise from fascia or muscle and are usually benign. They are associated with pregnancy and trauma and may be intra-abdominal or extra-abdominal. Intra-abdominal desmoids are diagnosed by MRI followed by incisional or core biopsy. Abdominal wall desmoids are treated by local excision with negative margins. Recurrence rates are very high but metastasis is rare.

III.B. Basal Cell Carcinoma

Basal cell carcinoma (BCC) is the most common form of skin cancer. It commonly involves the sun-exposed areas of the head and neck in older patients with light skin. Increased incidence has also been noted in immunosuppressed patients. Patients with xeroderma pigmentosum have significantly increased susceptibility to BCC and other types of skin cancer.

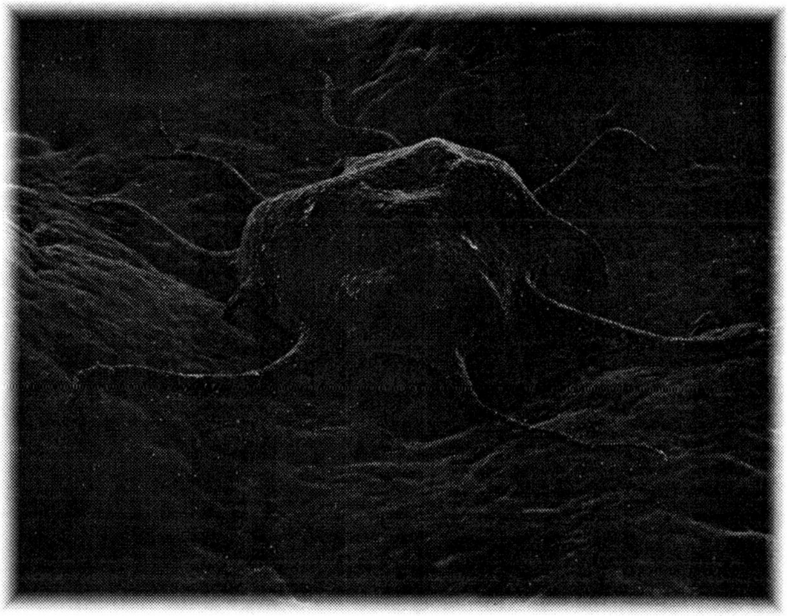

BCC lesions originate from basal epithelial cells in the epidermis and present as pink, pearly papules with rolled edges and central ulceration. They are classified based on their appearance and growth pattern: nodular, superficial spreading, pigmented, or morpheaform sclerosing. Nodular BCC is the most common type, has the classical appearance, and is historically called a "rodent ulcer." Superficial spreading BCC tends to be red and scaly, and grows horizontally without dermal invasion. Pigmented BCC contains melanin and is often confused with melanoma. Morpheaform sclerosing BCC resemble scars in appearance, have indistinct borders, and therefore tend to have positive margins or recur after excision.

BCC is generally locally invasive with low metastatic potential. Less than 0.1% of BCC metastasize to lymph nodes and other distant locations. The primary treatment for BCC is surgical excision with 3 to 5 mm margins. More aggressive lesions, particularly morpheaform sclerosing lesions with indistinct borders, may benefit from margins up to 7 mm. Cure rates for BCC is very high, although there is potential for recurrence; periodic surveillance is necessary. In recurrent cases, cure can usually be achieved with re-excision.

III.C. Squamous Cell Carcinoma

Squamous cell carcinoma (SCC) of the skin is the second most common form of skin cancer. Major risk factors include fair skin, sun exposure, immunosuppression, human papilloma virus, and carcinogens such as nitrates, arsenic, and hydrocarbons. SCC may also develop at the site of chronic wounds. In addition, there are several premalignant lesions that may undergo transformation into SCC. The most common of these lesions is actinic keratosis, which is a scaly, irregularly shaped maculopapular lesion. Actinic keratosis should be treated to prevent transformation into SCC; topical 5-fluorouracil or photodynamic therapy is sufficient in most cases.

SCC generally presents as nodular or papular indurated lesion with distinct borders with ulceration and necrosis over time. They are typically red-brown or erythematous, but may also appear similar to BCC. SCC is classified into verrucous type, ulcerative type, and Marjolin's ulcer. Verrucous SCC is an exophytic, slow-growing lesion with low metastatic potential. Ulcerative SCC is more aggressive and likely to metastasize. Marjolin's ulcers are metastatic lesions that develop in chronically inflamed tissue, particularly in burn scars after several decades.

In general, melanoma has higher metastatic potential than SCC, which has a higher metastatic potential than BCC. Wide local excision with adequate margins is recommended for treatment of most lesions. Margins vary from 4 to 10 mm, and depend on size, depth, location, and grade. Regional lymphadenectomy is indicated if there are palpable nodes or if the lesion is a Marjolin's ulcer. In cases of high-risk lesions without palpable nodes, sentinel lymph node biopsy may be considered. Radiation and chemotherapy are not indicated for primary treatment, but may play a role in recurrent disease or poor operative candidates. Overall cure rate with wide local excision is 95%. However, prognosis is worse with greater depth of invasion, in certain locations (ears, nostrils, scalp, and extremities), and for Marjolin's ulcers. SCC in an extremity with a positive node after node dissection carries a 35% 5-year survival rate.

III.D. Melanoma

Melanoma accounts for less than 5% of skin cancers, but results in 65% of the deaths from skin cancer. Major risk factors include fair skin and hair, sun exposure, history of sunburns, advanced age, immunosuppression, and positive family history. Males develop melanoma more commonly on the trunk, whereas women develop melanoma more commonly in the lower extremities. While blacks have a 10 to 20 times lower risk of developing melanoma, the prognosis is worse because of delayed diagnosis. Predisposing conditions include atypical mole syndrome or familial B-K mole syndrome, dysplastic and atypical nevi, large congenital nevi, and xeroderma pigmentosum.

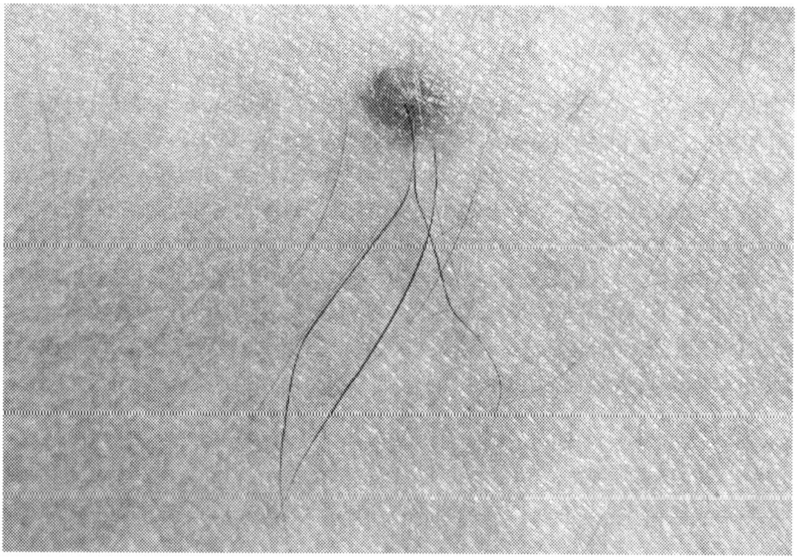

Melanoma originates from the neural crest cells or melanocytes in the basal layer of the epidermis. Early on, radial expansion occurs with little risk of invasion and metastasis. Metastatic potential increases dramatically as the lesion enters the vertical growth phase. Lesions are classically characterized by the ABCDs: asymmetry, border irregularities, color variation, and diameter > 6 mm. The mnemonic can be extended to E for evolution or change in the lesion's appearance.

Melanoma is classified into superficial spreading, nodular, acral lentiginous, and lentigo maligna types. Superficial spreading melanoma is the most common type and has the typical ABCD appearance. They usually arise from preexisting nevi and are of intermediate malignancy. Nodular melanoma is the most aggressive type, arising without a precursor lesion and starting with the aggressive vertical phase. This type of melanoma forms a dark, raised nodule with sharp margins. There is often invasion into deeper tissue with metastasis at the time of diagnosis. Acral lentiginous melanoma occurs on the palms, soles, subungual areas, and mucosa. It is relatively uncommon in whites, but comprises up to 60% of melanoma in African-Americans. The lesions are flat with irregular borders and colors, but are diagnosed late because of their obscure locations. This delay in diagnosis leads to this type of melanoma having the worst prognosis. Lentigo maligna melanoma is the least aggressive type, with a long radial growth phase as a flat pigmented precursor lesion prior to its vertical growth phase.

Melanoma is staged using the TNM (tumor node metastasis) system. Traditionally, primary tumors were described using the Clark levels, which indicate the histologic skin layer to which the tumor has invaded. Studies have shown, however, that tumor thickness (Breslow thickness) is a better indicator of prognosis. T0 lesions are confined to the epidermal layer, T1 lesions are up to 1 mm thick, T2 lesions are up to 2 mm thick, T3 lesions are up to 4 mm thick, and T4 lesions are greater than 4 mm thick. Tumors without and with ulceration are denoted by "a" and "b," respectively (e.g., T1 lesions with ulceration are T1b lesions).

Because melanoma treatment and prognosis is based so strongly on Breslow depth, diagnosis should be made based on biopsies that preserve depth information, and not shave biopsies. Wide local excision is the primary treatment modality, with horizontal margins dependent on depth of invasion. T0 lesions may be treated with 5 mm margins, T1 lesions with 1 cm margins, T2 or T3 lesions with 2 cm margins, and T4 lesions with 3 cm margins if possible. The deep margin should be superficial to the underlying fascia.

Sentinel lymph node biopsy (SLNB) is indicated for all tumors over 1 mm thick without palpable regional lymph nodes. If there are palpable lymph nodes or positive nodes on SLNB are found, complete regional lymphadenectomy is necessary. Adjuvant therapy is reserved for patients who are not surgical candidates and for palliation. Surveillance for recurrence is critically important. Prognosis for melanoma-in-situ is excellent with 5-year and 10-year survival of nearly 100%, while the presence of positive nodes (stage III) carries a 5-year survival of less than 70%. Metastasis (stage IV) is associated with a 5-year survival of less than 20%. The prognosis is significantly worse for black patients, ulcerated lesions, blue discoloration, and mucosal lesions.

Recurrent tumors are likely to be found at the site of excision. Metastasis is most frequently to the lung, brain, and liver. The most common type of tumor metastasis to the small bowel is from melanoma. If the metastasis is isolated to a single site, options for surgical resection should be explored.

Chemotherapy and adjuvant therapy are in the form of cisplatin, vinblastine, dacarbazine (CVD) with interferon alpha and interleukin 2. Long term survival benefits are questionable.

TABLE 12. Melanoma excision margins.

T Stage	Depth of Invasion	Excision Margin
T0	Epidermis	5 mm
T1	<1 mm	1 cm
T2	1 – 2 mm	2 cm
T3	2 – 4 mm	2 cm
T4	>4 mm	2 – 3 cm

Melanoma stages:

Stage 0: Melanoma in situ (Clark level I), 99.9% survival
Stage I/II: Invasive melanoma, 85-95% survival

- T1XN0M0, $T2^{a}$N0M0

Stage II: High risk melanoma, 40-85% survival

- T2BN0M0, T3XN0M0, T4XN0M0

Stage III: Regional metastasis, 25-60% survival

- TXNXM0

Stage IV: Distant metastasis, 9-15% survival

- TXNXM1

III.E. Merkel Cell Carcinoma

Merkel cell carcinoma is a rare and aggressive skin cancer originating from neuroendocrine cells. The firm, painless nodules are often found on the head, neck, and extremities. These nodules may be flesh-colored, red, or blue. Surgical excision is the primary treatment modality, but chemoradiation is frequently indicated as adjuvant therapy.

III.F. Paget Skin Disease

Paget disease of the skin is the development of an adenocarcinoma arising from the apocrine sweat glands. Treatment is with excision unless the tumor is invasive into deeper structures. Paget disease of the skin is associated with gastrointestinal cancer. Radiation therapy is beneficial.

III.G. Summary

- BCC tends to be locally invasive with low metastatic potential.
- The nodular form of BCC exhibits early vertical growth and deep invasion, whereas the superficial spreading form tends to grow horizontally without invasion. Pigmented BCC is often mistaken for melanoma. Morpheaform sclerosing BCC has indistinct borders and may benefit from a wider excision margin.
- Treatment of BCC is excision with 3-5 mm margins (consider 7 mm margins for morpheaform).
- SCC has higher metastatic potential than BCC, but lower metastatic potential than melanoma.
- Treatment of SCC is excision with 4-10 mm margins depending on size, depth, location, and grade. Sentinel lymph node biopsy may be considered in high risk cases without palpable regional nodes. Lymphadenectomy is indicated in the case of palpable regional nodes or positive sentinel nodes.
- Melanoma is less common than BCC or SCC, but accounts for most of the deaths.

- Melanoma can be identified by the ABCDs: asymmetry, border irregularities, color variation, and diameter > 6 mm.
- Superficial spreading melanoma has a long horizontal growth phase, nodular melanoma has an early vertically growth phase and is therefore more aggressive, acral lentiginous melanoma occurs in obscure locations and diagnosed late, and lentigo maligna melanoma is the least aggressive subtype.
- Treatment of melanoma is excision with margins based on depth of invasion. Sentinel lymph node biopsy is indicated for high risk lesions, including all lesions ≥ 1 mm thick. Lymphadenectomy should be performed if there are palpable regional nodes or positive sentinel nodes. There are few indications for adjuvant therapy.
- Prognosis with melanoma is worse for black patients, lesions with a blue color or ulceration, and mucosal lesions.

IV. Soft Tissue Tumors

IV.A. Sarcoma

1. Assessment of Sarcoma

The initial evaluation of a sarcoma typically reveals a slowly growing soft tissue mass over 5 cm. It is generally painless. A core biopsy or incisional biopsy should be performed to yield a tissue diagnosis. Tumors smaller than 3 cm can be excised en toto. Imaging should be completed with an MRI or CT, but the former is often preferred. Sarcomas tend to spread via a hematogenous route, so lymph node biopsy is typically not necessary. Staging is completed based on histology, size, and presence of metastatic disease.

2. Management of Sarcoma

The initial treatment pathway is to complete a margin-negative en bloc resection of the entire tumor; 2 cm margins are preferred. Chemotherapy is effective in Ewing sarcoma and rhabdomyosarcoma. Radiation therapy is also often used.

IV.B. Stewart-Treves Syndrome

Stewart-Treves syndrome is the development of angiosarcoma from prolonged lymphedema, commonly arising after a modified radical mastectomy with full axillary dissection leading to a disruption of lymphatic channels. Resection and radiation therapy is necessary but five year survival is low.

IV.C. Kaposi Sarcoma

Kaposi sarcoma is a tumor of the lymphatic endothelium. It arises especially in the setting of HIV/AIDS. HHV8 (human herpesvirus 8) is the responsible virus leading to these characteristic progressive purple plaques. It typically affects the skin but may also spread to the gastrointestinal and respiratory tracts. Antiviral therapy, chemoradiation, and excision are effective.

V. Clinical Topics in Oncology

V.A. Esophageal Cancer

Perioperative mortality with esophagectomy is 10% and risk factors are increased in older patients, with neoadjuvant therapy, elevated alkaline phosphatase, renal dysfunction, diabetes, alcoholism, and ascites. Wound dehiscence is higher with THE (transhiatal esophagectomy) while TTE (transthoracic esophagectomy) has higher lymph node yield. Neoadjuvant chemotherapy improves 3 year survival in patients with advanced tumors (T3+).

V.B. Colorectal Cancer Syndromes

HNPCC is associated with microsatellite instability and mutations in the MSH2 and MLH1 mismatch repair genes. Gardner syndrome occurs from APC mutations (TSR involved in apoptosis), followed by K-ras activation (transmembrane signal transduction), p53 inactivation (especially left colon and distal), and DCC (Deleted in Colon Cancer) inactivation. Prognosis from the position of the APC mutation is possible and predicts the occurrence of desmoid tumors. Node positive cancers should be treated with

FOLFOX (5-FU, leucovorin [folinic acid], and oxaliplatin), along with any perforating or obstructing tumor. 5-FU can improve survival in stage III cancers by 20%. Capecitabine (Xeloda) is converted to 5-FU but can be taken by mouth with less neutropenia but risk of hand-foot syndrome. Oxaliplatin is a topoisomerase I inhibitor. Bevacizumab (Avastin) is a monoclonal anti-VEGF antibody. Cetuximab (Erbitux) blocks HER-1/EGFR receptors.

V.C. Metastatic Colorectal Cancer

Patients with colorectal cancer metastatic to the liver are candidates for liver resection with 1 cm margins if there are no other lesions that cannot be resected. RFA is suitable only for patients who are not candidates for liver resection. PET CT eliminates patients who are not candidates for liver resection and so improves overall 5 year outcome data.

V.D. Biliary Cancers

Gallbladder adenocarcinoma that extends beyond the mucosa requires wedge hepatectomy, and regional lymphadenectomy. Implantation of the cancer at port sites (including the camera site) is a real problem and requires excision of the port sites. Cholangiocarcinoma that occurs near the hepatic duct requires lobar resection; if it occurs near the common duct, a pancreaticoduodenectomy is completed. Imaging studies include ultrasound and CT. ERCP or MRCP confirms the diagnosis. Tumor along the middle of the biliary tree can be treated with excision and a roux-en-y hepaticojejunal anastomosis.

V.E. GIST

GIST tumors often arise from the stomach or small intestine, and require gross resection with negative margins. Metastasis is hematogenous and lymphadenectomy is therefore not necessary. Gleevec (imatinib), a tyrosine kinase inhibitor, is used as an adjunctive therapy for unresectable or metastatic GIST; most tumor cells express the c-Kit receptor or PDGFRa receptor.

V.F. Epidermoid Anal Cancer

Epidermoid anal cancer responds well to the Nigro protocol: chemoradiation consisting of 50 Gy of radiation and 5-FU and mitomycin C (or cisplatin). Leucovorin can be combined with this therapy in rectal adenocarcinoma. The anal canal extends from the anal sphincter to the anal verge (located at the start of the perianal glabrous region). The dentate line is located at the midpoint of the anal canal. The valves of Houston are within the rectum.

V.G. Appendiceal Cystadenocarcinoma

The presence of a cystadenocarcinoma in the proximal one-third of the appendix or a malignant and invasive lesion in the distal appendix requires a right hemicolectomy.

V.H. Pediatric Tumors

The most common presacral neonatal solid tumor is teratomas. The most common abdominal tumor is neuroblastoma. Rhabdomyosarcoma tends to occur in the head and neck, GU tract, and arms and legs. Wilms tumor is a nephroblastoma and may present with thrombus formation. Ewing sarcoma affects the extremities and responds to chemotherapy.

V.I. Palliative Therapy for Breast Cancer

A patient with a history of breast cancer who presents with back pain needs an MRI for diagnosis of suspected metastatic disease. Radiotherapy is required, and it is urgent in cases of cord compression. High dose corticosteroids are also often given with radiotherapy. Bisphosphonates are used for lytic bone disease.

V.J. MALToma

MALToma (Mucosa-Associated Lymphoid Tissue lymphoma) is associated with H. pylori. Radiation may be administered if necessary; surgery is reserved only for more advanced cases.

V.K. GI Cancer Associations

TABLE 13. Common GI cancer associations.

Syndrome	Mutation	Locus	Notes
HNPCC	hMSH2, hMLH1, hMSH6		Right sided colon CA
FAP	APC	5q21	Thousands of polyps and early CA
Peutz-Jegher	STK11	19p3.3	GI polyps, bowel obstruction, and increased CA risk
Juvenile polyposis syndrome	SMAD4, BMPR1[a] (TGF-beta)		Increased GI malignancy w/ colon hamartomas
Cowden syndrome	PTEN		Hamartomas of skin and GI tract, microcephaly, thyroid dysfunction

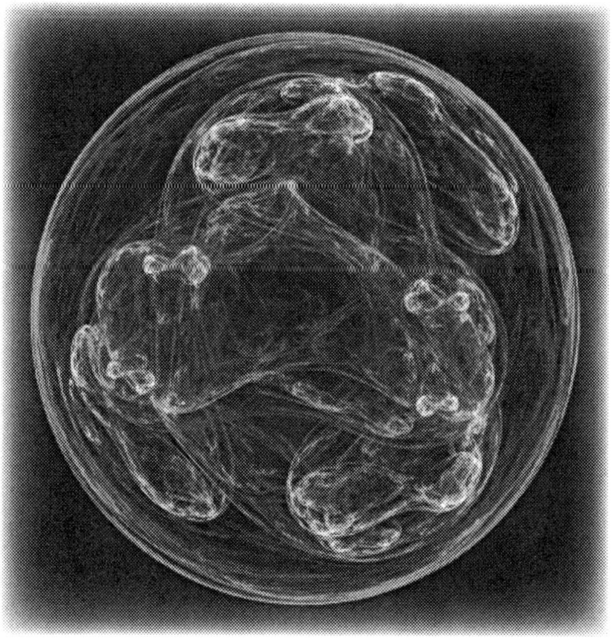

TRANSPLANT

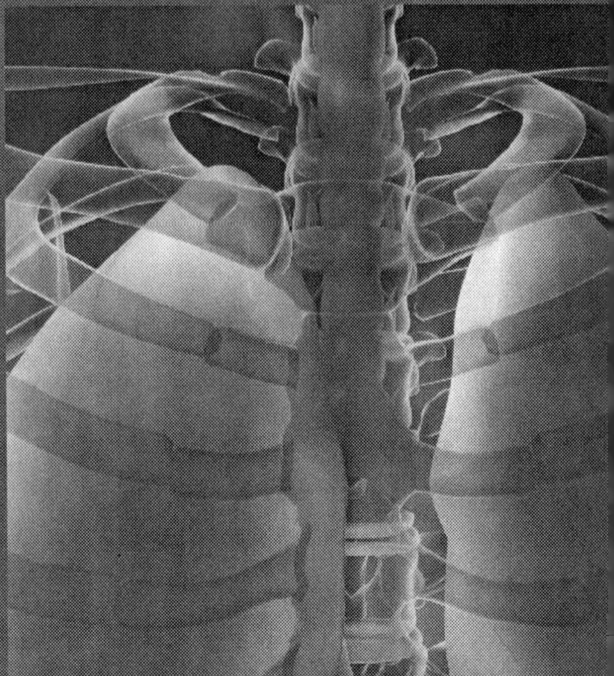

D'autre part, comme il est impossible de connaître parfaitement le tout, si l'on ne connaît dans une certaine mesure chacune de ses parties, il est impossible que celui-là soit bon médecin qui ignore absolument l'art de la chirurgie.

Henri de Mondeville
Die Anatomie (1304)

SURGISPHERE

TRANSPLANT SURGERY

Keri E. Lunsford, M.D., Ph.D. and Sapan S. Desai, M.D., Ph.D.

I. Transplant Immunology

I.A. General Concepts

The immune system acts as the barrier for the body from the outside world. It functions to recognize "self" from "non-self" for the purpose of isolating or removing foreign particles. It most-commonly functions against "non-self" pathogens and microorganisms, including bacteria, fungi, and viruses. In the case of malignancy, mutated "self" cells are recognized as "non-self" and are eradicated. Under some circumstances, "self cells" are recognized as "non-self" and are attacked by the immune system, resulting in autoimmune disease.

The immune system is broadly divided into the innate and adaptive branches. The innate immune system immediately recognizes foreign peptides and cell surface molecules in a non-specific fashion. It is present from birth, and immune response mounted does not require prior exposure to antigens. Components of the innate immune system include complement and the cellular components neutrophils, macrophages, natural killer cells, and eosinophils. Innate immune effectors are active early upon encountering foreign peptides, but they have no memory, so the response to antigens is the same each time it is encountered.

In contrast, the adaptive immune system relies on effector cells that are clonally selected to recognize specific foreign antigenic peptides. Cells are present from birth but are initially naïve to foreign antigen. Components include CD4+ T cells, CD8+ T cells, B cells, and antibodies. They become clonally selected to differentiate "self" and "non-self.'" To avoid self-reactivity, cells that are reactive against "self" molecules undergo anergy and clonal deletion during maturation. Those that are not reactive to self circulate in blood and lymphoid tissue until they encounter foreign peptides presented in conjunction with Major Histocompatibility Complex (MHC) on Antigen Presenting Cells (APC). Once encountered, adaptive immune cells become specifically activated against the presented foreign peptides to form effector cells and antibodies. After the immune response has subsided, the activated immune cells differentiate into memory cells. Memory cells have been previously primed against foreign antigens and can mount a rapid response the next time the antigen is encountered. Memory cells in conjunction with preformed circulating antibodies impart long-lasting immunity.

I.B. Components of the Immune System

1. Innate Immunity

The innate immune system provides the body's initial defense against invading pathogens. It is rapidly activated after encounter with foreign antigen, and it is also phylogenetically the oldest branch of the immune response. Its components react primarily to structures that are not present in normal mammalian cells, including those unique to microbes. These include dsRNA present in replicating viruses, LPS from gram negative bacteria cell walls, unmethylated CpG nucleotides present in bacterial DNA, N-formylmethionyl peptides of bacterial proteins, mannose-rich glycans of microbial glycoproteins or glycolipids, and phosphorylcholine present in microbial membranes. Unlike the adaptive immune system, which undergoes somatic rearrangements, the receptors of the innate immune system are encoded in the germline, and thus have limited diversity. The innate immune system comprises the epithelial barrier to invading pathogens, circulating effector proteins, and effector cells (Table 293).

2. Epithelial Barriers

The intact epithelial barriers form a physical barrier to pathogen entry into the host. This is comprised of an intact barrier of skin, gastrointestinal mucosa, and respiratory mucosa. The epithelial barriers are further enhanced by the production of peptides with intrinsic antimicrobial properties, such as defensins, which increase in response to pro-inflammatory cytokines. In addition, epithelial barriers contain intraepithelial T-lymphocytes, B-1 subset B cells with limited diversity, as well as Mast cells which may respond rapidly to penetration of the epithelial barrier.

3. Effector Proteins

Many plasma proteins are involved in innate immune recognition and effector function, including the complement system, mannose binding lectin, C-reactive protein, and cytokines. The complement system serves to recognize microbes, activate inflammation, and trigger their destruction (Table 1). Complement activation via the classical pathway uses protein C1 to bind to surface antibodies, mainly IgG and IgM. Complement activation via the alternative pathway utilizes direct recognition of certain microbial cell surface elements. Activation of either pathway stimulates a cascade of complement proteins which are proteolytically cleaved to either be covalently bound as opsonins or to act as chemokines for the recruitment of phagocytes. The cascade ultimately cleaves protein C5 into C5a, which attracts and activates neutrophils, and C5b which becomes bound to the complement complex on the target cell. C5b subsequently recruits and binds C6, C7, C8, and C9 which form and Membrane Attack Complex (MAC). This MAC forms a pore in the target cell membrane resulting in cell lysis.

Mannose binding lectin is a plasma protein that binds carbohydrates with terminal mannose or fructose molecules that are typical of bacterial membranes. It acts as an opsonin for binding of a macrophage receptor, called the C1q receptor, resulting in subsequent phagocytosis C-reactive protein is another plasma protein which may act as an opsonin by binding bacterial phospholipids. It subsequently may either bind C1q or induce phagocytosis by interacting with phagocyte FcgR.

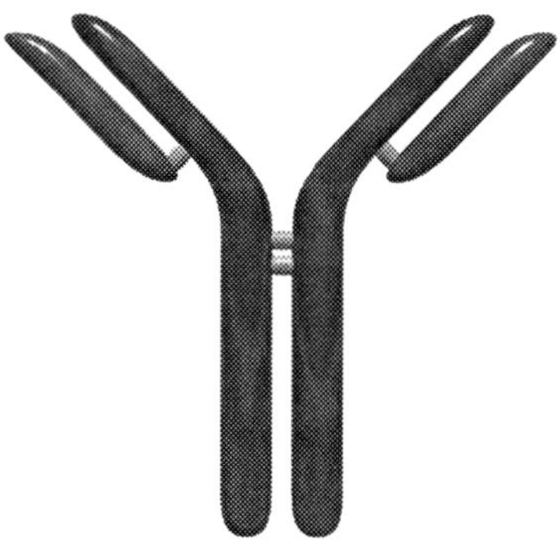

TABLE 1. Complement

Type	Function
C1	Binds to antigen-antibody complex. C1q binds the Fc portion of antibody induces classical complement pathway with target cell death. C1q may also act as an opsonin binding the C1q Receptor on Macrophages inducing phagocytosis
C2	Binds to antigen-antibody complex / activated.
C3	Binds to microbial cell surface to serve as an opsonin. Component of C3 and C5 convertase. Broken down into C3a and C3b. Activated by C3 convertase (C3b/Bb – alternative pathway or C4b/C2a – classical pathway)
C3a	Weak neutrophil chemotactic agent, anaphylatoxin, stimulates inflammation.
C3b	Combines with C2a and C4b (classic pathway) or combines with Bb (alternative pathway) to form C5 convertase which activates the late steps of the complement pathway
Bb	Alternative pathway. Serine protease and the active enzyme in C3 and C5 convertase.
C4	Cleaved by C1 to form C4a and C4b
C4a	Anaphylatoxin, stimulates inflammation
C4b	Binds to surface of cell where antibody is bound and complement is activate. Combines with C2a and C3b in the classical pathway to form C5 convertase
C5	Broken down into C5a and C5b by C5 convertase
C5a	Strong neutrophil chemotactic agent.
C5b	Membrane attack complex.
C6	Membrane attack complex.
C7	Membrane attack complex.
C8	Membrane attack complex.
C9	Membrane attack complex.
DAF	Found on surface of cells to prevent complement-deposition and activation.

4. Effector Cells

Neutrophils, macrophages, and NK cells are the major components of cell-mediated innate immunity. Their functions are summarized in Table 293.

Neutrophils or polymorphonuclear leukocytes (PMNs) are the most abundant circulating leukocyte class. They are the first cells to response to an inflammatory response. Their main effector function is the secretion of cytolytic and proteolytic enzymes from cytoplasmic granules or the phagocytosis of opsonized cells.

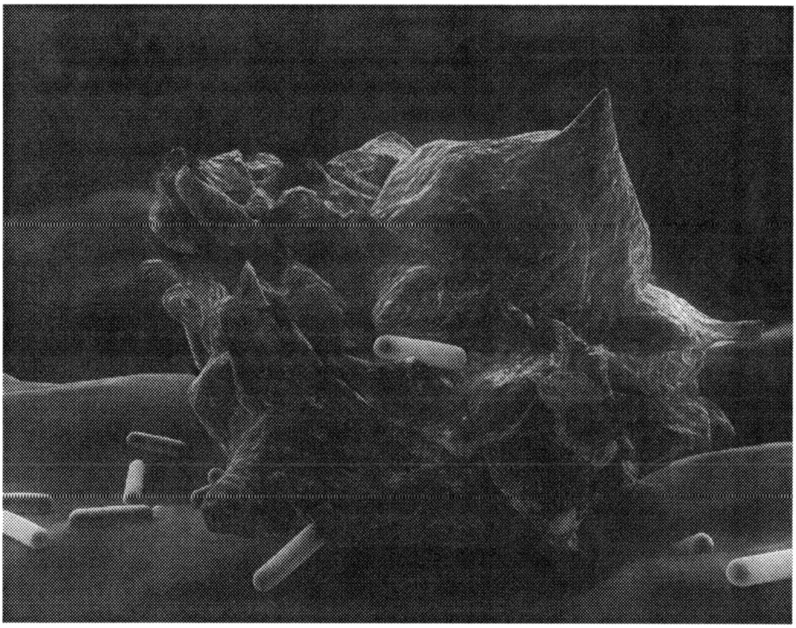

Macrophages constitute the majority of resident immune cells within tissues. They are thus poised to be early responders to inflammation, and their functions overlap greatly with those of neutrophils. However, unlike neutrophils, macrophages are not terminally differentiated, and they thus persist much longer during the inflammatory response than do neutrophils. They function to secrete cytotoxic agents, phagocytose opsonized cells, and to recruit lymphocytes to the site of inflammation through the secretion of various chemokines and cytokines.

NK cells are a subset of lymphocytes that are not MHC restricted and that do not acquire memory. They principally act as defense against viral infections and intracellular pathogens via direct cell lysis and via antibody-dependent cell mediated cytotoxicity through interaction of antibody coated cells with surface Fc receptors on NK cells.

Table 2. Effector cells of the immune system.

	Cell Type	Selected Surface Proteins	Function
Innate Immune Effector Cells	Neutrophils (PMNs)	FcgR1 Mannose Receptor IL8-R	-Circulate in blood until recruited to a site of inflammation -Secrete cytotoxic granules filled with degradative enzymes such as lysozyme, collagenase, and elastase -Secrete reactive oxygen intermediates and NO to kill extracellular microbes -Phagocytosis of microbes and opsonized particles -Mediate the earliest phases of the immune response -Terminally differentiated- Life span of only six hours then undergo programmed cell death if not recruited to site of inflammation
	Macrophages	MHC II, Mac-I FcgR1 C1qR TLRs	-Resident immune cells in connective tissue, parenchymal interstitial, vascular linings of spleen and liver, and lymph node sinuses -Phagocytosis of antigens at sites of entry to the host -Activated early in the immune response but longer-lasting response than neutrophils -Present phagocytosed antigen to T cells via MHC to activate the adaptive immune response -Secrete reactive oxygen intermediates and NO to kill extracellular microbes -Secrete chemokines and cytokines, including TNF-ab, IFN-a, IFN-b, and IL-12 as effectors of cell-mediated immunity and recruiters of leukocyte migration. -May divide in tissues (i.e. not terminally differentiated) -Specialized Macrophages are found in tissues including liver (Kupffer cells), Skin (Langerhans cells), bone (Osteoclasts), and brain (Microglia).

	NK cell	CD16 MHC I TLRs	-Lymphocyte subset which does not acquire memory -Principle function in defense against viruses and intracellular microbes -Lyse target cells via antibody-dependent cell-mediated cytotoxicity -Recognize and lyse cells lacking MHC I, such as tumor cells -Produce IFN-g -Expansion and cytolytic properties stimulated by IL-15 and IL-12
Adaptive Immune Effector Cells	B-cell	CD19, CD20 IgM MHC I MHC II	-Antibody production (Humoral immunity). -Activated B cells form plasma cells which secrete large amounts of antibody and form a clonal population. -Memory B-cells – long-lasting humoral immunity with ability to rapidly form a clonal population when reactivated. -Act as antigen-presenting by presenting foreign antigen in conjunction with MHC II for T cell activation
	CD8+ T cell	CD3, CD8 TCR	-Naïve CD8+ T cells recognize antigen in conjunction with MHC class I -Activated CD8+ T cells become cytotoxic T lymphocytes which directly attack target cells presenting "non-self" antigen on MHC class I, such as virally infected cells, by excretion of cytotoxic granules and perforin -Induce cell death of target cells via interaction of Fas and Fas Ligand
	CD4+ T cell	CD3, CD4, CD28 TCR	-Naïve CD4+ T cells recognize antigen in conjunction with MHC class II present on Antigen Presenting Cells -Activated CD4+ T cells differentiate into Th1 or Th2 phenotypes which predominantly secrete cytokines for the activation and recruitment of effector cells -Th1 subset activates predominantly cell-mediated responses through secretion of IFN-gamma and IL2. -Th2 subset activate predominantly humoral responses through secretion of IL-4 and IL-10

5. Cytokines

Cytokines and chemokines are proteins produced by cells of the innate and adaptive immune system that mediate the activation, recruitment, and effector function of these cells. Certain cytokines are intrinsic within the innate immune response. These include IL-1, IL-6, IL-12, IL-15, IFN-a, IFN-b, TNF-a/b, and IFN-g. The function of these cytokines is reviewed in Table 294. Briefly, the cytokines IL-1, IL-6, and TNF-a/b are important early cytokines produced during the innate immune response. TNF is the principle mediator of the acute inflammatory response. In high doses, it enters into circulation to mediate many of the systemic complications associated with sepsis. IFN-a and IFN-b are important in the activation and anti-viral function of NK cells. IL-12 increases the cytolytic activity of NK cells, and IL-15 stimulates NK cell proliferation. IFN-g is important in increasing activation of macrophages and enhancing antigen expression on MHC.

Table 3. Selected cytokines.

Type	Features	Notes
IL-1	Produced by macrophages, endothelial cells, and some epithelial cells (e.g. skin). Activates acute phase reaction and inflammation. Activates endothelial cells. Stimulates fever in the hypothalamus. Stimulates production of acute phase proteins by the liver.	Increases body temperature (resets hypothalamus temperature regulation) and increases adhesion factor expression by cells (promotes extravasation of immune mediators). IL-1 receptor antagonist is used for the treatment of RA.
IL-2	Produced by T-cells and stimulates T-cell response.	Used as adjunctive therapy in cancer, especially malignant melanoma and renal cell carcinoma. IL-2R antagonist used as induction agent for transplantation
IL-6	Produced by macrophages, endothelial cells, and T cells. Activates acute phase reaction and inflammation. Stimulates production of acute phase proteins by the liver. Stimulates antibody production by B cells	Very high levels following trauma, burns, and tissue damage. Stimulates osteoblasts to stimulate osteoclasts. Estrogen inhibits IL-6 and so can theoretically be used for the treatment of osteoporosis. Induces fever. Works through gp130.

IL-10	Produced by macrophages and T cells (mainly Th2 cells). Inhibits IL-12 production and expression of MHC class II and costimulatory molecules by macrophages	
IL-12	Produced by macrophages and dendritic cells. Induces IFN-g production and increases cytolytic activity by NK cells and T cells. Stimulates differentiation into Th1 lineage by CD4+ T cells	
IL-15	Produced by macrophages. Stimulates proliferation of NK cells and T cells	
IL-18	Produced by macrophages. Induces IFN-g production by T cells and NK cells	
IFN-a, -b	Produced by macrophages and fibroblasts. Activates NK cells. Up regulates expression of MHC class I and II.	Inhibit viral protein synthesis providing resistance to viral infection
IFN-g	Increase MHC I and MHC II expression by cells to increase antigen-processing. Activates macrophages and enhances microbial killing	Used in treatment of hairy cell leukemia.
TNF-a/b	Produced by macrophages and T cells. Major role in inflammation and acute phase response. Released by leukocytes during inflammation and by endothelium upon damage. Strong chemotactic and activating agent for neutrophils. Induces IL-1 production. Increases insulin resistance. Stimulates synthesis of acute phase proteins by the liver, Induces fever by action on the hypothalamus. Induces catabolism of muscle and fat. In large quantities, inhibits myocardial contractility and vascular smooth muscle tone resulting in shock. Induces endothelial cell expression of tissue factor and inhibits thrombomodulin, which activates coagulation.	Synthetic forms used for the treatment of autoimmune disorders.

I.C. Adaptive Immunity

The adaptive immune system provides activation of a wide diversity immune responses that are antigen-specific but not self-reactive. The responses are self-limited allowing for initiation of new antigens when encountered while maintaining memory for previously encountered antigens. The adaptive immune response can be further divided into humoral and cellular immunity. Humoral immunity encompasses B cells, which produce antibodies in response to antigens. CD4+ and CD8+ T cells are the major effectors of cellular adaptive immunity.

1. Major Histocompatibility Complex

The crux of the adaptive immune system revolves around antigen presentation on the Major Histocompatibility Complex or MHC. Cellular peptide molecules are processed by the cell and presented in a groove on the MHC. Interaction of the MHC occurs with only a few amino acid residues of the presented peptide allowing a large number of peptides to be presented on each MHC. Human MHC genes are known as human leukocyte antigen (HLA). These genes are located on the short arm of chromosome 6 and thus have a low recombination frequency. Thus, each child will inherit 1 haplotype from each parent, and genetic siblings will have a 25% chance of being HLA identical. There are three classes of MHC genes (Table 295).

Class I MHC consists of a single polymorphic alpha chain that associates with a single beta-2 microglobulin molecule. Class I MHC is expressed on all nucleated cells. It presents self-peptides and intracellular foreign peptides such as viruses and intracellular microbes. There are three class I loci in humans, HLA-A, -B, and -C.

Class II MHC consists of a polymorphic alpha chain associated with a polymorphic beta chain. It is presented only on antigen presenting cells as well as thymic epithelium, but expression can be up-regulated on endothelial cells and other somatic cells during periods of extreme inflammation. Peptides of phagocytosed cells and microbes are processed and presented in conjunction with MHC class II. There are three polymorphic co-dominant MHC class II loci in humans, HLA-DP, -DQ, and -DR.

The Class III MHC genetic loci encode a number of molecules that are not directly involved in antigen presentation but that are involved in the inflammatory response. These include molecules such as heat-shock proteins, cytokines, and complement. They are not polymorphic and are thus conserved across individuals of a given species.

A number of peptides produced by the genome are polymorphic but are not involved in the generation of the immune response. These are termed minor histocompatibility antigens. In the case of transplantation, these minor histocompatibility antigens can be processed and presented in conjunction with self-MHC to elicit an allograft rejection response. However, the rejection response elicited by minor antigens is generally slower or weaker than that elicited by major histocompatibility antigens.

Transplant Surgery

Table 4. MHC domains.

Types	Function	Notes
MHC-I	Involved in the generation of immune response to host cell infected by bacteria, virus, or transformed cells. Binds to T cell receptor in conjunction with CD8+ on CD8+ (cytotoxic) T-cells HLA Domains: -A, -B, -C	Found on all nucleated cells and platelets within the body. A single transmembrane alpha chain associated with beta-2-microglobulin. Loads cytoplasmic proteins in the rough endoplasmic reticulum. Loci also encodes HLA-X, -E, -J, -H, -G, and –F, which are class I like genes with unknown function or no known immunologic function
MHC-II	Involved in generation of immune response to phagocytosed cells, bacteria, and viruses. Binds to T cell receptor in conjunction with CD4+ on CD4+ (helper) T-cells HLA Domains: -DP, -DQ, -DR	Found on antigen presenting cells (macrophages, B cells, and dendritic cells) and on thymic epithelium. Composed of polymorphic alpha and beta chains. MHC-II region also encodes HLA DM and TAP1 and TAPII which are involved in MHC processing and loading
MHC-III	Encodes Complement, Cytokines, Heat-Shock Proteins	Encodes C4B, C4[a], Factor B, C2, HSP-70, LT-b, TNF, and LT

2. Antigen Presenting Cells

Certain cells in the immune system are defined by their ability to process and present antigen on MHC, in conjunction with adhesion molecules and costimulatory molecules, to generate a strong immune response to foreign antigen. These cells are known as antigen presenting cells (APCs). They include dendritic cells, macrophages, and B cells.

Dendritic cells constitutively express both MHC class I and class II as well as costimulatory molecules B7-1 and B7-2. These cells are found in tissues and are highly effective at ingesting and processing antigen for presentation. In response to inflammation, they will traffic to nearby lymphoid depots to present antigen to naïve T cells in conjunction with adhesion and costimulatory molecules to activate the adaptive immune response. They also produce cytokines that can aid in lymphocyte activation and function.

B cells take up antigens through interaction with the membrane IgM or IgD to be processed and presented on MHC class II. In response to inflammation, B cells will up regulate the expression of costimulatory molecules on its surface to facilitate T cell activation. Antigen presentation by B cells to T cells can serve to coordinate the immune response to a given antigen between the humoral and cellular branches of the adaptive immune system.

Macrophages up-regulate the expression of MHC class II and costimulatory molecules in response to inflammation. As previously discussed, these cells are highly efficient phagocytes and may produce cytokines to aid in the direction of activation of the adaptive immune response. Both macrophages are B cells are more efficient activators of differentiated effector cells than of naïve T cells.

3. T Lymphocytes

T cells are one of the two main effector cell types of the adaptive immune response and are specifically the effectors of cell-mediated immunity. The "T" refers to thymus-derived lymphocytes. All T cells express the cluster of differentiation (CD) CD3. Phenotypically, they are divided into two main subsets based on their expression of CD proteins in conjunction with the T cell receptor (TCR). These are CD4+ and CD8+ T cells.

CD8+ T cells. CD8 interacts only with MHC class I to allow antigen recognition through the TCR and subsequent CD8+ T cell activation and differentiation. Activated CD8+ T cells develop into cells with primarily cytolytic function known as cytolytic T lymphocytes (CTLs). CTLs kill target cells through the release of cytotoxic granules (granzymes) directly into cells through transmembrane pores formed by the protein perforin. Alternatively, CTLs can induce target cell apoptosis though the binding of Fas ligand on CD8+ T cells with Fas on target cells.

CD4+ T cells. CD4 interacts only with MHC class II to allow antigen recognition through the TCR and subsequent CD4+ T cell activation and differentiation. Activated CD4+ T cells develop into cells with primarily helper function (helper T cells) that produce cytokines important in B cell growth and differentiation, CD8+ T cells activation, and macrophage activation.

All lymphocytes of T cell lineage originate in the bone marrow as bone marrow stem cells. They then traffic to the thymus where they undergo somatic gene rearrangement of their TCR gene to produce diversity in antigen recognition. Subsequently, they undergo positive selection through interaction of TCR with MHC expressed on thymic epithelial cells. Only cells whose TCR weakly binds self epithelial antigens continue to maturity; whereas, those that do not bind undergo apoptosis. Positively selected T lymphocytes then transit to the thymic medulla where they interact with dendritic cells. Cells that have high affinity for self-peptides encountered on self-MHC are negatively selected and undergo apoptosis. The remaining cells are released into circulation as mature naïve T lymphocytes. These cells generally recognize self-MHC, but they will not react with self-peptides.

Naïve T lymphocytes must undergo activation in order to become effector T cells. This is hypothesized to require two signals. Signal one is the antigen specific interaction of the TCR with self MHC presenting foreign antigen. The signal is transduced to intracellular proteins by the CD3 protein associated with each TCR. The extracellular CD4 or CD8 interacts with MHC II or I, respectively, to restrict each specific cell type to its given MHC. Cell surface proteins known as costimulatory molecules proved signal 2 for T cell activation. Costimulatory molecules are found on the surface of activated APCs. The best characterized of these are the costimulatory molecules B7-1 (CD80) and B7-2 (CD86), which interact with CD28 found on T cells. CD40L (CD154) on T cells may also receive costimulatory signals through interaction with CD40 found on APCs. In the absence of costimulation, T cells undergo anergy or apoptosis. In response to signals 1 and 2, T cells become activated to proliferate and differentiate into effector T cells.

The functional response of antigenically stimulated T cells only persists for a few days or weeks. As the antigen is eliminated, the response wanes, and the effector T cells are eliminated in the absence of continuous antigen exposure. However, some T cells survive as memory T cells. This subset of circulating cells can rapidly respond and proliferate upon reencountering a specific antigen resulting in an accelerated secondary immune response. These memory cells survive in blood without the need for continuous antigen exposure.

4. B Lymphocytes

B cells, the other of the two main effector cell types of the adaptive immune response, are the effectors of humoral immunity and the producers of antibody. The "B" refers to the bursa of Fabricius in birds were these cells were first found to mature. In humans, there is no bursa equivalent. Instead, B cells mature in the bone marrow. The clonally distributed B cell receptor is membrane-expressed immunoglobulin (Ig). Ig is composed of two heavy (a, d, g, e, or m) and two light chains (k or l), which are covalently linked via disulfide bonds. The variable amino terminal is the Fab fragment and binds antigen. Immunoglobulins have constant regions at their carboxy terminal, known as the Fc fragment. Ig molecules are either membrane expressed as the B cell receptor or are secrete by activated B cells as antibodies.

Similar to T cells, in the bone marrow B cells undergo positive selection for cells expressing functional Ig molecules. Resultant immature B cells express antigen-specific membrane IgM composed of a membrane-bound m heavy chain in association with either k or l light chains. These cells do not proliferate or differentiate in response to antigen. Instead, cells encountering self-antigen in the bone marrow apoptosis or anergy as the process of negative selection. The resultant mature naïve B cells express functional membrane IgM and IgD are then released to circulate in blood and lymphoid tissue.

Upon entering blood and lymphoid tissue, naïve B cells become activated upon encountering foreign antigen for which their membrane IgM and IgD are specific. Similar to T cells, B cells require two signals for activation. The first is provided by interaction of the membrane IgM or IgD with foreign antigen. This results in intracellular signal transduction through membrane-bound invariant Iga and Igb. Signal 2 is provided by complement breakdown products, such as C3d, interacting with the complement receptor 2 (CR2). Signal 2 initiates an intracellular phosphorylation cascade through CD19 and CD81, which are complexed with CR2.

B cell activation results in proliferation, clonal expansion, differentiation into plasma cells that actively secrete antibody or into memory B cells that will circulate and persist after resolution of the initial immune response. B cells destined to differentiate into plasma cells enter into the cell cycle, become larger, and increase their intracellular organelles for antibody production. Simultaneously, there is an increased expression of costimulatory molecules B7-1 and B7-2 for function in T cell activation. In addition, cytokine receptor expression is increased to allow for further activation and antibody class switching. Anti-apoptotic protein expression (e.g. Bcl-X) is up-regulated in order to increase the survival of mature activated B cells. However, in order to fully mature, activated B cells require help from helper T cells in the form of cell-cell interactions (e.g. CD40-CD40L) or cytokine production (IL-2, IL-4, IL-5, IL-6, IFN-g, and TGF-b). This initiates class switching and clonal expansion. The activated plasma cells subsequently produce antibodies for the humoral immune response.

Similar to the response of activated T cells, the functional response of antigenically stimulated B cells only persists for a few days or weeks. Antibodies produced during the response persist and circulate in blood. In addition, some B cells survive as memory B cells, which can rapidly respond and proliferate upon reencountering a specific antigen resulting in an accelerated secondary immune response.

5. Antibodies

The primary antibody response of activated B cells to foreign antigen is the production of IgM (and to a lesser extend IgD). Upon further B cell activation, class switching occurs. Through this process, the heavy chains a, g, and e may be induced for the production of IgA, IgG, and IgE, respectively. The class of antibody is influences by the cytokine milieu the B cell is exposed to, and the result is production of antibodies with specific effector function. The antibody subclasses and their function are reviewed in Table 296.

TABLE 5. Antibody classes.

Type	% Antibody	Isotype-Specific Effector Function	Key Differences
IgG	65%	-Opsonization of antigens for phagocytosis -Activation of classical complement cascade -Antibody-dependent cell-mediated cytotoxicity -Neonatal immunity: maternal IgG cross the placenta and gut to transfer maternal antibodies to fetus. -Feedback inhibition of B cell activation	-Crosses placenta -Fixes complement -Longest half-life -4 subclasses (IgG1-IgG4)
IgA	20%	-Mucosal immunity: secreted in the lumens of the GI and respiratory tracts and lungs as well as tears and saliva -Neonatal Immunity: secreted in breast milk -May form dimers	-Mucosal immunity -Secreted in Breast Milk -Forms dimmers -2 Subclasses (IgA1, IgA2)
IgM	10%	-Activation of classical complement cascade -Antigen receptors on naïve B cells. -Secreted IgM may form pentameres.	-First antibody produced -Naïve B cell receptor -Fixes complement -Pentameres
IgD	1%	-Antigen receptor on naïve B cells	-Naïve B cell receptor
IgE	1%	-Antibody-dependent cell-mediated cytotoxicity involving eosinophils -Induce Mast cell degranulation for induction of Type I hypersensitivity reaction (anaphylaxis) -Response to parasitic infections	-Anaphylaxis -High levels in parasitic infection -Heat labile

I.D. IMMUNE-MEDIATED DISEASES

Although the adaptive immune response functions to provide effective defense against microbes and other pathogens, it may also function to cause tissue injury and disease. These include hypersensitivity reactions and autoimmune diseases.

1. Hypersensitivity Reactions

Hypersensitivity diseases are classified based on the effector mechanism responsible for causing tissue and cell injury into four classes. These are a heterogeneous group of disorders that occur when effector mechanisms of the normal adaptive immune response result in tissue injury and disease. The four types of hypersensitivity reactions and their disease are reviewed in Table 297.

TABLE 6. Hypersensitivity reactions.

Type	Immune Mechanism	Mechanism of Tissue Injury	Diseases
Type I: Immediate Hypersensitivity	IgE mediated response that leads to activation of mast cells and granulocytes.	Rapid immediate response due to degranulation of mast cells, releasing histamine, proteoglycans such as heparin, serine proteases, prostaglandin D2 (vasodilatation), cytokines, and leukotriene C4.	-Allergic reactions (hives, wheals, flares, urticaria, and pruritus) -Anaphylaxis
Type II: Antibody Mediated Hypersensitivity	IgG and IgM mediated response against cell surface or extracellular matrix proteins.	-Direct antibody-mediated cell opsonization and phagocytosis -Complement and Fc Receptor-mediated recruitment and activation of leukocytes	Autoimmune hemolytic anemia, erythroblastosis fetalis (Rh disease), Goodpasture, rheumatic fever, Graves Disease, bullous pomphigoid.
Type III: Immune Complex Mediated Hypersensitivity	Immune complexes of circulating IgM and IgG deposit in tissues	Complement and Fc receptor mediated recruitment and activation of leukocytes	Serum sickness, Arthus reactions, fungal infections of the lung, PAN, SLE, PSGN, and RA.
Type IV: T cell Mediated Hypersensitivity	Activation of CD4+ T cells (delayed-type hypersensitivity) and CD8+ T cells (T cell mediated cytolysis)	-Cytokine-mediated inflammation -CD4+ T cells cause macrophage activation -CD8+ T cells direct cell lysis	TB test, contact dermatitis, Type I Diabetes Mellitus, Rheumatoid Arthritis, Inflammatory Bowel Disease. Myocarditis

2. Autoimmune Disease

Autoimmune diseases are a heterogeneous group of disorders identified as the activation of immunity against self-antigens. Owing to positive and negative selection, immature T and B-cells are not generally self-reactive. However, failure or break-down of self-tolerance may result in the activation of the cellular and humoral immune response against organs and tissues. In some cases, this is a result of immunologic abnormalities in lymphocytes and APCs. In other cases, specific genes and HLA haplotypes may predispose an individual to the activation of immunity against self-antigens. Autoimmune diseases may result in systemic diseases through the formation of circulating antigen-antibody complexes and there deposition in tissues. Alternatively, cell-mediated or humoral immune responses against tissues-specific antigens may result in organ-specific injury. Certain antigen targets with resultant autoantibody production have been identified in autoimmune diseases. These autoantibodies are reviewed in Table 298.

TABLE 7. Autoantibodies.

Type	Disease
c-ANCA	Wegener's granulomatosis
Centromere	CREST
Mitochondrial	Primary biliary cirrhosis
nAChR	Myasthenia gravis
Neutrophil	Vasculitis
pANCA	Polyarteritis nodosa
Scl-70	Scleroderma
Smooth muscle	Autoimmune hepatitis
Thyroid peroxidase	Hashimoto thyroiditis
TSH-R	Graves disease
VGCC	Lambert-Eaton syndrome

II. Liver Transplant

II.A. Preoperative Evaluation

1. Preoperative Workup

Patients who are candidates for liver transplant require a thorough preoperative evaluation with pertinent consultation of specialists for any comorbid conditions. The preoperative workup requires a thorough history and physical examination, evaluation of all comorbid conditions, and confirmation that the patient is of sufficient health to tolerate a major surgical procedure. Specific evaluation of the anatomy is also undertaken for preoperative planning.

2. Indications for Surgery

The decision to complete a liver transplant is a multifactorial process. The most important indication for surgery is end stage liver disease with imminent fulminant liver failure. As discussed previously in the Hepatopancreatobiliary Surgery chapter (page 285), the MELD score is the best studied model that predicts whether a liver transplant in a patient with liver disease will be beneficial. The MELD score is based on creatinine, INR, and bilirubin. The worse these values, the higher the MELD score. Patients with a MELD score over 17 are likely to benefit from a liver transplant.

Critically ill patients with symptomatic liver failure may be prioritized. Those with severe hepatic encephalopathy and require a higher level of care may receive preference due to the immediate danger to life from their liver disease.

Specific indications for surgery include severe alcohol-induced liver disease and cirrhosis, hepatitis B or C, biliary atresia, Budd-Chiari syndrome, primary biliary cirrhosis, nonalcoholic steatohepatitis, primary sclerosing cholangitis, various metabolic disorders, limited hepatocellular carcinoma, type IV and V choledochal cysts, and acute fulminant liver failure. Severe disease leading to compromise of the liver and a MELD score over 17 is necessary for many of these conditions. For hepatocellular carcinoma, disease localized to the liver with no evidence of extracapsular spread is necessary. Most centers will consider transplantation for stage I or stage II disease; the overall tumor size should be less than 5 cm. Transplantation should also be considered for other liver cancers, particular hepatoblastoma in children and limited cholangiocarcinoma.

3. Patient Selection Criteria

Careful selection of patients is necessary to maximize outcome following a liver transplant. Significant barriers that may preclude a liver transplant exist, but are always changing as the level of care we can provide to our patients improves. There are few absolute contraindications, but among them are comorbid conditions that are incompatible with survival following a major operation; for example, severe cardiac or pulmonary disease that render a patient unable to tolerate anesthesia or shifts in intravascular volume may negate any survival advantage of transplant. Severe bleeding or thrombotic disorders may also be major contraindications to the safe completion of this type of surgery. Severe sepsis and metastatic cancer are also absolute contraindications.

An individualized approach is necessary as part of the selection process for liver transplantation. Patients with portal vein thrombosis, juvenile-onset diabetes, HIV, neurologic compromise, and substance-abuse disorders all need to be examined closely. In the setting of a satisfactory support network and clinical resources, even these barriers can be overcome in carefully selected patients.

II.B. Surgical Procedure

1. Perfusion

The University of Wisconsin is the most widely used perfusion solution used for the preparation of the donor organs. The solution functions as an isotonic bath that stops cellular function and stabilize cell membranes. High energy precursors in the form of phosphate, amino acids, and carbohydrates are part of the solution. Potassium lactobionate prevents cellular swelling. The University of Wisconsin solution can permit cold ischemia times over 24 hours, but all attempts to minimize this time are vital for the prevention of postoperative complications such as biliary stricture formation.

The University of Wisconsin solution consists of 100 mmol of potassium-lactobionate, 30 mmol of phosphate and sulfate intermediaries (KH2PO4 and MgSO4), 30 mmol of carbohydrates in the form of raffinose, 8 mmol of amino acids (adenosine and glutathione), 100 U of insulin, 8 mg of dexamethasone, 1 mmol of allopurinol, and a small dose of penicillin.

2. Donor Operation

The donor operation typically occurs in a deceased cardiac donor who is brought to the operating room with a beating heart. A large midline incision extending from the suprasternal notch to the pubic bone is made. Entry into the mediastinum is made to permit access to the heart and lungs, and also to facilitate removal of these organs if suitable for transplant. A large cruciate incision is also made in the abdomen to permit ready access to the liver, kidneys, pancreas, and intestines. Following isolation of the major vascular structures to each of the organs of interest, the University of Wisconsin solution is infused rapidly while the right atrium of the heart or supradiaphragmatic inferior vena cava is transected. The organs are fully dissected free, with care taken to avoid damage to replaced or recurrent arteries.

3. Recipient Operation

The recipient procedure can be broken into two major parts. The first part involves resection of the native liver. The primary incision is a large subcostal incision. The ligamentum teres is ligated and the portal triad isolated. The hepatic artery should be tracked to ensure that any aberrant anatomy is not present. The portal vein should be followed until a widely patent section is identified. The constituents of the portal triad are freed and ligated. Patients with portal vein thrombosis should undergo thrombectomy via eversion endarterectomy prior to freeing up the portal vein. The liver is then mobilized by dividing the falciform and right and left triangular ligaments. Care is taken to avoid damage to the inferior vena cava during retraction of the liver. The draining hepatic veins are ligated proximally during this process.

The second part of the procedure is the anhepatic phase, during which transplantation of the donor organ is being completed. Stable patients can undergo clamping of the inferior vena cava and portal vein. A dramatic decrease in cardiac filling pressure will occur during this process. Patients that do not tolerate clamping can undergo venovenous bypass between the inferior vena cava and superior vena cava. The native organ is resected out of the body and the donor organ introduced.

A series of primary side-to-side anastomoses are made between the donor organ and the recipient vasculature starting with the vena cava. The hepatic veins are attached either together or separately to the inferior vena cava. The portal vein and hepatic artery are then reanastomosed, followed by the biliary anastomosis via a choledochocholedochostomy. Alternatively, a Roux-en-Y choledochojejunostomy can be performed if insufficient duct remains.

Living donor liver transplantation can be completed using an adult liver that will be transplanted into a child. Split graft transplantation where one large adult liver is divided into two and transplanted into two patients can also be done. Living donor transplantation has been successful and is becoming more common. However, split graft transplantation has so far been shown to be inferior to conventional transplantation and will need advances in technique and preparation prior to becoming more common.

4. Surgical Considerations

There are several unique considerations for liver transplant patients in the intraoperative period. First, rapid sequence intubation (RSI) is necessary as many patients will not have a suitable nil per os (NPO) period prior to surgery. Precautions to avoid aspiration during induction are therefore necessary. Second, there are major shifts in intravascular volume from fluid losses, bleeding, and intravenous resuscitation. This leads to the development of various coagulopathies that should be carefully monitored during surgery. Patients with severe liver disease may have hepatic congestion leading to splenomegaly. Infusion of platelets may be necessary due to the subsequent thrombocytopenia.

II.C. Postoperative Management

1. Goals of Postoperative Management

Patients who successfully complete a liver transplant may develop a fibrinolytic state as the new liver is perfused and flushed of various metabolites it has accumulated during its ischemic state. Treatment with aminocaproic acid may be necessary in severe instances; its use should be carefully monitored due to the potential for intravascular thrombosis.

2. Immunosuppression

The burden of immunosuppression is lower in the liver than it is for other organs, for reasons that are incompletely understood. Further, the liver is more resistant to hyperacute rejection from preformed antibodies against ABO groups, and so permits ABO-incompatible transplantation in properly selected patients. HLA crossmatching is therefore not mandatory with liver transplantation.

The relative ease of a satisfactory plane of immunosuppression in liver transplant patients compared to kidney transplant or small bowel transplant has dramatically reduced the risk of acute cell-mediated rejection, most common within a month of surgery. Careful monitoring of liver function on a regular basis after transplant permits early identification of rejection.

Chronic rejection occurs over years and presents with loss of hepatic bile ducts due to immune-mediated destruction. The only treatment for end stage chronic rejection is retransplantation.

3. Outcomes

Mortality within the first year of liver transplant is about 10% and decreases to about 3% per year thereafter. Children do better than adults. Mortality is worse for patients who had a transplant for hepatic cancer and cirrhosis from alcohol or hepatitis. Survival also appears to be better in high volume centers.

4. Complications

a) Primary Nonfunction

Nearly 5% of patients will have primary nonfunction and require urgent retransplantation. Primary nonfunction is thought to be secondary to ischemic damage in an otherwise fragile liver. Such patients are classified as status 1 and receive priority for any upcoming compatible organs in the region.

Primary nonfunction is diagnosed in the setting of rapid, fulminant liver failure leading to compromise of multiple body systems. Factor V levels can be followed as a sensitive indicator of new liver function.

b) Bile Leak

Bile leak can occur in nearly 25% of patients and is due to relative ischemia of the biliary tree following transplant. ERCP and or percutaneous transhepatic cholangiography are completed to confirm the diagnosis and to rule out thrombosis or stenosis; a biliary stent can then be placed to assure patency and to exclude the leak. All bilomas should be drained. Severe disease may require a return to the operating room for a Roux-en-Y hepaticojejunostomy.

c) Bleeding

Postoperative hemorrhage affects about 10% of patients and typically presents as anuria following transplantation. Any coexistent coagulopathy should be corrected first. Continuing bleeding may require reoperation.

d) Thrombosis

Thrombosis of the biliary anastomosis or hepatic artery can occur in up to 10% of patients. Biliary thrombosis can sometimes be corrected with ERCP and stent placement, but may need a Roux-en-Y hepaticojejunostomy for definitive repair. Hepatic artery thrombosis presents about a week after surgery and is diagnosed by ultrasound or arteriography. An early sign is sudden liver failure. The treatment is thrombectomy. Thrombosis is more common in pediatric hepatic transplants due to the smaller caliber vessels. A difficult postoperative course also contributes to thrombosis due to lower pressures and a greater inflammatory state.

Portal vein thrombosis occurs in less than 5% of patients after liver transplant and presents with the development of ascites and portal hypertension. The condition is diagnosed by ultrasound, MRI, or arteriography. Treatment with a transhepatic portography and stent placement can be completed. Thrombectomy can also be pursued.

III. Kidney Transplant

III.A. Preoperative Evaluation

1. Preoperative Workup

Similar to that for liver transplantation, a complete history and physical examination with evaluation of all comorbid conditions is necessary. Clearance for surgery must be obtained and all existing renal diseases fully explored.

The living-related donor requires a thorough workup and evaluation of the contralateral kidney. The ideal donor must be free of comorbid conditions that impact renal function, such as hypertension, diabetes, and other renal disease. An intravenous pyelogram or renal arteriogram is done to evaluate the donor anatomy prior to surgery. Due to the longer renal vein, the left kidney is preferred.

Procurement from patients who are donors by cardiac death (DCD) or following a terminal neurologic condition is termed cadaveric donation. All attempts to minimize ischemia time should be made to maximize organ function and avoid delayed graft function.

2. Indications for Surgery

The ideal surgical candidate is a patient with progressive, terminal renal disease who has not yet started dialysis. The most common patients are those who are nearing end stage renal disease (ESRD) secondary to hypertension and diabetes. Other common diseases include a variety of glomerulonephritides, polycystic kidney disease, systemic lupus erythematosus, fulminant renal failure, and a variety of immunologic conditions.

3. Patient Selection Criteria

Selection criteria for potential recipients are similar to that of liver transplantation. The major absolute contraindications include inability to survive the operation, metastatic cancer, and severe sepsis. Patients with a history of cancer should have their operation delayed by 3-5 years to ensure a satisfactory cancer-free interval and thereby minimize the risk of recurrent disease.

A thorough evaluation of the renal and genitourinary anatomy should be completed for operative planning and to ensure that there are no conditions that may complicate the operation. Voiding cystograms and urodynamic studies are completed in patients with congenital defects to ensure that the potential for postrenal obstruction is minimized.

III.B. Surgical Procedure

1. Living-Related Donor Operation

A living-related donor operation is typically completed via laparoscopy and has been demonstrated to have a shorter hospitalization and fewer postoperative pain-related complications. Either a transperitoneal or retroperitoneal approach may be used. The left kidney is preferred due to the longer renal vein and slightly easier access. The renal artery is ligated and transected, followed by the renal vein. The ureter is then ligated and transected as close to the bladder as possible.

2. Cadaveric Donor Operation

The cadaveric donor operation has been described in the section on liver transplantation (page 441).

3. Recipient Operation

The recipient kidney is implanted extraperitoneally within the iliac fossa. A generous curvilinear incision along the iliac fossa is made extending from the anterior superior iliac spine to the pubic symphysis. Following satisfactory exposure, the retroperitoneal iliac vasculature is identified. The graft is placed into the field and an end-side anastomosis made between the renal vessels and the external iliac vessels. The ureter is then anastomosed with the bladder via an extravesicular approach with oversewing of the bladder around the anastomosis to minimize reflux. A Carrel patch can be used in patients with multiple renal arteries to ensure a widely patent anastomosis.

4. Surgical Considerations

Most kidneys will begin to function immediately upon anastomosis of the renal artery and will begin to produce urine. However, nearly 25% of all transplants will have a delayed graft function, particularly with the use of deceased donor kidneys. This is a diagnosis of exclusion and requires ruling out of thrombosis, acute rejection, and postrenal obstruction.

III.C. Postoperative Management

1. Goals of Postoperative Management

Immediate postoperative management centers on adequate fluid resuscitation. A postsurgical diuresis is common and requires matching of intravenous intake to avoid hypovolemic oliguria. This is particular important in patients with immediate graft function, as a delay in fluid resuscitation can lead to perfusion limited flow to the new kidney and damage to an already sensitive organ. Patients with delayed graft function should have fluid restriction and started on dialysis if they experience a hyperkalemia, uremia, or fluid overload.

2. Complications

Any decrease in urine output in the postoperative period requires a search for thrombosis, acute rejection, and postrenal obstruction. The Foley catheter should be irrigated and ruled out as a source of obstruction. A renal biopsy may be necessary to evaluate for rejection. Central venous pressure monitoring may be necessary to ensure satisfactory perfusion of the new kidney. Ultrasound can be used to evaluate for ureteral or vascular obstruction. Nuclear scans can also be done to evaluate renal function.

Specific complications associated with renal transplantation are similar to that for liver transplant. However, complications after renal transplant are significantly lower. Renal artery thrombosis affects only 1% of all grafts and presents with sudden anuria. Renal artery stenosis affects about 10-15% of patients and leads to uncontrollable hypertension; treatment with stent placement or reoperation can be done for refractory cases. Renal vein thrombosis is typically secondary to technical error or the formation of a lymphocele and should be treated with thrombectomy or removal of the graft if the thrombosis involves the renal parenchyma.

Pseudoaneurysms from technical errors may be treated with stenting or operative repair. Rapidly expanding aneurysms may be mycotic in nature and require antibiotics and excision of the graft. A urine leak may occur in about 10% of patients and presents with a drop in urine output and a rise in creatinine. Ureteral stent placement may be therapeutic. Stricture formation should be treated with surgery. The polyoma virus has been associated with ureteral stricture formation.

3. Immunosuppression

The kidney is considerably more sensitive to differences in HLA and ABO compatibility compared to the liver. A satisfactory negative crossmatch is necessary in most instances prior to proceeding with transplantation. However, secondary to long wait times and progressive disease, experimental ABO incompatible transplants have been done with some success.

Immunosuppression is a key mediator in maintaining renal function. Acute rejection should be treated urgently and vigilant monitoring is necessary for early diagnosis. However, the level of immunosuppression required for renal transplantation is fraught with infectious complications. The patients are at particular risk for pneumonia, urinary tract infections, and CMV activation. CMV infection becomes evident about 1 month after transplant and presents with pneumonia and renal dysfunction. Prophylaxis with ganciclovir is necessary in seronegative recipients who receive an organ from a donor with CMV. Various opportunistic infections can also occur, such as Candidiasis and P. carinii – both can be avoided with prophylactic antibiotics (fluconazole and TMP-SMX, respectively). Infection with the BK virus is of concern and can lead to loss of the graft; treatment is typically by reducing the level of immunosuppression.

Significant immunosuppression has also lead to an increase in carcinogenesis. Skin cancer is the most common type of cancer after renal transplantation, and nearly half of all patients who have had a kidney transplant will develop squamous cell or basal cell carcinoma. Non-Hodgkin lymphoma is also relatively common.

4. Outcomes

Outcomes are superior for patients that undergo transplant prior to the initiation of dialysis. Living-related donors have gained favor as a means to avoid additional morbidity in patients with progressive renal disease, and the number of such procedures rivals that of cadaveric donor transplants. Living-related kidney transplants are superior to cadaveric transplants. Extended criteria kidneys from patients that are older, have hypertension, a slight increase in creatinine, or cerebrovascular accident also do somewhat poorly and have a greater incidence of delayed graft function compared to standard criteria donors.

The specific outcome is related to the number of antibody mismatches such that zero-mismatched donor-recipient combinations are given national priority.

IV. Pancreas Transplant

IV.A. Preoperative Evaluation

1. Indications for Surgery

Indications for pancreas transplantation are patients with type I diabetes and carefully selected patients with type II diabetes at particular risk for diabetes related complications. The majority of patients have end stage renal disease when they are considered for pancreatic transplant, hence the reason that simultaneous kidney-pancreas transplants are favored.

A simultaneous kidney-pancreas transplant permits a single operation to correct the diabetes and renal failure, and has a superior outcome due to the greater sensitivity of the kidney to rejection that permits earlier detection and correction of graft rejection. Living kidney and living pancreas donor operation, or living kidney and deceased pancreas donor operations can also be completed with a similar outcome. Nearly 10% of living pancreas donors will experience major complications related to pancreatitis and leak.

A pancreas after kidney transplant permits a functional kidney to be implanted while the patient awaits the availability of a suitable pancreas. The hazard occurs with the second operation and relative difficulty with assessing pancreas graft function and early diagnosis of pancreas rejection.

Patients who do not have concomitant renal dysfunction are candidates for a pancreas-only transplant. Candidates often have progressive secondary complications related to their diabetes.

2. Preoperative Workup

The preoperative evaluation for patients who are candidates for pancreas or islet-cell transplantation is similar to that for liver and kidney transplantation. Patients must be satisfactory candidates for surgery without any major restrictive comorbid conditions that could seriously compromise their perioperative recovery. Completion of a pancreas or islet-cell transplant in carefully selected patients will lead to autogenous glucose control. The best results are those in patients who receive a simultaneous kidney-pancreas transplantation compared to pancreas alone or pancreas after kidney transplantation.

A thorough cardiac evaluation is necessary, particularly in patients with demand ischemia or other symptomatic disease. The peripheral vascular disease complications associated with diabetes should also be thoroughly reviewed; correction of critical limb ischemia should be completed prior to transplantation. Evaluation for malignancy should be completed as part of the pre-transplant workup.

IV.B. Surgical Procedure

1. Pancreas Donor Operation

The procurement of a pancreas is a uniquely critical step that profoundly affects the success of the transplanted organ. Great care must be taken to avoid injury to the organ during retrieval, as any trauma to the organ dramatically increases the risk of complications such as leak and pseudocyst formation.

The procedure begins with the Kocher (duodenal mobilization) and Cattell-Brash maneuvers (right colon mobilization). The major vascular structures are identified and isolated, and attention is then turned to mobilization of the pancreas via the lesser sac. The pancreas is removed in conjunction with the duodenum, jejunum, and spleen. Preparation of the pancreas for transplantation involves dissecting the pancreas free of the spleen and ensuring adequate length for all of the vessels.

2. Islet Cell Donor Operation

Transplantation of beta-cells (insulin-producing cells) of the pancreas can be completed in selected candidates and avoids the need for a major operation. Extensive histologic manipulation of the cells can be completed prior to transplantation, permitting improved survival and decreased immune reactivity. Donor pancreas not suitable for direct transplantation is procured and islet cells are harvested via enzymatic digestion and mechanical isolation.

3. Pancreas Recipient Operation

The pancreas transplantation procedure is similar to kidney transplantation in that the organ is placed within the iliac fossa. The portal vein remnant is anastomosed to the external iliac vessels via an end-to-side anastomosis. Connection to the portal circuit is possible in lieu of systemic drainage by completing an end-to-side anastomosis between the portal vein remnant to the superior mesenteric vein. Bladder drainage is preferred with the iliac crest transplantation and permits monitoring of pancreatic function by measuring urine amylase. Enteric drainage has the benefit of reducing the rate of UTIs.

4. Islet Cell Recipient Operation

Patients with adult-onset insulin-dependent diabetes mellitus are selected who are failing maximum medical management. Transplantation is minimally invasive and proceeds with injection of the purified islet cell mix into the portal vein via a laparoscopic approach.

IV.C. Postoperative Management

1. Immunosuppression

Immunosuppression is especially important in pancreas transplantation due to the extensive immunologic component within the gland. A combination of agents is used to maximize immunosuppression and also because monitoring the success of immunosuppression is difficult; these drugs include steroids, calcineurin inhibitors, and antiproliferative agents (i.e. cellcept).

Immunosuppression for islet cell transplantation involves cellcept for primary immunosuppression and tacrolimus for maintenance.

2. Outcomes

The success of simultaneous kidney-pancreas transplantation is superior to pancreas after kidney transplantation due to the ability to simultaneously correct dysfunction in two organ systems, monitor and treat rejection, and reduce the morbidity of a repeat operation and induction therapy. Simultaneous transplants survive in about 90% of patients after 1 year and nearly 70-80% of patients after 5 years. Graft survival is higher for the kidney than it is for the pancreas. Simultaneous transplant offers a superior longevity and quality of life compared to continued dialysis or isolated kidney transplantation.

Graft survival in a pancreas after kidney transplantation is about 80% after 1 year and 50% after 5 years. Isolated pancreas transplantation has a graft survival similar to pancreas after kidney transplantation. It remains controversial whether pancreas-only transplantation significantly improves survival.

3. Complications

Complications following pancreas transplantation include thrombosis from reperfusion injury, bleeding in about 5-10% of patients, and leak. The most susceptible anastomosis is the duodenal and can lead to peritonitis. Chronic rejection is manifest as gland fibrosis and atrophy.

The most common complication following islet cell transplantation is bleeding from the portal vein secondary to the anticoagulation necessary to prevent portal vein thrombosis. The usual complications of immunosuppression also apply.

V. Intestinal Transplant

V.A. Preoperative Evaluation

1. Indications for Surgery

The majority of patients who are on the waiting list for an intestinal transplant are under 6 years of age. The most common cause is short gut syndrome and dependence on total parental nutrition (TPN). Due to the long term morbidity and mortality associated with chronic TPN dependence, intestinal transplantation has slowly gained favor as an alternative modality. A variety causes can lead to short gut syndrome (reviewed on page 225). Specific complications associated with long-term TPN include metabolic derangements, sepsis from catheter-related infections, thrombosis, and progressive fulminant liver failure after TPN for more than 5 years.

2. Patient Selection Criteria

Patients who are on TPN who do not have other ongoing threats to life are candidates for intestinal transplant if they are otherwise able to tolerate the surgery and immunosuppression.

3. Preoperative Workup

The preoperative evaluation involves a thorough history and physical examination, all pertinent laboratory testing in preparation for a major operation, and evaluation of baseline liver function. If any liver dysfunction is suspected, a biopsy may be necessary to rule out concomitant liver disease. All steps to minimize line infections in the preoperative period should be undertaken. A valid crossmatch is necessary – ABO-identical transplants have the best outcome with this highly immunogenic organ. Evaluation of the donor gastrointestinal tract via contrast studies and/or endoscopy should be completed to rule out any existing pathologies and for anatomic evaluation.

V.B. Surgical Procedure

1. Donor Operation

A standard transplant incision should be used with wide exposure of the abdomen. Adequate exposure of the aorta is necessary to permit infusion of the University of Wisconsin (UW) solution. The small bowel should be fully mobilized before infusion, exsanguination, and cooling. Mobilization of the small intestine should be completed, followed by transaction of the ileum at the ileocecal valve. A total colectomy is completed followed by exposure of the mesenteric vessels at the root. The proximal jejunum is transected at the ligament of Treitz. Care is taken to preserve the vascular supply to the resected small bowel. Perfusion of the UW solution occurs at this point and infuses the small bowel via the superior mesenteric vessels.

2. Recipient Operation

In the recipient, a wide exposure and lysis of all adhesions is performed first. The vascular anastomosis will occur with the abdominal aorta and inferior vena cava, and adequate exposure is necessary. The proximal and distal targets for the small bowel anastomosis are identified and prepared. The arterial and venous anastomoses are created in an end-to-side manner, followed by the small bowel anastomosis. A diverting loop ileostomy permits endoscopic monitoring of the transplanted organ. Closure of the abdominal wall should be attempted if a tension-free closure can be achieved. In more extreme circumstances, an abdominal wall transplant can also be completed for primary closure. A feeding G-tube is also implanted.

V.C. Postoperative Management

1. Goals of Postoperative Management

Monitoring of the implanted bowel can be done by monitoring serum lactate levels to assess for bowel viability. Standard postoperative labs should also be drawn to monitor for bleeding. Diet is advanced slowly following a return of GI function. GI function is initially delayed due to the dysmotility of the transplanted organ; this dysmotility can be aggravated by pre-existing dysmotility syndromes in the recipient.

2. Immunosuppression

Induction therapy is necessary in many patients to permit satisfactory immunosuppression. This is achieved by either a monoclonal antibody (i.e. daclizumab) or polyclonal antibodies (i.e. thymoglobulin). Maintenance with tacrolimus along with sirolimus and steroids are used. Cellcept is not commonly used due to its gastrointestinal effects. Prostaglandin E1 can be used to maintain gastrointestinal blood flow. Intravenous antibiotics for at least 1 week are used.

3. Outcomes

Intestinal transplant has a 1 year survival of about 75% and a 5 year survival of 50%. These rates have steadily improved with advances in immunosuppression therapy and postoperative management. The most common cause of death after intestinal transplant is sepsis.

4. Complications

The most common complication is infection, which is the most common cause of loss of the transplanted organ. The remaining causes are attributed to rejection. Posttransplant lymphoproliferative disease (PTLD) can lead to degeneration of the transplanted organ, destruction of the mucosal barrier, and bacteremia. More severe cases can lead to sepsis. Viral infections in particular also raise the risk of infection-mediated graft failure. The most common agents are EBV and CMV.

VI. Heart Transplant

VI.A. Indications for Surgery

Patients who are satisfactory candidates for heart transplantation have end-stage heart failure secondary to a progressive cardiac process. The most common causes are high grade coronary artery disease, congenital heart disease, and cardiomyopathy. Patients with high grade pulmonary disease, end stage renal disease, high grade diabetes, active infection, or cancer are not candidates for surgery.

VI.B. Perioperative Period

Maximum medical management of the existing cardiac dysfunction should be undertaken. Most patients should be treated with beta blockers, anticoagulants, and afterload reduction to maximize cardiac function and decrease the risk of thrombosis. Extraordinarily ill patients who are candidates for transplantation may benefit from mechanical afterload reduction via an intraaortic balloon pump (IABP), or even with a ventricular assist device (VAD). The use of a VAD as a bridge to transplantation can be an effective means to sustain a person until a heart becomes available. Left ventricular (LVAD), right ventricular (RVAD), and biventricular (BiVAD) devices are all available.

VI.C. Outcomes

The best outcomes following heart transplantation are found in patients with ischemia times less than 4 hours. Immunosuppression with steroids, antiproliferative, and calcineurin inhibitor are used for optimal outcome. Graft survival after 1 year is about 80%; 5 year survival is about 65%.

VI.D. Complications

The most common complication associated with heart transplantation stems from the underlying immunosuppression. Infection can lead to rejection of the graft, sepsis, and death. Physiologically, the transplanted heart has no innervation and can therefore lead to bradycardia from the loss of sympathetic beat-by-beat control. Most patients will respond to theophylline, a beta agonist. Arrhythmias can be controlled with amiodarone.

Long term survivors may eventually succumb to diffuse atherosclerosis leading to cardiac failure – this is a combination of continuing coronary vascular disease and chronic rejection. Malignancy and PTLD also become issues with prolonged immunosuppression.

VII. Lung Transplant

VII.A. Indications for Surgery

Patients with end stage pulmonary disease with an expected life expectancy of only a few years are the best candidates for lung transplantation. Specific indications include end stage emphysematous and bullous disease of the lung, idiopathic pulmonary fibrosis, cystic fibrosis, alpha-1-antitrypsin deficiency, and pulmonary hypertension. Patients under 60 are candidates for bilateral transplant; those under 65 are candidates for a single lung.

The standard contraindications to transplant surgery apply for lung transplants as well. Further, due to the challenge of finding suitable donors, patients with chronic diseases poorly controlled with medical management, those over the age of 65, and those with significant heart disease are typically ruled out as suitable recipients.

VII.B. Perioperative Period

Donor organs can be evaluated with plain films of the chest and bronchoscopy. Donor organs with limited infiltrates can be used as part of a bilateral lung transplant, and most donor organs are deemed to harbor some type of infection at the time of transplant. However, purulent discharge is almost always an absolute contraindication for transplant. Rapid deterioration of arterial blood gasses is another frequent reason for rejecting a donor lung. Suitable organs are matched based off patient height.

Similar to the heart, the lungs are very susceptible to ischemic injury. Ischemic times under six hours are preferable, and prostaglandin E is often infused into the lung to assist with limiting ischemic injury. Attempts to minimize reperfusion injury are also made, due to the unique susceptibility of the lungs.

VII.C. Outcomes

There is a growing body of evidence that single lung transplantation is a suitable procedure in patients over 50 years of age. The major contraindication to this approach is in patients with pulmonary hypertension, in whom a bilateral transplant leads to improved cardiopulmonary function.

One year graft survival following lung transplant is 75%; five year survival is 50%. Few patients survive past seven years.

VII.D. Complications

Complications from lung transplant can be divided into perioperative complications and postoperative complications. Perioperative problems include transaction of the recurrent laryngeal or phrenic nerves, myocardial infarction, and technical difficulties with creating the anastomoses. Postoperative complications include graft failure (most common), heart failure, and dehiscence of the airway anastomosis. Chronic rejection leads to obliterative bronchiolitis. Infection by a variety of organisms, most commonly S. aureus, also leads to considerable morbidity.

Transplant Surgery

CRITICAL CARE

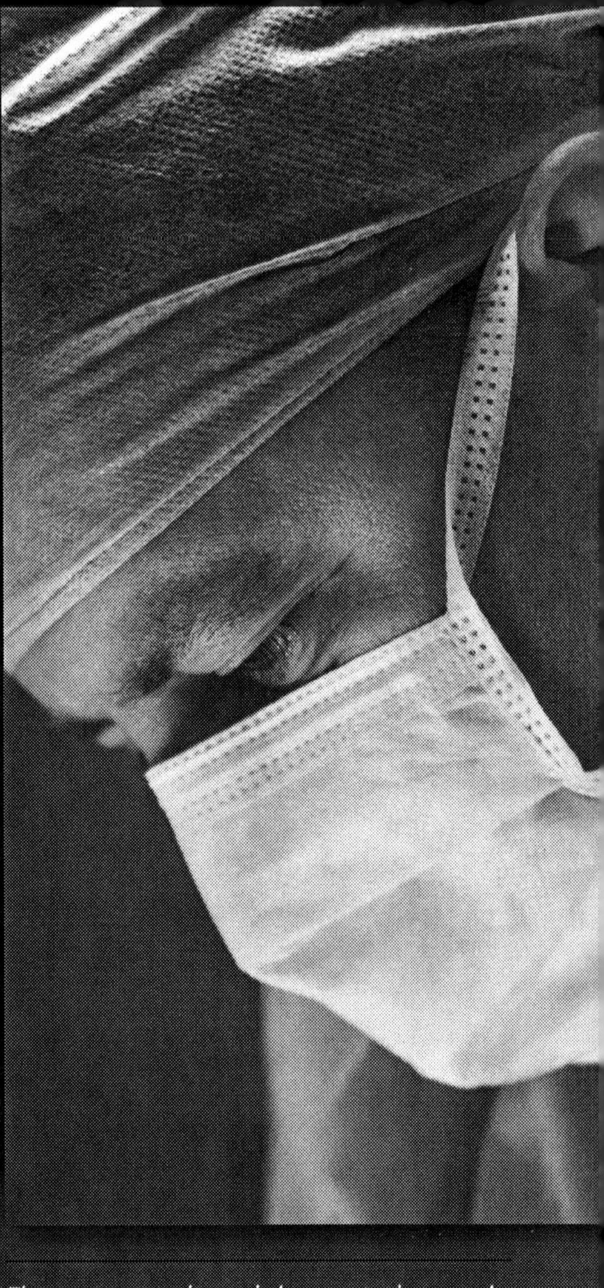

The more complicated the surgical case, the simpler the anesthesia.

Unknown

SURGISPHERE

SURGICAL CRITICAL CARE

Sapan S. Desai, M.D., Ph.D. and Mark D. Williams, M.D.

I. Sepsis, Shock and Resuscitation

I.A. Postoperative Fever

1. Postoperative Days 1 and 2

The most common cause of postoperative fever depends on when the pyrexia occurs. Fevers that occur by postoperative day two are from atelectasis; this can be minimized with incentive spirometry. Deep inspiration has a more positive effect than inducing cough. Mechanical ventilation and chest procedures increase the risk of atelectasis. It is for this reason that an epidural can be beneficial as part of the treatment for flail chest.

2. Postoperative Days 3 through 5

Urinary tract infection is the most common cause of fever from postoperative days three through five. Prophylactic measures can be taken in patients who are more susceptible to UTI. This population includes patients who have indwelling Foley catheters and a history of UTI. Prophylactic antibiotics such as trimethoprim are used to prevent UTI in immunocompromised transplant patients.

3. Postoperative Days 4 through 6

Deep vein thrombosis is the most common cause of postoperative fever on days four through six, and can lead to sudden death from pulmonary embolism. Low-dose subcutaneous heparin, sequential compressive devices (SCD), and early ambulation reduce the incidence of DVT. The patient population most at risk of DVT is those who have undergone abdominal, pelvic, or orthopedic procedures, and trauma patients.

4. Postoperative Days 5 through 7

Surgical wound infections are most common postoperative days five through seven. However, surgical wound infections in deep wounds may not present for 2-3 weeks.

5. Postoperative Days 7 and Beyond

Fevers that occur after postoperative day seven can be from medications. The surgeon must first rule out causes of fever from the operation. Medication-induced fever is not typically associated with tachycardia.

6. Summary

- Wind – Atelectasis
- Water – UTI
- Wound – Surgical wound infection
- Walking – Thromboembolism
- Wonder Drug – Medication fever

I.B. Systemic Inflammatory Response Syndrome

1. Etiology and Pathophysiology

Systemic inflammatory response syndrome (SIRS) is the presence of two or more of the following:

- Fever / Chills: > 38°C or < 36°C
- Tachycardia: > 90 bpm
- Tachypnea: > 20 breaths per minute or a $PaCO_2$ < 32 mmHg
- Leukocytosis: > 12,000/µL or < 4,000/µL or > 10% bands

SIRS can be due to bacteremia (sepsis) and can progress to end-organ damage (severe sepsis). SIRS should be thought of as a global inflammatory state with a pronounced cytokine cascade activation leading to multiple organ dysfunction syndrome (MODS). The proinflammatory state includes numerous acute phase reactants and release of vasoactive cytokines. The more end organs affected, the higher the risk of mortality.

2. Presentation and Diagnosis

With lactic acidosis, change in mental status, decreased urine production, or other signs of organ dysfunction, MODS develops with SIRS. If the etiology is bacteremia, the sepsis becomes severe sepsis. The addition of hypotension to sepsis (SIRS due to bacteremia) is septic shock. Systolic BP < 90 mmHg or a need for vasopressors is septic shock.

3. Treatment

SIRS is treated with admission to the ICU, antibiotics if infection is suspected, and supportive therapy. Fluid sequestration and third space fluid losses can be large; thus fluid resuscitation is necessary. A pulmonary artery catheter (PAC) can be used to monitor cardiac function, however their use for monitoring resuscitation is becoming rare as there is little clinical data showing that their use leads to a better clinical outcome. There are newer technologies now becoming available that can monitor cardiac function noninvasively.

Activated protein C (Xigris) leads to fibrinolysis and reduces inflammation but can lead to bleeding. Aggressive fluid resuscitation with correction of central venous PO_2, serum lactate, base excess, urine output, and blood pressure must be done. Intravenous steroids are often used not only in patients with adrenal dysfunction but also in septic shock patients who are not responding. Patients in septic shock who otherwise do not have adrenal dysfunction cannot mount the massive adrenal response necessary and steroids need to be added. Tight glucose control has been shown to be beneficial. If the etiology of SIRS (usually infection) is not discovered and treated, the patient will progress to severe sepsis, MODS, and septic shock.

I.C. Sepsis

1. Etiology

Sepsis is SIRS with bacteremia. The most common cause of sepsis is from gram negative bacteremia. The most common source is genitourinary, followed by respiratory and abdomen.

2. Pathophysiology

Diversion of blood flow from the central circulation to the peripheral vessels occurs due to increased heat production from hypermetabolism. Without fluid repletion, ischemia of central tissues occurs. Further, there is a diffuse increase in microvascular permeability secondary to the inflammatory response taking place. Left uncontrolled, the end result is decreased urine output from renal hypoperfusion, hypotension from diversion of intravascular volume, and warming of the extremities from decreased systemic vascular resistance (SVR). Cardiac output increases to compensate for the hypotension. Sepsis causes decreased oxygen consumption and exerts its effects on the mitochondria of cells. In sepsis with a pronounced inflammatory response and cytokine activation, no matter how much oxygen is delivered to the cells, they do not use it well. Sepsis also causes microthrombosis at the capillary level which produces shunting of oxygenated blood from the pre-capillary arterioles to post-capillary venules without the oxygen being used by the tissue. APC works by preventing this microthrombosis. This decreased oxygen consumption produces an increase in mixed venous oxygen content.

3. Presentation and Diagnosis

Proof that infection is the etiology of the SIRS can be elusive, but sepsis has a source of infection. If organ dysfunction is evident, the sepsis is severe sepsis. Numerous general symptoms are often present. Fever and mental status changes are common. The source of infection must be diligently sought. IV lines should be immediately tested and changed, especially central lines. A complete physical exam should be done to identify any source of infection. If tachypnea is one of the features of the SIRS, respiratory alkalosis is often present. Virtually any uncontrolled infection or significant disease process can lead to SIRS.

Almost anything can cause SIRS: an amusement part thrill ride often makes people tachycardic and tachypneic. Many disease processes can cause SIRS and organ dysfunction yet that is not sepsis unless an infection is involved. For instance, sterile fulminant pancreatitis can cause SIRS, MODS and even death without sepsis.

Glucocorticoid release in shock leads to insulin resistance. The resulting hyperglycemia is the earliest sign of impending sepsis and may occur up to 24 hours preceding hypotension, low SVR, high CO, and warm extremities. Respiratory alkalosis, hyperventilation, and altered mental status are other early signs of sepsis. Sepsis is associated with an increase in IL 6. Late sepsis will progress with worsening hypotension, a decrease in cardiac output from poor filling pressures (low CVP and BV), increased PVR, cold extremities, conversion to lactic acidosis with metabolic acidosis, and hypoventilation.

4. Treatment

Supportive therapy and maintaining organ perfusion are essential to decrease morbidity and mortality. Infection by IV lines may be treated with imipenem, meropenem, cefoperazone, cefepime, or vancomycin. APC (Xigris) used in the treatment of sepsis leads to fibrinolysis, but has strict criteria for use.

I.D. Shock

1. Septic Shock

a) Assessment

Septic shock is sepsis with shock and causes hypoperfusion of end organs. Tachypnea and abnormalities in the WBC are typically present. Distributive shock is the early stage of septic shock and results with uneven fluid distribution (third space fluid sequestration and diversion of blood from central organs to the periphery) throughout the body. This is secondary to release of acute phase reactants and a gross systemic inflammatory reaction. This inflammation is commonly secondary to infection by gram negative organisms and subsequent production of endotoxins. Unopposed activation of TNF commonly occurs as the initiator of this inflammatory cascade. With continued hypoperfusion, the period of warm septic shock with shunting of blood to the periphery is replaced with late shock and leads to a state of global hypoperfusion and imminent cardiovascular collapse.

b) Management

Treatment for septic shock requires correction of the underlying septic source, fluid resuscitation, and the use of pressors. End organ dysfunction must be corrected as quickly as possible to avoid long term damage. Steroids may have some role to help mitigate the immune response. Septic patients with end organ failure who meet APACHE II criteria may be candidates for APC (Xigris).

In Summary

Septic shock = sepsis + shock

Shock = hypoperfusion of end organs, systolic blood pressure < 90mmHg, or the need for vasopressors

Severe sepsis = sepsis + MODS

MODS = multiple organ dysfunction syndrome

Sepsis = SIRS + infection

SIRS = two or more of the following:

- Fever: > 38°C or < 36°C
- Tachycardia > 90 bpm
- Tachypnea > 20 bpm or PaCO2 < 32 mm Hg
- WBC >12,000/µL or < 4,000/µL or >10% bands)

If the infecton causing the SIRS is not treated, it will advance to severe sepsis, MODS, and septic shock.

2. Hypovolemic Shock

a) Assessment

Severe hypovolemia can overwhelm the body's ability to generate sufficient vasoconstriction and cardiac output. Hypovolemic shock is the most common type of shock and can occur secondary to hemorrhage, burns, dehydration, abuse of diuretics, vomiting, and diarrhea. The initial response is increased peripheral vasoconstriction and cardiac contractility, tachycardia and cool extremities. The renin-angiotensin-aldosterone axis is stimulated, ANP release by the heart is inhibited to decrease diuresis, and the desire to drink fluid is stimulated.

b) Management

Hypovolemia requires replacement of the intravascular volume. Typically, lactated ringers is given as a bolus. In the adult when hemorrhage is thought to be the etiology of the shock, if two liters of ringers lactact does not correct the shock or if the hemorrhage continues, packed red blood cells should be infused. Correction of the inciting events leading to the hypovolemia (stop the hemorrhage!) is the first priority. Admission to an ICU and use of invasive pressure monitoring may be required.

3. Cardiogenic Shock

a) Assessment

Cardiogenic shock is due to compromised function of the heart, such as with heart failure following a myocardial infarction, arrhythmia, cardiomyopathy, or high-grade congestive heart failure. Sustained hypotension leading to hypoperfusion is the result even with satisfactory filling pressure of the left ventricle. Cardiogenic shock therefore presents with prerenal failure, mental status changes, and cool extremities. Jugular venous distention and pulmonary edema are other findings. Pericardial tamponade, saddle pulmonary embolus, and tension pneumothorax must be ruled out as they can produce symptoms similar to cardiogenic shock.

b) Management

Following diagnosis, most practitioners will consider the use of a pulmonary artery catheter to help guide resuscitation and tailor therapy according to the available cardiac function. Inotropic agents such as dobutamine are often necessary to augment cardiac function. If the left heart failure is poignant, an intra-aortic balloon pump may be necessary to reduce afterload and augment cardiac function. Failing this, a left ventricular assist device or heart transplantation may be required.

4. Anaphylactic Shock

a) Assessment

Widespread vasodilation in response to excess histamine release leads to anaphylactic shock. It is secondary to a severe type I hypersensitivity reaction. Systemic vasodilation occurs and overwhelms the ability of the heart to generate sufficient output. There are a variety of causes, including bee stings and allergic reaction to various medications. Anaphylactic shock is induced by IgE. Severe swelling of the face and throat can occur and lead to obstruction of the airway.

b) Management

Anaphylactic shock requires immediate supportive therapy due to the risk of respiratory arrest. Epinephrine is used to forestall the collapse of the airway and stimulate the cardiovascular system.

5. Neurogenic Shock

a) Assessment

Neurogenic shock occurs secondary to acute disruption of central nervous system pathways, typically at the level of the spinal cord from acute trauma. Loss of background sympathetic activity leads to hypotension, bradycardia, and peripheral vasodilation.

b) Management

Treatment of neurogenic shock requires supportive therapy and stabilization of any fractures leading to compromise of the spinal cord. A significant amount of fluid resuscitation may be necessary. Atropine may be used for symptomatic bradycardia. Pressors may be required. If the neurogenic shock is due to trauma, hemorrhagic shock must first be ruled out (stop the bleeding!) as the source of the shock.

6. Endocrine Shock

Endocrine shock may occur secondary to profound hypothyroidism, thyrotoxicosis, or adrenal insufficiency. A combination of hypovolemic and cardiogenic shock may occur. Treatment is to support the endocrine function. Endocrine shock may contribute to septic shock as an inadequate adrenal response to septic shock has been recognized and steroid supplementation may be needed.

II. Acid-Base Management

II.A. Arterial Blood Gas

The ABG is used to measure oxygenation of the blood and to determine the nature of hypoxia. ABG measures five values: pH, $PaCO_2$, PaO_2, HCO_3^-, and O_2 saturation, while the base excess is automatically calculated. Normal ranges for these values are presented on page 134. Acidosis or alkalosis is determined by the pH. Hypoxemia is determined by the PaO_2. Compensation for any potential metabolic acidosis or alkalosis is measured by $PaCO_2$ and HCO_3^-. The change is pH due to a change in the PCO_2 (hyper or hypoventilation) can be calculated:

$$\text{Corrected } HCO_3^- = \text{measured } HCO_3^- + (\text{anion gap} - 12)$$

$$\text{Anion gap} = (Na^+ + K^+) - (Cl^- + HCO_3^-)$$

$$\text{Expected } PaCO_2 = (1.5 \times HCO_3^-) + (8 \pm 2)$$

$$\text{Acute respiratory acidosis: pH} = 0.08 \times [(PaCO_2 - 40) / 10]$$

$$\text{Chronic respiratory acidosis: pH} = 0.03 \times [(PaCO_2 - 40) / 10]$$

$$\text{Acute respiratory alkalosis: pH} = 0.08 \times [(40 - PaCO_2) / 10]$$

$$\text{Chronic respiratory alkalosis: pH} = 0.03 \times [(40 - PaCO_2) / 10]$$

A corrected HCO_3^- is calculated to determine whether there is also a metabolic acidosis or alkalosis. Because the measured bicarbonate may be normal due to a changed anion gap. This correction is relatively straightforward:

The normal corrected HCO_3^- should be approximately 24. Significant variation indicates a complex metabolic disturbance – HCO_3^- more than 24 indicates a coexisting metabolic alkalosis, while an HCO_3^- less than 24 indicates a coexisting non-anion gap metabolic acidosis.

The expected respiratory compensation for a metabolic acidosis can be calculated with Winter's formula. This is due to a linear relationship between changes in HCO_3^- and compensation by the lung to change in $PaCO_2$.

Metabolic acidosis causes hyperventilation and a drop in $PaCO_2$ as respiratory compensation. Variation outside of the range specified by Winter's formula indicates a concurrent respiratory disturbance and not just compensation for a metabolic acidosis. Winter's formula can only be used for metabolic acidosis; it does not predict the respiratory compensation in response to a metabolic alkalosis. With metabolic alkalosis, the respiratory response is hypoventilation and a $PaCO_2$ above 40 but less than 50, and alkalotic pH above 7.42.

TABLE 1. Acid-base changes and compensation

Metabolic acidosis = gain in H^+ or loss of HCO_3^- = drop in HCO_3^-, drop in pH	Respiratory compensation = hyperventilation, drop in $PaCO_2$ = acidic (low) pH to normal
Metabolic alkolosis = loss of H^+ or gain of HCO_3^- = rise in HCO_3^-, rise in pH	Respiratory compensation = hypoventilation, rise in $PaCO_2$ = alkalotic (high) pH to normal
Respiratory acidosis = hypoventilation, rise in $PaCO_2$, drop in pH	Metabolic compensation = rise in HCO_3^- = acidic (low) pH to normal
Respiratory alkolosis = hyperventilaton, drop in $PaCO_2$, rise in pH	Metabolic compensation = drop in HCO_3^- = alkalotic (high) pH to normal

TABLE 2. Arterial Blood Gas Interpretation

Variable	Normal Range	Notes
pH	7.35 - 7.45	Determines acidosis vs. alkalosis, the presence of mixed disorders, and compensation.
PCO_2	35 - 45	PCO_2 is determined by ventilation. A high PCO_2 with low pH indicates respiratory acidosis. A low PCO_2 with high pH indicates respiratory alkalosis. PCO_2 > 60 may indicate the need for mechanical ventilation.
PO_2	75 - 100	PO_2 < 60 may indicate the need for mechanical ventilation.
HCO_3^-	22 - 30	Indicates the presence of a metabolic derangement. A low HCO_3^- indicates metabolic acidosis; high values indicate metabolic alkalosis.
Base excess	-2 - +2	Negative base excess indicates acidosis. Positive values indicate alkalosis.

II.B. ACID-BASE

1. Metabolic Acidosis

a) Anion Gap Metabolic Acidosis

An anion gap metabolic acidosis means that the metabolic acidosis is due to hydrogen ions not measured by the laboratory standard chem 7. It is commonly due to lactic acidosis (commnly from hypoperfusion of end organs, shock) ketoacidosis (but not ketone bodies), uremia in chronic renal failure, and ingestion of toxins such as aspirin, ethylene glycol, methanol, and paraldehyde. Anion gap metabolic acidosis is diagnosed by the presence of ketoacids (as in alcoholic ketoacidosis, diabetic ketoacidosis, paraldehyde poisoning, starvation, high-fat diet, and isopropyl alcohol poisoning) or ketoacids being absent (as in renal failure, lactic acidosis, methanol poisoning, ethylene glycol poisoning, and aspirin poisoning). The indications for dialysis include acidosis, hyperkalemia, symptomatic uremia, drug filtration, and fluid overload.

b) Non-Anion Gap Metabolic Acidosis

A non-anion gap metabolic acidosis means that the metabolic acidosis is due to hydrogen ions measured by the chem 7. It is a disturbance common in renal tubular acidosis (RTA), diarrhea, GI tract fistulas, pancreatic disease, use of carbonic anhydrase inhibitors, acid ingestion, dilution of alkali, ileostomy, and various medications (beta-blockers, spironolactone). Treatment is to correct the underlying etiology but to avoid hypernatremia, fluid overload, and excessive bicarbonate infusion.

c) Renal Tubular Acidosis

(1) *Assessment*

RTA type I is known as distal RTA, and occurs with medications such as amphotericin, lithium, and NSAIDs, and in diseases such as nephrolithiasis, sickle cell anemia, infection, and autoimmune disorders. RTA type I presents with inability to acidify urine with secondary hyperaldosteronism, hypokalemia, nephrolithiasis, and nephrocalcinosis.

RTA type II is known as proximal RTA, and occurs with Wilson disease, Fanconi syndrome, amyloidosis, vitamin D deficiency, hypocalcemia, hepatitis, and autoimmune diseases. RTA type II leads to basic urine in the early stage until the bicarbonate is lost, then subsequent urine acidification. RTA type II also leads to hypokalemia, osteomalacia and rickets.

RTA type IV is known as hypoaldosteronism RTA, and occurs from a decrease in aldosterone or insensitivity to angiotensin II, diabetes, Addison disease, sickle cell disease, and renal insufficiency. RTA type IV presents with hyperkalemia and hyperchloremic non-anion gap metabolic acidosis.

(2) *Management*

RTA type I is treated with oral bicarbonate and potassium replacement. RTA type II is treated with potassium replacement and volume depletion to enhance bicarbonate reabsorption. Thiazide diuretics are also useful. RTA type IV is treated with fludrocortisone, a mineralocorticoid.

2. Metabolic Alkalosis

a) Assessment

Metabolic alkalosis is an increase in pH, increased bicarbonate, and compensatory hypoventilation with an increase in $PaCO_2$ (the opposite of metabolic acidosis). Chloride-responsive metabolic alkalosis has a urine chloride of less than 15, and is commonly due to vomiting, pyloric stenosis, laxative abuse, diuretics, and hypercapnia. Chloride-resistant forms have a urine chloride more than 15, and are commonly a result of severe potassium or magnesium deficiency (as in diuretic abuse), increased mineralocorticoids, Bartter's syndrome, chewing tobacco, and licorice consumption.

b) Management

Neuromuscular excitability, hypokalemia, and hypovolemia are commonly found on exam, and treatment involves correcting the underlying disorder. KCl is sometimes given to correct significant electrolyte abnormalities. Potassium must be corrected first in chloride-resistant metabolic alkalosis.

3. Respiratory Acidosis

a) Assessment

Respiratory acidosis is due to hypoventilation and produces a compensatory increased bicarbonate. Causes of respiratory suppression include COPD, airway obstruction, pneumothorax, myasthenia gravis, muscular dystrophy, nervous system disorders (such as Guillain-Barré syndrome), botulism, tetanus, organophosphate poisoning, and central depression of the respiratory system (as in narcotic abuse or general endotracheal anesthesia). Presenting signs include confusion leading to stupor and coma, and encephalopathy.

b) Management

Respiratory acidosis is managed by treating the underlying cause, and using artificial ventilation to decrease CO_2 retention. Oxygenation of COPD patients who are chronically hypoxic and depend on hypoxia for respiratory stimulation, may lead to depression of the respiratory drive, so only the minimum amount of oxygen via nasal cannula should be provided to maintain oxygenation of the blood.

4. Respiratory Alkalosis

a) Assessment

Respiratory alkalosis is elevated pH, because of hyperventilation (decrease PCO_2), and a compensatory decrease in bicarbonate. It is commonly a result of anxiety causing hyperventilation but may also be a consequence of shock, pulmonary disease, pregnancy, cirrhosis, hyperthyroidism, and aspirin poisoning. Presentation is with rapid, deep breathing, anxiety, chest pain, and circumoral paresthesia.

b) Management

Treat respiratory alkalosis by minimizing anxiety in the patient, breathing into a paper bag to increase PCO_2, and decreasing minute volume if the patient is artificially ventilated.

The SAFE study and Australian ICU study, two of the best studies of the plethora of research over decades that have compared crystalloid to colloid, have indicated that crystalloid administration for hypotensive patients is as effective as colloids or blood unless the patient is anemic and has a specific indication for transfusion.

III.B. Electrolyte Disturbances

1. Hyponatremia

a) Etiology and Pathophysiology

Hyponatremia = serum $Na^+ < 135$ mEq/L

- Hypotonic
  - Hypovolemic
    - Diuretics, salt wasting syndromes, vomiting, diarrhea, burns
    - Third-space losses (pancreatitis, peritonitis)
  - Isovolemic
    - Renal failure, SIADH, glucocorticoid deficiency, hypthyroidism, various medications
  - Hypervolemic
    - Cirrhosis, CHF, nephrotic syndrome
- Isotonic
  - Excessive isotonic infusions with glucose or mannitol, pseudohyponatremia
- Hypertonic
  - Hyperglycemia 100 mL/dL > normal causes Na^+ decrease of 1.6 mEq/L
  - Hypertonic infusions of glucose or mannitol

b) Presentation and Diagnosis

The severity of symptoms depends for a large part on how quickly the soidum level dropped.

— Moderate hyponatremia

- Confusion, lethargy, anorexia, and myalgia

— Severe hyponatremia

- Coma or seizures

Diagnosis is made by examining the osmolarity, carefully assessing the patient for objective signs and symptoms (i.e. tachycardia, dehydration), and measuring serum glucose. Pseudohyponatremia is diagnosed with normal or elevated osmolarity that does not match the calculated osmolarity; common causes include multiple myeloma and hypertriglyceridemia that increase the protein or lipid fraction in the plasma. The sodium deficit can be calculated because 60% of body weigh is fluid and 140 mEq/L is the normal Na^+ concentration:

c) Treatment

The treatment for hyponatremia is to slowly correct the serum sodium with half corrected in the first 24 hours. A rate no faster than 1 mEq/hr should be used to avoid central pontine myelinolysis (CPM), seizure, and increased intracranial pressure (ICP). Hypovolemic hyponatremia is corrected with 0.9% normal saline (NS); hypervolemic hyponatremia is corrected with sodium and water restriction and ACE-inhibitors may be beneficial. CPM tends to occur in severe hyponatremia and presents with stupor, confusion, lethargy, and quadriparesis. Some patients recover from CPM over a period of weeks. Conservation of sodium is done through an ADH-independent reabsorption.

2. Hypernatremia

a) Etiology and Pathophysiology

Hypernatremia, $Na^+ > 145$ mEq/L

- Hypovolemic
  - Water loss from diuretics, GI, respiratory, and skin
- Isovolemic
  - Decreased TBW with decreased ECF, DI, skin losses, central defects in osmolarity
- Hypervolemic
  - Increased TBW with increased Na^+, hypertonic fluid, excess salt intake, Conn or Cushing syndrome

b) Presentation and Diagnosis

Just as in hyponatremia, the severity of symptoms is due largely to how quickly the hypernatremia develops. Hypernatremia presents with fatigue, confusion, and lethargy that can progress to seizures and coma.

c) Treatment

Hypovolemic hypernatremia is treated with NS given at 2 mOsm/kg/hr. Isovolemic hypernatremia is treated with 0.45% NaCl (½ NS) with half the water deficit corrected over the first day. No more than 1 mEq/L/hr should be given in an acute setting. DI is treated with vasopressin. Hypervolemic hypernatremia is treated with ½ NS and loop diuretics.

3. Hypochloremia

Hypochloremic alkalosis should be treated with potassium. Vomiting will lead to hypochloremic metabolic alkalosis.

4. Hypokalemia

a) Etiology and Pathophysiology

Hypokalemia is K+ < 3.5 mEq/L

- Decreased intake
  - Especially in the elderly or in those receiving total parenteral nutrition
- Increased losses
  - Diuretics, mineralocorticoids, hyperaldosteronism, osmotic diuresis, excess urine flow, and gastrointestinal losses from diarrhea)
  - Vomiting: loss of volume and gastric acid causes extracellular Na^+ shift (volume) in exchange for K^+ plus renal reabsorption of Na^+ with loss of K+
- Intracellular shift
  - Acute insulin therapy for hyperglycemia
  - B12, ß-blockers, digibind, and alkalosis (each 0.1 pH increase leads to a shift of 0.5 mEq/L of K^+).

b) Presentation and Diagnosis

Hypokalemia presents with hypertension if the underlying cause is primary hyperaldosteronism or licorice ingestion, while hypotension may suggest laxative abuse, Bartter syndrome, or bulimia. Hypokalemia may also present with flaccidity, muscle weakness, and loss of deep tendon reflexes (DTRs). Arrhythmia can also occur.

c) Treatment

Prevent further potassium loss and replenish the stores to treat hypokalemia. Most K^+ is intracellular so serum K^+ may underestimate the replenishment needed. No more than 10 mEq/hr can be infused via peripheral lines due to venous irritation. A maximum of 40 mEq/hr can be infused through central lines in emergent situations.

5. Hyperkalemia

a) Etiology and Pathophysiology

Hyperkalemia is the result of increased intake of potassium, impaired excretion of potassium, or a shift from the intracellular to extracellular space. Decreased excretion is commonly due to potassium-sparing diuretics, ACE-inhibitors, NSAIDs, type IV RTA, and renal failure. Hyperkalemia is common in hospitalized patients, rhabdomyolysis, and diabetes. The adrenocortical syndromes pertaining to 21-hydroxylase deficiency and 11-beta hydroxylase deficiency are other causes. Mortality occurs with the development of fatal arrhythmias in very high potassium titers.

b) Presentation and Diagnosis

Identifying the etiology of hyperkalemia is done by renal function tests to identify renal insufficiency. Obtain: urine K^+ urine osmolality, serum K^+, serum osmolality, and EKG. Hyperkalemia causes EKG changes including peaked T waves, PR interval prolongation, QRS widening, disappearance of the P wave, and sinus arrest. Bradycardia may also be present.

c) Treatment

Treatment involves correcting toxicity caused by the hyperkalemia, removing excess sources of potassium, and shifting potassium intracellularly with glucose and insulin administration. Bicarbonate and ß-blockers can be used to correct the metabolic acidosis and to decrease extracellular potassium. Potassium excretion can be facilitated with fluorohydrocortisone and stopping potassium-sparing diuretics and ACE-inhibitors. GI excretion can be increased with potassium-binding resins such as Kayexalate. Dialysis is an option in emergency situations.

6. Hypocalcemia

a) Etiology and Pathophysiology

Hypocalcemia occurs with serum calcium level less than 8.5 mg/dL. Loss of calcium regulation by vitamin D, parathyroid hormone (PTH), calcitonin, hypomagnesemia, and hyperphosphatemia account for the majority of hypocalcemic presentations. Other causes include pancreatitis, sepsis, rhabdomyolysis, and exposure to toxins such as fluoride, ethanol, phenytoin, citrate, and cimetidine. Since 50% of the calcium is bound to albumin, hypoalbuminemia produces a low serum calcium but the ionized calcium concentration (the physiologically active form) remains normal.

b) Presentation and Diagnosis

Symptomatic hypocalcemia may lead to circumoral paresthesia, Chvostek sign (facial spasm after tapping on the facial nerve anterior to the tragus), and Trousseau sign (spasm of the wrist after stopping forearm blood flow with a blood pressure cuff). Diagnosis is made by electrolyte panels and EKG findings positive for a prolonged QT interval. Albumin levels should be checked and the Ca^{2+} value corrected:

Corrected $Ca^{2+} = Ca^{2+} -$ albumin + 4. The ionized Ca^{2+} can be measured instead.

c) Treatment

Treatment of hypocalcemia includes identifying PTH deficits, giving vitamin D or calcitriol along with thiazide diuretics to prevent excess Ca^{2+} excretion, correcting hypomagnesemia, restricting phosphate, oral Ca^{2+} supplementation, and infusion in emergent situations. Calcium carbonate is useful as an oral supplement. Calcium chloride infusion requires a central line, while calcium gluconate can be given via a peripheral line.

7. Hypercalcemia

a) Etiology and Pathophysiology

Hypercalcemia is diagnosed with a serum Ca^{2+} level more than 10.5 mg/dL. Half of the Ca^{2+} is bound to albumin, which must be measured in order to determine the amount of free ionized calcium, unless the lab can provide free ionized Ca^{2+} concentrations. Hypercalcemia primarily affects the kidneys and CNS and leads to fatigue, depression, personality changes, confusion, somnolence, and even coma and death. Nephrolithiasis, positive inotropy, arrhythmia, constipation, and anorexia are other manifestations. The vast majority of cases are due to hyperparathyroidism or malignancy from metastatic cancer to the bone or parathyroid hormone related peptide (PTHrP) secretion by lung cancer. Other conditions include vitamin A or D excess and renal failure.

b) Presentation and Diagnosis

Dehydration is common in hypercalcemia, and metastatic calcifications in other tissues are common in more severe cases (termed calciphylaxis), particularly if phosphorus is also high. PTH levels should be measured and a search for malignancy should be undertaken. A shortened QT interval may be present on EKG. Always check albumin levels.

c) Treatment

Treatment involves volume repletion, mobilization, reducing GI Ca^{2+} absorption with prednisone and oral phosphate, preventing bone resorption with biphosphonates such as pamidronate, etidronate, risedronate, and alendronate, and administering calcitonin. Dialysis may also be used in more serious cases. A surgical option includes a partial parathyroidectomy. Hypercalcemia with diarrhea should begin a search for MEN syndrome; gastrin levels should be measured as the diarrhea may be a sign of a gastrinoma.

8. Hypophosphatemia

a) Etiology and Pathophysiology

Phosphate levels less than 2.5 mg/dL qualify as hypophosphatemia. Causes for hypophosphatemia include poor intake, increased excretion, or a shift from the extracellular to intracellular space. Alcoholics, patients with eating disorders, Crohn disease, vitamin D deficiency, RTA, antacids that bind to phosphate, hyperparathyroidism, hypokalemia, hypomagnesemia, volume expansion, respiratory alkalosis, and acetazolamide are other causes for hypophosphatemia.

b) Presentation and Diagnosis

Hypophosphatemia presents with rhabdomyolysis, seizures, coma, hemolytic anemia, and platelet dysfunction. The urine phosphate content is measured. Deficits less than 100 mg/d imply gastrointestinal loss or redistribution of phosphate; greater deficits are due to Fanconi syndrome. High Ca^{2+} with hypophosphatemia implies primary hyperparathyroidism or malignancy as the chief cause. Low Ca^{2+} with hypophosphatemia indicates 2° hyperparathyroidism, rickets, renal failure, and familial causes. Hypophosphatemia leads to decreased cardiac output, increased RBC destruction, depletion of 2,3 DPG, and left shift in the oxygen-hemoglobin curve. There is also increased difficulty weaning from a ventilator.

c) Treatment

Treatment for hypophosphatemia includes oral repletion in minor cases or IV administration if severe. Vitamin D supplementation is given. Primary or secondary hyperparathyroidism may require a parathyroidectomy.

d) Refeeding Syndrome

Hypophosphatemia following refeeding presents as respiratory failure and prolonged dependence on a mechanical ventilator. Refeeding syndrome is due to phosphorylation of glucose intermediaries and leads to decreased phosphate available for ATP generation. Failure of ATP production occurs. The most appropriate therapy is to replete phosphate.

9. Hyperphosphatemia

a) Etiology and Pathophysiology

Hyperphosphatemia = phosphate > 5 mg/dL in the serum. Excess intake can occur with vitamin D intoxication. Decreased clearance can occur with hypoparathyroidism or renal failure. A shift from the intracellular to extracellular space occurs in rhabdomyolysis and tumor lysis syndrome.

b) Presentation and Diagnosis

Hyperphosphatemia presents with hypocalcemia and calciphylaxis. Most patients are asymptomatic, but muscle cramps, perioral paresthesia, uremic symptoms, and general malaise can occur.

c) Treatment

Hyperphosphatemia is treated by temporizing renal failure, dietary restriction of phosphate, binders such as calcium carbonate, insulin and glucose infusion as a temporary measure, and dialysis in more serious cases.

10. Hypomagnesemia

a) Etiology and Pathophysiology

Hypomagnesemia is Mg < than 1.8 mg/dL. It is commonly due to malabsorption, poor dietary intake, excess excretion, or redistribution within the body. Causes of excess excretion include diarrhea, diuretic abuse, ATN, hypokalemia, hypercalciuria, or endocrine disturbances. Redistribution in the body can occur with hypoalbuminemia, pancreatitis, glucose and insulin administration.

b) Presentation and Diagnosis

Hypomagnesemia presents with weakness, hyperreflexia, seizures, hypokalemia, and hypocalcemia. EKG changes include prolonged QT and PR, flattened T waves, atrial fibrillation, and torsade de pointes.

c) Treatment

Treatment of hypomagnesemia is by oral magnesium oxide supplements or IV magnesium sulfate. Cardiac dysfunction must be addressed.

11. Hypermagnesemia

a) Etiology and Pathophysiology

Hypermagnesemia = Mg > 2.5 mg/dL. It is due to renal failure with decreased excretion, abuse of antacids, tumor lysis syndrome, rhabdomyolysis, DKA, pheochromocytoma, and toxicity from lithium.

b) Presentation and Diagnosis

Hypermagnesemia presents with decreased DTR, hypotension, paresthesia, coma, and specific EKG changes. EKG changes are opposite of those found with hypomagnesemia.

c) Treatment

Reverse EKG changes in hypermagnesemia with IV calcium. If necessary, dialysis may be used to regain normal magnesium homeostasis.

IV. Nutrition

IV.A. Nutritional Requirements

Familiarity with nutritional requirements and energy content of various sources of intake are an important component of providing appropriate nutritional care to the surgical patient. The major source of protein turnover is skeletal muscle, which becomes especially significant in prolonged starvation and acute injury.

Table 3. Energy Content

Energy Content	
Carbohydrate	3.4 kcal / g
Protein	4 kcal / g
Lipid	9 kcal / g

The Harris Benedict equation is used to determine basal energy expenditure. Various modifications are used to determine the estimated caloric needs for patients. The equation varies for men and women. The average caloric need for a 70 kg male is about 1700 kcal/day. The average caloric need for a 70 kg female is slightly less. The metabolic cart can also be used to calculate overall nutritional status and the respiratory quotient. Indirect calorimetry works by calculating CO_2 production. The respiratory quotient is calculated as the ratio between CO_2 produced to O_2 consumed.

The respiratory quotient is a unitless number calculated as the ratio between the amount of carbon dioxide produced and the amount of oxygen consumed. This value typically correlates to the caloric value for each liter of carbon dioxide produced.

Surgical Critical Care

Table 4. Respiratory Quotient

Process	Respiratory Quotient
Carbohydrate oxidation	1
Fat oxidation	0.7
Protein breakdown	0.8
Lipogenesis	> 1.0
Normal	0.8

Table 5. Energy Requirements

Energy Requirements	
Protein requirement	0.9-1.5 g/kg/day of protein (normal requirements)
	2-3 g/kg/day of protein (severe burn or sepsis)
	Limit total intake to 40-50 g/day in hepatic failure.
Nitrogen balance	Nitrogen: non-protein calories = 1:100-1:200

IV.B. Enteral and Parenteral Nutrition

1. Enteral Nutrition

Enteral feeding provides the advantage of a decreased risk of sepsis through line infection, induction of the immune system through small intestine production of IgA, and maintenance of the gastrointestinal tract. This leads to increased integrity of the GI tract with decreased spontaneous bacterial translocation across the cell wall. Gastrin induction increases insulin release and anabolism. Enteral nutrition, however, has a decreased rate of absorption in the immediate postoperative period. Tube feeding does not improve longevity or quality of life in nursing home residents. Nonocclusive bowel necrosis may occur within two weeks of starting enteral feeds and present with pneumatosis and necrosis. Treatment is reversion to TPN.

2. Parenteral Nutrition

Parenteral nutrition has specific indications due to the significant morbidity and mortality associated with TPN. TPN has a proven benefit with enterocutaneous fistulae and improves their closure rate, decreases the incidence of renal failure in ARF, improves morbidity with short gut syndrome and severe burn patients when enteral feeding would be insufficient, and may induce remission of Crohn disease. TPN has also been used to mitigate symptomatic pneumatosis intestinalis when surgery is not indicated. TPN should be stopped slowly over a period of time to avoid hypoglycemia. The rate of TPN should initially be reduced to 50 ml/hr for several hours, and then stopped. Sudden discontinuation of TPN should be treated with a solution of D10W.

Table 6. TPN Composition

TPN Composition	
Protein content	1 g/kg/day (1 g nitrogen = 6.25 g protein)
Caloric content	4 cal/g x 1g x wt (kg)
Non-protein content	25 cal/kg/day
Water	30-40 mL/kg/day
Total energy	30-60 kcal/kg/day
Amino acids	1-2 g/kg/day
Essential minerals	Acetate/gluconate, calcium, chloride, chromium, copper, iodine, magnesium, manganese, phosphorus, potassium, selenium, sodium, zinc

3. Essential Amino Acids

Arginine is an essential amino acid that augments the immune system. Glutamine is the amino acid most abundant in circulation. Glutamine levels following intestinal surgery are decreased due to an increase in utilization by the intestinal cells.

IV.C. Malnutrition and Obesity

1. Obesity

a) Assessment

Obesity is an epidemic in the United States, affecting over a quarter of the population. It is especially common in American Indians, Hawaiians, Hispanics, and African Americans. Obesity is defined as having a body mass index (BMI) over the 85th percentile or more than 30 kg/m^2, calculated as weight (kg) divided by height (m^2).

Obesity has a genetic inheritance, but changes in society, poor diet, and lack of exercise all contribute. Complications of obesity include obstructive sleep apnea (OSA), pseudotumor cerebri, liver dysfunction, cardiovascular disease, hypertension, hypertriglyceridemia, arthritis, diabetes, and cancer. Other factors that can contribute to obesity include Prader-Willi syndrome, Down syndrome, Turner syndrome, growth hormone deficiencies, pseudo-hypoparathyroidism, hypothyroidism, polycystic ovarian syndrome, and medications such as antidepressants and oral contraceptives.

b) Management

Treatment of obesity requires major lifestyle changes; thus treatment is multifaceted and must include reducing other risk factors (such as smoking or alcohol abuse), and treating any concomitant disorders such as DM, HTN, CVA, and heart disease. The last resort is surgical intervention in the form of bariatric surgery – this is typically used in patients with a BMI exceeding 40. Expanded criteria for surgery are used at centers of excellence due to experience.

2. Malnutrition

a) Etiology and Pathophysiology

Malnutrition may present as:

- Kwashiorkor: protein starvation, significant edema
- Marasmus: both protein and caloric starvation, cachexia

Deficiencies in multiple vitamins and significantly poor diet are commonly implicated for malnutrition. There are systemic effects with significant cognitive and physical retardation, and diminished immune activity. Severe malnutrition is rare in the United States; nearly 150 million children worldwide are affected by malnutrition.

b) Presentation and Diagnosis

Malnutrition presents with weight loss, trailing off the normal growth curves, and behavioral/cognitive changes. Physical exam detects anasarca with kwashiorkor. Cheilosis, angular stomatitis, fatty hepatomegaly, and skin hyperpigmentation with peeling are present. Thin and brittle hair is commonly found. Iron deficiency presents with constitutional symptoms, anemia, decreased cognition, headache, glossitis, and koilonychia.

Iodine deficiency presents with goiter and physical and mental retardation. Albumin is not recommended for acute monitoring due to its long half-life; pre-albumin and transferrin are better markers for nutrition due to their shorter half-lives.

c) Treatment

Treatment involves identifying the particular dietary inadequacies and having a full replacement of missing proteins, calories, vitamins, and minerals. Up to 150 kcal/kg/d may be necessary to regain weight.

3. Vitamin Deficits

a) Vitamin A Deficiency

Retinol deficiency is primarily due to poor diet and excessive rice consumption, and secondarily due to malabsorption syndromes and malnutrition syndromes. Vitamin A deficiency presents with growth retardation, night blindness, xerophthalmia, hair changes, keratomalacia, follicular hyperkeratosis, and Bitot spots with foamy patches in the conjunctiva.

b) Vitamin C Deficiency

Vitamin C deficiency is due to poor diet, pregnancy, thyrotoxicosis, inflammatory disease, after surgery, burns, and diarrhea. Scurvy presents with splinter hemorrhages in the nail bed, swollen and friable gums, loss of teeth, breakdown of old scars, poor healing, spontaneous hemorrhage, petechiae, and hyperkeratotic hair follicles. A dietary deficiency as the etiology of scurvy amongst their sailors was proven by a surgeon in the British Navy. The British are referred to as 'limeys' as they carried and consumed limes (a good source of vitamin C) on their long sea voyages by sail and prevented their sailors from becoming 'scurvy dogs.'

c) Vitamin D Deficiency

Vitamin D deficiency is primarily due to poor sunlight exposure or poor intake of calcium or phosphorus. Secondary causes include hypoparathyroidism, hereditary diseases, and poor absorption. The effect of vitamin D deficiency is rickets in children and osteomalacia in adults. Treatment is adequate intake of calcium, phosphorus, and vitamin D supplements.

d) Vitamin E Deficiency

Tocopherol deficiency is a natural state in infants but may present later in life with poor intake, malabsorption syndromes, or genetic causes. Vitamin E deficiency presents with hemolytic anemia, reticulocytosis, hyperbilirubinemia, abetalipoproteinemia, neuropathy such as spinocerebellar ataxia and loss of DTRs, and retinopathy.

e) Vitamin K Deficiency

(1) *Etiology*

Vitamin K is a lipid soluble vitamin essential for the formation of clotting factors. It is produced by colonic bacteria. Terminal ileum disease or resection prevents normal vitamin K production and absorption as there is an enterohepatic circulaton of vitamin K from intestine, ileal absorption, portal venous system, liver, bile back to intestine.

Deficiency may occur from cirrhosis, malabsorption syndromes, biliary disease, various medications (coumadin, INH, rifampin, barbiturates, and others), lupus, DIC, polycythemia vera, cystic fibrosis, and leukemia.

(2) *Pathophysiology*

Vitamin K helps to form coagulation factor II (prothrombin), factor VII (proconvertin), factor IX (Christmas factor), and factor X (Stuart factor). Protein C, protein S, Protein Z, and several bone matrix proteins reliant on glutamic acid residue conversion by vitamin K are also modified by vitamin K. Coumadin is used as a therapeutic anticoagulant because it interferes with vitamin K metabolism which causes a deficiency in the vitamin K dependent clotting factors

(3) *Presentation*

Vitamin K deficiency presents as hemorrhagic disease of newborns (HDN) or as a bleeding diathesis in adults. Vitamin K deficiency, if severe enough, presents as complaints of significant hemorrhage following mild trauma. Ecchymoses, petechiae, hematomas, and oozing of blood are common. GI bleeds, hematuria, menorrhagia, epistaxis, and mucosal bleeds occur frequently. PT and aPTT are elevated. Des-gamma-carboxy prothrombin is present in the absence of vitamin K.

(4) *Treatment*

Treatment for vitamin K deficiency involves correcting the cause of the underlying deficit and providing vitamin K supplements. FFP is necessary in severe disease to prevent hemorrhage. Subcutaneous injections of phylloquinone (vitamin K1) can be given; menadione (vitamin K3) can be given orally in malabsorption syndromes. Phytonadione can also be directly injected in severe disease. Green leafy vegetables and oils provide a good source of vitamin K.

f) Vitamin B1 Deficiency

Primary thiamine deficiency is due to decreased intake especially in a high-rice diet. Secondary deficiency is due to hyperthyroidism, pregnancy, fever, malabsorption syndromes, diarrhea, and liver disease. Alcoholism impairs utilization. Thiamine deficiency presents as dry beriberi with peripheral neurologic symptoms including distal extremity paresthesias, cramps, and pain, CNS symptoms including Wernicke-Korsakoff syndrome, and cardiovascular symptoms including high output cardiac failure with tachycardia, diaphoresis, warm skin, and lactic acidosis.

Korsakoff syndrome presents first with confusion and confabulations, Wernicke encephalopathy happens last and consists of nystagmus, ophthalmoplegia, and coma. Shock can occur and death ensues rapidly if treatment is not started in time. Magnesium sulfate is given with thiamine to reduce peripheral resistance to thiamine. Electrolyte replacement is also be necessary.

g) Vitamin B2 Deficiency

Riboflavin deficiency is due to decreased intake of milk and animal products; secondary deficiency is due to malabsorption syndromes, diarrhea, liver disease, and alcoholism. Riboflavin deficiency presents with pallor, mucosal ulceration such as angular stomatitis and cheilosis, and linear fissures in the skin commonly infected by *Candida*. A red tongue is present, and cutaneous lesions leading to erythema and acanthosis may occur. Keratitis may lead to lacrimation and photophobia.

h) Nicotinic Acid Deficiency

Niacin, vitamin B3, deficiency is due to excessive maize consumption, amino acid imbalances, malabsorption syndromes, cirrhosis, and alcoholism. Pellagra may occur and present with a photosensitive rash, red stomatitis, glossitis, bloody diarrhea, and CNS changes. Desquamation, keratosis, edema of the tongue and other mucous membranes, GI discomfort, confabulations, cogwheel rigidity, and psychiatric changes occur in severe cases. Tryptophan deficiency may present in a similar manner. Deficiency is treated with niacinamide along with replenishment of other lacking vitamins.

i) Vitamin B6 Deficiency

Pyridoxine deficiency is rarely a primary deficiency; secondary causes include oral contraceptive use, use of hydralazine, cycloserine, or penicillamine, and increased metabolic activity. Seborrheic dermatosis, cheilosis, glossitis, peripheral neuropathy, lymphopenia, seizures, and anemia develop with worsening deficiency.

j) Biotin Deficiency

Biotin deficiency occurs in raw egg consumption or long term total parenteral nutrition (TPN). Biotin deficiency presents with alopecia, keratoconjunctivitis, immunologic deficiencies, and retardation of development.

4. Mineral Deficiency

Chromium deficiency may lead to hyperglycemia after prolonged TPN. Selenium deficiency may lead to myalgia and cardiomyopathy. Like most mineral nutrients, iron from digested food or supplements is almost entirely absorbed in the duodenum. Iron deficiency may occur following a pancreaticoduodenectomy.

5. Vitamin Toxicity

a) Vitamin A Toxicity

Excessive vitamin A causes thickening of hair and increased hair loss throughout the body. As the toxicity worsens, pseudotumor cerebri, headache, and weakness may develop. Hepatosplenomegaly is also seen.

b) Vitamin D Toxicity

Vitamin D toxicity leads to anorexia, nausea, vomiting, polyuria, polydipsia, pruritus, azotemia, proteinuria, metastatic calcifications from hypercalcemia, and anxiety. Acidifying the urine and administering corticosteroids are treatment options.

c) Vitamin E Toxicity

Tocopherol toxicity can decrease the effectiveness of vitamin K, which may lead to spontaneous hemorrhage in patients on warfarin.

d) Vitamin K Toxicity

Vitamin K toxicity is rare, but very high doses of its precursor, menadione, may lead to hemolytic anemia and kernicterus.

e) Vitamin B6 Toxicity

Excessive vitamin B6 consumption may lead to sensory ataxia and decreased lower extremity proprioception.

V. Hemostasis and Coagulation

V.A. General Concepts

1. Thromboxane A_2

Thromboxane A_2 is a vasoconstrictor and increases platelet aggregation. It is released by activated platelets. The formation of TxA_2 is inhibited by aspirin. Plavix leads to inhibition of platelet aggregation by inhibiting ADP. Plavix should be stopped five days prior to surgery.

2. Prostacyclin

Prostacyclin is an inhibitor of platelet aggregation. It is released from the endothelium and also promotes vasodilation, thereby antagonizing the effects of TxA_2.

3. Antithrombin III

Antithrombin III is an inhibitor of thrombin, and factors IX, X, and XI. It is bound by heparin and this binding produces the anticoagulant effect of heparin. Antithrombin III deficiency is treated by FFP. Thrombin converts fibrinogen to fibrin and leads to the activation of platelets and factors V and VIII. Fibrin forms split products which work with platelets to form a hemostatic plug. Fibrin crosslinking relies on factor XIII.

4. Plasmin

Plasmin plays a role in anticoagulation and is activated by tissue plasminogen activator released by the endothelium. It leads to the destruction of the platelet plug through degradation of factors V and VIII and fibrin. Plasmin is inhibited by alpha-2 antiplasmin.

5. Blood Products

Cryoprecipitate is used as a therapy for von Willebrand disease due to the high concentration of vWF and fibrinogen. FFP contains all factors, proteins C and S, and antithrombin III. Factors VIII and vWF can be released by the endothelium through the administration of DDAVP and is a suitable intervention in vascular surgery patients who may be bleeding slightly following an arteriovenous fistula placement for dialysis access.

6. Blood Transfusion

A negative crossmatch is required between donor blood cells and recipient serum, in addition to satisfactory ABO compatibility. Postoperative transfusion criteria include a symptomatic low hematocrit or hypovolemia such that resuscitation with crystalloid would produce anemia. The earliest intraoperative sign of blood mismatch is hypotension. The goal of a blood transfusion is to maintain oxygen carrying capacity when an increase in oxygen saturation alone would not be sufficient.

Most practitioners will wait for hemoglobin below 7 or hematocrit below 21 before transfusing a healthy person. However, there are studies that show that transfusing at a lower hematocrit would also be permissible. Blood transfusions for a hematocrit above 22 in most patients, or transfusing to a goal (i.e. hematocrit of 30) has increased morbidity.

Massive blood transfusions, such as following severe trauma, can lead to hypothermia, hypocalcemia, hyperkalemia, loss of platelets and clotting factors leading to additional coagulopathy, and metabolic alkalosis.

V.B. Transfusion Reactions

1. Etiology and Pathophysiology

Transfusion reactions occur due to immune reactions against antigens in donated blood. Serious reactions can lead to death, and rapid identification and reversal are necessary. Antibodies against major blood groups (AB) can lead to death through intravascular hemolysis. Non-ABO antibodies result in extravascular reactions and are milder. Nonimmune reactions occur with damage to the donated RBCs and cause hemoglobinuria and hemoglobinemia.

Cytokines in donated blood can precipitate acute phase reactants and lead to constitutional symptoms. Immune reactions can present as severe anaphylaxis. Multiparous women are more likely to have symptoms. The most common cause of a transfusion reaction is clerical error.

TABLE 7. Transfusion reactions and infections.

Transfusion Reactions and Infections
CMV most likely infectious risk
Hepatitis C 1/500,000
HIV 1/2,000,000
Allergic reaction 1/300
Non-fatal immune reaction 1/10,000
Anaphylaxis 1/50,000
Fatal reaction 4/1,000,000

2. Presentation and Diagnosis

TABLE 8. Signs of a transfusion reaction.

Signs of a Transfusion Reaction
Early: fever hypotension, flushing, anxiety, wheezing
Late: DIC
nonhemolytic: fever with mild hypotension and mild constitutional symptoms
Allergic reactions: maculopapular rash and pruritus
Anaphylactic reactions: dyspnea, wheezing, anxiety, bronchospasm, and hypotension

In transfusion-related acute lung injury (TRALI), SOB, hypoxia, and orthopnea with cardiac decompensation may be present due to clotting within the pulmonary capillaries. Diagnosis is made by a direct Coombs test. Dilutional thrombocytopenia may also occur after massive transfusion.

3. Treatment

Stop the transfusion and carefully observe. Prophylaxis against renal failure and DIC are necessary. Diuresis may be necessary. Acetaminophen is used for fever, diphenhydramine for mild allergic reactions, and epinephrine for anaphylactic reactions. Severe symptoms may require admission to ICU and supportive therapy. A workup for sepsis may be necessary. Transfusion of over 1–1.5 L of hetastarch (Hextend) can lead to an increased risk of bleeding.

V.C. Anticoagulants and Thrombolytics

Topical thrombin activates the fibrin glue used in surgery. Absolute contraindications to the use of fibrinolytics include a CVA within 2 months or active internal bleeding. Recent surgery, peptic ulcer disease, or trauma are major relative contraindications. See page 498 for a list of commonly used anticoagulants and thrombolytics.

VI. Patient Care

VI.A. ICU Admission

Emergency ICU admission is correlated with the development of a pressure ulcer, which is correlated to increased mortality.

VI.B. Venous Catheter Infection

Venous catheter infection is diagnosed if blood drawn from the catheter has five times as many colony-forming units compared to blood simultaneously drawn via venipuncture. Subclavian vein catheters have a lower risk of infection compared to internal jugular access, but have a higher risk of causing pneumothorax.

VI.C. Stress Ulcer Prophylaxis

Indications for stress ulcer prophylaxis include intubation, head injury, and coagulopathy with less than 50,000 platelets or elevated INR/PTT.

VI.D. Beta Blockade

High risk patients undergoing surgery should have perioperative beta blockade. Patients with unstable angina or other urgent indication for CABG are the only people who should have preoperative CABG completed. High risk patients: age > 65, hypertension, diabetes, hyperlipidemia, smoking history, ischemic heart disease, or renal insufficiency.

Table 9. Anticoagulants and Thrombolytics

DRUG	INDICATIONS	MECHANISM OF ACTION
Heparin	Anticoagulation	• Antithrombin III potentiation leading to prevention of clot formation • Inhibits factors II, IXa, Xa
LMWH		Factor Xa inhibition
Warfarin		Inhibits epoxide reductase in liver to prevent formation of factors II, VII, IX, X, protein C, and protein S
Abciximab	Anticoagulation in PTCA	Prevents platelet aggregation and thrombus formation
Streptokinase	Fibrinolytic	Cleaves plasminogen to produce plasmin and breakdown clots
tPA	Fibrinolytic	Serine protease forms plasmin to breakdown clots
Clopidogrel	Hypercoagulability	Prevents platelet aggregation through ADP receptor blockade on platelets
Aspirin	• Hypercoagulability • Fever	• Increased bleeding time by impaired platelet release, inhibition of COX, and decreased thrombus formation • Irreversible effects

VII. Anesthesia

VII.A. Arterial Line

Invasive measurement of arterial blood pressure is required with the infusion of vasoactive medications or the need for continuous pressure monitoring. An Allen test must be completed prior to placement. Major complications include thrombosis and infection. Sterile technique is required.

COMPLICATIONS	CONTRAINDICATIONS	NOTES
• HIT (early is benign; late is IgG mediated); treat with danaparoid sodium or lepriludin due to risk of thrombosis • Can lead to white clot syndrome	• Existing bleeding disorder • Safe in pregnancy	• Follow aPTT time • Give protamine sulfate as antidote (beware of hypotension) • Half-life: 90 mins • Test factor VIII function if intrinsic elevation in PTT
	Cleared renally	PTT is not followed
• Interacts with numerous medications (P-450) • GI bleed • Limb necrosis	• Existing bleeding disorder • Avoid in pregnancy • Can lead to skin necrosis from lack of protein C – treat with heparin	• Must monitor therapeutic index via PT/INR • Half-life: 40 hours
TCP	Existing bleeding disorder	GPIIb/IIIa Ig inhibitor; similar to ticlodipine
• Allergic reaction on subsequent doses • Bleeding	Hemorrhagic disorder	• Usually given only once following MI • Intrinsic elevation = malignancy
Bleeding	Hemorrhagic disorder	Used in MI and stroke within the first six hours of symptom onset
• Neutropenia • TTP • Hemorrhage	Safe in pregnancy	• Plavix, MI and stroke risk • Similar to ticlodipine
		• Stop 7-10 days before surgery • Prostacyclin inhibits platelet aggregation

VII.B. Central Venous Line

When there is need to monitor central vascular pressure (to monitor volume status and/or cardiac function), infusion of high concentrations of potentially irritating drugs, or total parenteral nutrition, a central venous line is necessary. Major complications include placement into an artery, pneumothorax, thromboembolism, and arrhythmia. Placement and dilation in a major artery requires an arteriogram and potential surgical repair.

Pneumothorax requires tube thoracostomy.

- Central venous lines permit measurement of central venous pressure (CVP), which is an indicator of volume atatus and right heart function.
- Ventilator inspiration = increased thoracic pressure = increased CVP, less right heart filling
- Ventilator expiraton = decreased thoracic pressure = decreased CVP, more right heart filling
- Spontaneous inspiration = decreased thoracic pressure = decreased CVP, more right heart filling
- Spontaneous expiration = increased thoracic pressure = increased CVP, less right heart filling

Expiration in patients on a ventilator leads to an overall drop in right heart pressure unless there is a significant amount of PEEP. Overall, the negative intrathoracic pressure generated during spontaneous inspiration leads to increased venous return via the vena cavae to the right heart. The right ventricle then fills during diastole and bulges into the left heart from the excess systemic return. This leads to impaired filling of the left ventricle, and therefore, a lower cardiac output.

VII.C. Pulmonary Artery Catheter

A pulmonary artery catheter, also known as a Swan-Ganz catheter, is indicated when information about cardiac function and vascular pressures is required. A PAC provides information about left heart pressure and volume status indirectly via measurements across the pulmonary capillary bed. Estimates of cardiac function can be derived from these pressure-volume recordings. Apart from the complications associated with central venous catheter placement, there is a unique risk for a potentially fatal pulmonary artery rupture. There is data questioning the utility of a PAC.

VII.D. Pneumonia

1. Etiology and Pathophysiology

Pneumonia is commonly the result of infection by community-acquired sources such as *Streptococcus pneumoniae* or *Haemophilus influenzae*, or hospital acquired sources such as *Pseudomonas aeruginosa*, *Staphylococcus aureus*, and enteric organisms. Atypical sources of pneumonia include *Chlamydia pneumoniae*, *Legionella pneumoniae*, and *Mycoplasma pneumoniae*. A common cause of pneumonia in alcoholics, the elderly, and with blood products includes *Klebsiella*, especially if currant jelly sputum is present. Patients with chronic bronchitis are likely to be infected by *Haemophilus influenzae*. Immunocompromised (IC) patients are likely to be infected by *Pneumocystis carinii* pneumonia (PCP). *Streptococcus pneumoniae* presents with rust-colored sputum. It is also the likely cause of a complicated pneumonia arising after influenza.

2. Etiology in Immunocompromised States

— HIV

- CD4 > 200: Mycobacterium
- CD4 < 200: *P. carinii, Histoplama, Cryptococcus neoformans*
- CD4 < 50: CMV, MAC

— Neutropenia: *Pseudomonas aeruginosa*, enteric bacteria
— Splenectomy: Encapsulated bacteria
— Steroid abuse: *Mycobacterium tuberculosis, Nocardia*
— Alcoholics: *Klebsiella, S. pneumonia, Haemophilus influenza*

3. Presentation and Diagnosis

Pneumonia generally presents with fever, productive cough, and pleuritic chest pain. Pneumonia is equally likely to present with atypical symptoms, such as dry cough, constitutional symptoms, and generalized GI symptoms. On physical exam, rales and tactile fremitus are present. Diagnosis is made by telltale CXR signs including a lobular or segmental infiltrate (upper lobe if TB or *Klebsiella*), cavities (small in TB, large in others), and bilateral infiltrates (in PCP and TB). Gram stains are done on sputum samples. Encapsulated organisms may be detected, including *Streptococcus pneumoniae*, *Haemophilus influenzae*, *Klebsiella*, and *Neisseria meningitidis*. Elevated LDH is indicative of PCP. No bacteria on smear may be indicative of *Legionella* and *Mycoplasma* spp.

4. Treatment

Inpatient treatment is necessary for patients at extremes of age, residents of nursing homes, hypotension, tachypnea, tachycardia, $PaO_2 < 60$, and pleural effusions. Treatment consists of penicillins, cephalosporins, and quinolones. Atypical pneumonias get coverage with erythromycin; hospital-acquired pneumonias are covered for *P. aeruginosa*; and pneumonia in immunocompromised patients gets PCP coverage. Aspiration pneumonia is treated with nasotracheal suction and PEEP.

VII.E. Endotracheal Intubation

Indications for intubation include any patient unable to protect their airway, combative patients whose safety is threatened, and patients with falling GCS scores in the 7-9 range. Any patient undergoing general anesthesia or a major respiratory procedure requires intubation. Serious failure in accessing the airway by way of intubation may require a surgical airway, such as a tracheostomy or cricothyroidotomy.

VII.F. Mechanical Ventilation

1. Pressure-Regulated Volume-Control Ventilation

PRVC ventilation is used with respiratory failure. Pressure-control inverse-ratio ventilation requires paralysis and is used for severe lung injury, to generate hypercapnia (to reduce barotrauma), and to generate auto-PEEP. It is achieved by increasing inspiratory time and decreasing expiratory time. Pressure-support ventilation is used to permit spontaneous breathing. Airway pressure release ventilation uses CPAP alternating with relaxation and permits spontaneous respiration.

2. Assist-Control Ventilation

Assist-control provides a set volume or pressure-controlled breath initiated by the patient. A minimum respiratory rate is set. Pressure or volume assist-control ventilation helps to wean a patient from a ventilator. Assist-control is contraindicated in patients with respiratory alkalosis due to the increased respiratory drive; SIMV is a better alternative. Assist-control is otherwise the mechanical support method of choice for most patients.

3. Synchronized Intermittent Mandatory Ventilation

SIMV provides pressure- or volume-limited breaths a certain number of times over a fixed interval. The patient is permitted to initiate that fixed number of breaths over the interval. SIMV with pressure-support helps to wean a ventilator by decreasing the respiratory rate.

4. Pressure-Support Ventilation

Pressure-support ventilation provides a patient breathing spontaneously through a high-resistance endotracheal tube with sufficient support to take a normal breath. Pressure-support is appropriate for patients who are comfortable, awake, and candidates for extubation.

5. Continuous Positive Airway Pressure

CPAP decreases the work of breathing and decreases cardiac work in heart failure. CPAP relies on the patient to initiate all breaths and is used as a means to augment respiration. CPAP is similar to positive end-expiratory pressure (PEEP) in that it provides a baseline elevated pressure to keep alveoli patent during expiration. This decreases respiratory resistance and improves ventilation, primarily through improvement of the functional residual capacity (FRC). High PEEP can cause respiratory trauma through disruption of the alveoli. PEEP decreases venous return to the right heart. It is specifically indicated if a PaO_2 of 60 cannot be reached with an FiO_2 of 60%. PEEP forces blood flow to the kidney cortex.

Table 10. Anticholinergics – Nicotinic Antagonists

DRUG	INDICATIONS	MECHANISM OF ACTION
Succinylcholine	• Muscle paralysis • Mechanical ventilation	• Rapid onset, short duration with decrease in excitatory potential; noncompetitive • Initial stage: prolonged depolarization > fasciculations, muscle pain. • Second stage: repolarization but blockade of receptors.
Cisatracurium, Vecuronium		Nicotinic receptor blockade
Rocuronium	Facilitate tracheal intubation	Competes for cholinergic receptor at motor end-plates
Dantrolene	NMS and malignant hyperthermia	Interferes with calcium ion release by sarcoplasmic reticulum
Sildenafil	• ED • Pulmonary HTN • Raynaud phenomenon	PDE-5 blocker that increases cGMP

6. High Frequency Oscillatory Ventilation

HFOV uses continuous pressure wave through high frequency respirations to generate a fixed low pressure volume at alveoli to ensure their patency in respiratory failure. Gas exchange is thereby permitted to occur without other confounding factors related to respiratory failure.

7. Emergency Surgery

Any emergency surgery in the elderly, fluid shifts, and vascular procedures place patients in a high-risk category for cardiac complications. Carotid endarterectomy is intermediate-risk for cardiac complications.

VII.G. Anesthetics and Analgesics

1. Epidural Analgesia

Contraindications to epidural analgesia include bleeding disorders, active infection, hemodynamic instability, and ileus. Epidurals are preferred with

CONTRAINDICATIONS	NOTES
• Malignant hyperthermia with halothane • Avoid in patients with increased ICP, burns, DMD, crush injury, MS, and hyperkalemia. • May lead to arrhythmia and bradycardia.	• Depolarizing NM agent • Use neostigmine as second stage antidote. No antidote for first stage. • Directly competes with acetylcholine.
No cardiac effects with vecuronium; pancuronium leads to tachycardia	• Use cisatracurium with renal or liver failure due to its Hoffman degradation.
	• Nondepolarizing NMJ agents. • Reverse with neostigmine or edrophonium.
Active hepatic disease, OPD	Calcium channel blocker
• Vasodilation • Priapism • MI • Arrhythmia	• MI w/ nitrates • Do not use if Hx of MI, hypotension, renal or hepatic disease, and retinal disorders

flail chest due to improved tidal volume, larger inspiratory force, and better pain control; there is no effect on FRC.

2. Anticholinergics – Nicotinic Antagonists

Malignant hyperthermia is a disorder of calcium metabolism with decreased reuptake by the sarcoplasmic reticulum leading to increased intracellular calcium. Increased end tidal CO_2 ($ETCO_2$) is an early sign of disease. The first physical finding is the presence of spasms in the masseter. $ETCO_2$ may also increase in the setting of pulmonary embolism, or air embolism experienced during laparoscopic surgery.

During general anesthesia, the muscle that is the last to be paralyzed and the first to recover is the diaphragm. A risk of general anesthesia in diabetes mellitus is hypoglycemia. Etomidate has few cardiovascular side effects. Use of nitric oxide permits lower concentrations of other anesthetics; it should not be used in patients with bowel obstruction or pneumothorax due to diffusion into closed spaces. Neostigmine can reverse muscular blockade. Flumazenil reverses benzodiazepines. Narcan reverses opioid overdose. Dantrolene treats malignant hyperthermia.

3. Sedatives and Hypnotics

Table 11. Sedatives and Hypnotics

DRUG	INDICATIONS	MECHANISM OF ACTION	COMPLICATIONS	NOTES
Midazolam	Preanesthetic		Myocardial depression	Short-acting
Diazepam	Preanesthetic			Long-acting
Flumazenil	Reversal of sedative effects of benzodiazepines	Competitively inhibits benzodiazepine receptor site	Seizures	Leads to amnesia, no analgesia

4. Anesthetics – Inhaled

Table 12. Inhaled Anesthetics

DRUG	INDICATIONS	COMPLICATIONS	NOTES
Halothane	Anesthesia	Bradycardia, hepatitis, malignant hyperthermia, arrhythmia, respiratory depression, increased ICP, cardiac and hepatic toxicity	
Sevoflurane	Anesthesia	Bradycardia, respiratory depression, increased ICP	Rapid onset
Nitrous oxide	Anesthesia	Minimal	Lowest potency, combined with other agents
Desflurane	Anesthesia	Airway irritation, coughing, respiratory depression, increased ICP	Most rapid onset

5. Anesthetics – Intravenous

TABLE 13. Intravenous Anesthetics

DRUG	COMPLICATIONS	NOTES
Midazolam	Respiratory depression, amnesia	Benzodiazepine; reverse w/ flumazenil
Ketamine	CV, hallucinations, ICP	Amnesia, analgesia, muscle relaxation
Morphine	Substance abuse and dependence, respiratory depression (brainstem CO2 response), miosis, CNS depression, constipation, N/V (CTZ)	Opioid, good analgesia No tolerance to miosis or constipation.
Fentanyl	Muscle rigidity at high doses that impedes ventilation	Opioid, good analgesia. Tolerated in large doses due to lack of histamine response.
Propofol	Hypotension	No cumulative effects, strict aseptic technique must be maintained.

Visceral pain is carried by C-fibers. Nociceptive stimuli are carried via afferent nerves of the spinothalamic tract. Ketamine may lead to hypertension in normal patients, and hypotension in patients in shock; it is a dissociative anesthetic and should not be used in patients with head injury. Meperidine is occasionally used due to its ability to prevent shivering. Morphine is preferred as it has no negative cardiovascular side effects and improves venous capacitance. Fentanyl is used in patients with respiratory disorders as it does not cause bronchospasm. Propofol should not be used in obstetrical anesthesia due to neonatal complications. The major side effect is hypotension. Prolonged use can lead to bradycardia or asystole, rhabdomyolysis, metabolic acidosis, and renal failure. As a result, propofol should not be used for more than 48 hours and avoided in patients with CNS disease.

6. Anesthetics – Local

TABLE 14. Local Anesthetics

DRUG	COMPLICATIONS	NOTES
Lidocaine	Toxicity signs: lightheadedness, dizziness, metallic taste, tinnitus, circumoral paresthesia, numbness, seizure, arrhythmia, cardiac collapse	• Greater amounts needed in infected tissue (acidic tissue) • Smaller fibers affected first, so pain is lost first, then touch • Give with epinephrine to increase local effects
Bupivacaine	CV toxicity	• No allergic cross reactivity between esters and amides. Long duration.

Spinal anesthetics are contraindicated when ICP is increased. Esters have a higher chance of causing a hypersensitivity reaction compared to amides. Use of local anesthetic leads to decreased pain in the postoperative period. The maximum safe dose for lidocaine is 3-5 mg/kg and should not exceed 300 mg. Epinephrine with lidocaine permits a dose of up to 7 mg/kg. Bupivacaine can be used up to 2.5 mg/kg, or 3.0 mg/kg with epinephrine. Intravenous lidocaine may lead to cardiac arrest, but intraarterial injection has few side effects at low doses. Early signs of toxicity include metallic taste, vasovagal response, tinnitus and lightheadedness, followed by numbness, seizures, and loss of consciousness. Cardiopulmonary depression may then occur. Treat with oxygen, atropine, and ephedrine first, followed by midazolam or other benzodiazepines to stop seizure activity. A lipid rescue is possible with immediate administration of lipids such as TPN.

7. Anxiolytics – Typical

TABLE 15. Typical Anxiolytics

DRUG	INDICATIONS	CONTRAINDICATIONS	NOTES
Clonazepam	Absence seizures	LFTs, glaucoma, pregnancy	Intermediate-acting
Diazepam	Sedation	Glaucoma, pregnancy, children	Longest acting Three active metabolites
Midazolam	Sedation Anesthesia		Shortest-acting benzodiazepine

Lorazepam is a long-term sedation. Dexmedetomidine is used as a bridge for extubation due to low respiratory suppression. Droperidol is an anxiolytic and antiemetic drug with cardiac side effects. Midazolam is an anxiolytic, sedative, and amnestic agent and is preferred over diazepam as the latter leads to accumulation of metabolites.

8. Barbiturates

TABLE 16. Barbiturates

DRUG	INDICATIONS	MECHANISM OF ACTION	COMPLICATIONS
Phenobarbital	• Anxiolytic • Hypnotic • Sedative	Facilitates $GABA_A$ and increase length of chloride channel opening to decrease neuronal firing	• Induce tolerance • Low therapeutic index • Respiratory depression • Myocardial suppression

9. Analgesics – NSAIDS

TABLE 17. NSAIDs

DRUG	MECHANISM OF ACTION	COMPLICATIONS	NOTES
Ibuprofen	Reversible inhibition of COX-1 and COX-2	Nephrotoxicity, aplastic anemia, PUD	Block prostaglandin synthesis
Indomethacin		Nephrotoxicity, aplastic anemia, PUD	Also used to close a PDA
Acetaminophen	Reversible inhibition of COX in CNS	Hepatic necrosis in OD, glutathione depletion	• Peripheral inactivation • NOT an anti-inflammatory • Treat OD with N-acetylcysteine
Aspirin	Irreversible COX-1 and COx-2 inhibition inhibits prostaglandin formation	PUD, Reye syndrome, tinnitus, reflex acidosis from reflex hypoventilation due to initial hyperventilation	• No effect on PT or PTT • Low doses decrease uric acid secretion • High doses decrease uric acid reabsorption

Surgical Critical Care

Aspirin irreversibly blocks COX-1 and COX-2; it should be stopped 4 days prior to surgery. Plavix and Ticlopidine block ADP-mediated platelet aggregation; the latter can lead to pancytopenia. Plavix should be stopped for at least 5-7 days prior to surgery. Abciximab blocks the GP IIb/IIIa receptor and is used in percutaneous angioplasty; the major complications are bleeding and pancytopenia. Cilostazol (Pletal) is a phosphodiesterase III inhibitor that leads to vasodilation and inhibits platelet function; it is indicated in claudication and needs to be stopped about a week before any surgery. NSAIDs inhibit COX-1 via thromboxane. LMWH works via AT III and inactivates factor Xa. Fondaparinux is a synthetic version with a similar mechanism of action but does not bind to PF IV and thereby has a negligible risk of HIT.

Factor VII binds to tissue factor and leads to activation of IX and X with thrombin production. Coagulation is enhanced. As a result, synthetic VII can be used as a treatment for hemophilia A and B, and also to reverse warfarin anticoagulation – especially in the presence of a head bleed or in other emergency situations.

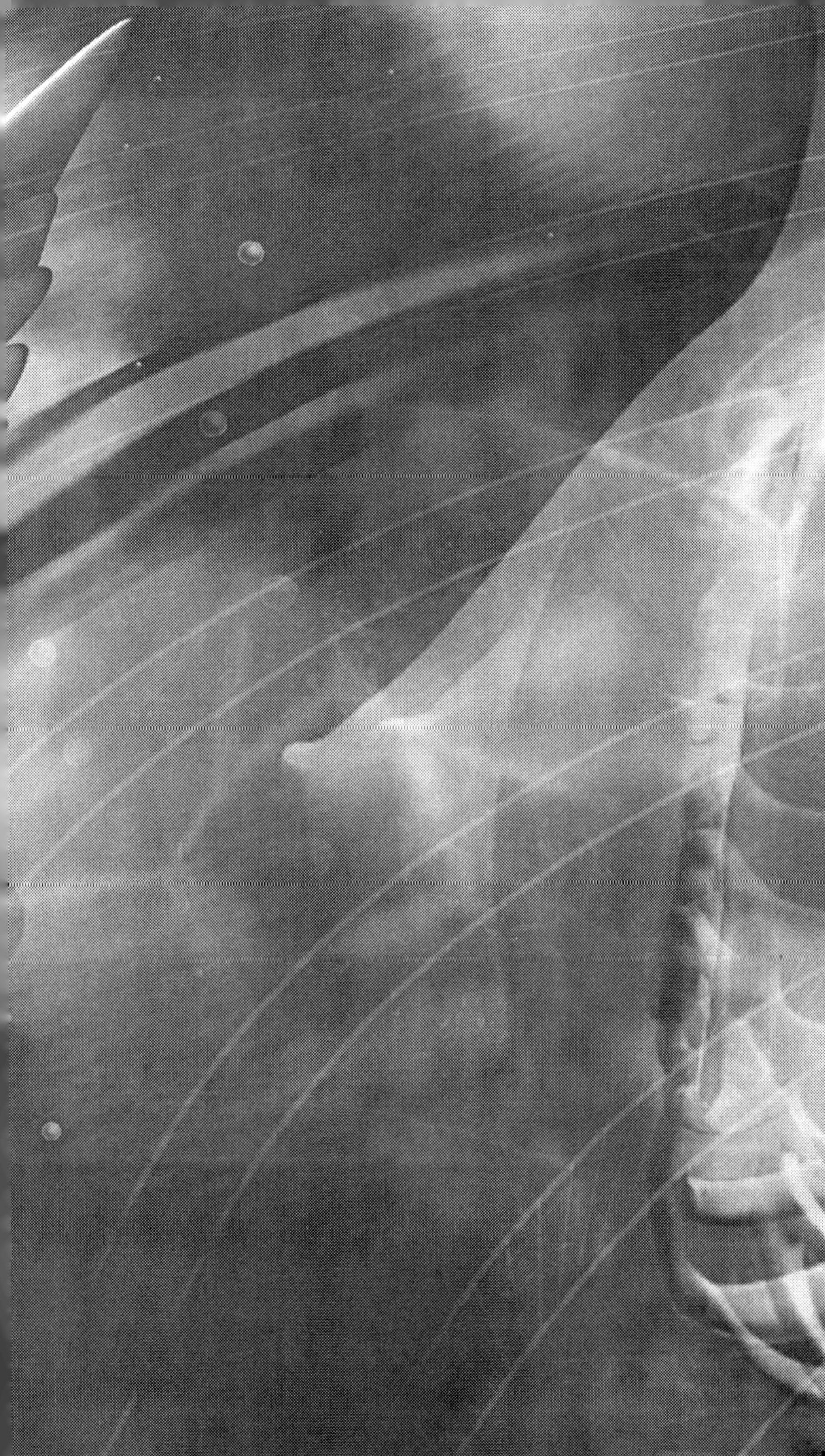

Surgical Critical Care

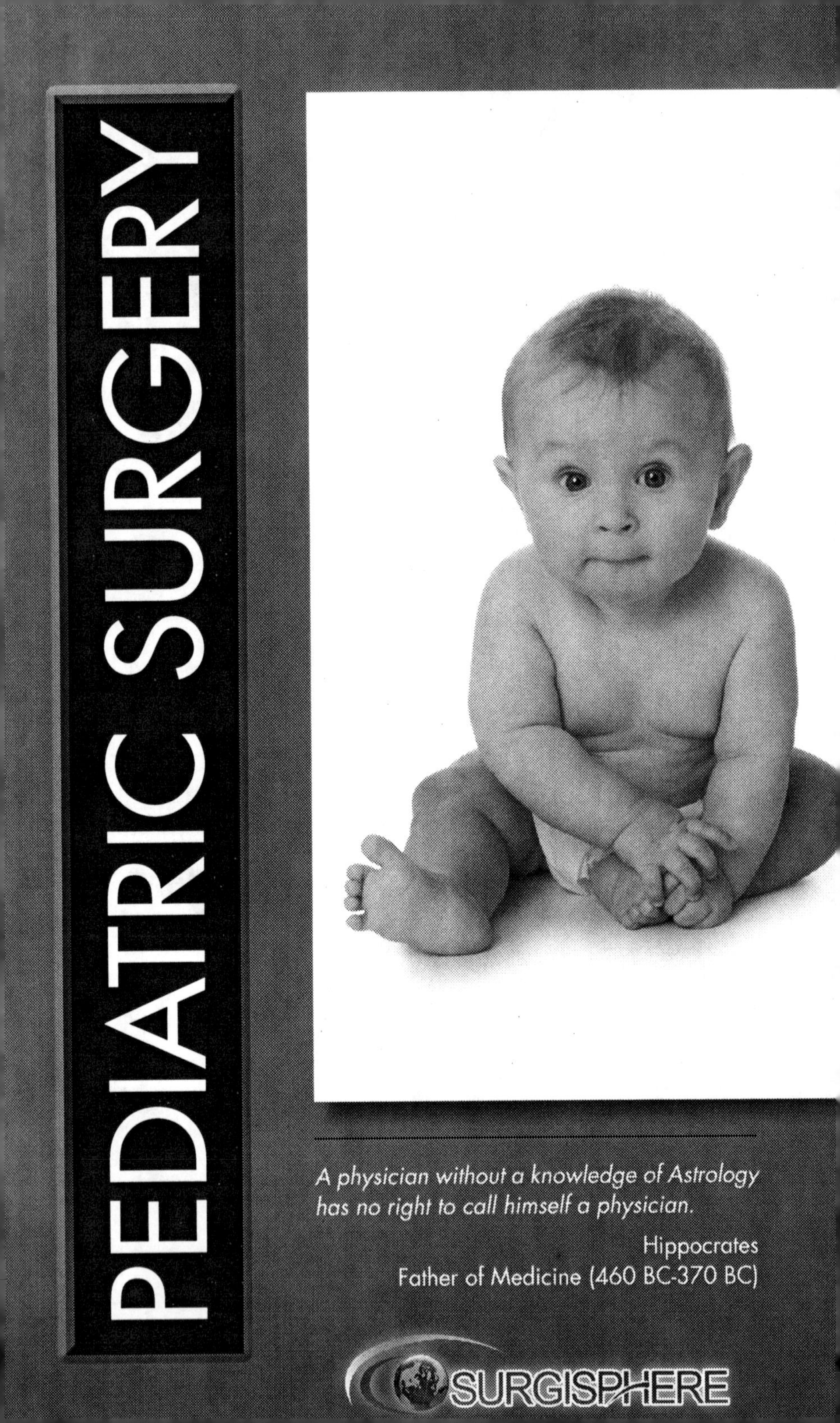
PEDIATRIC SURGERY
A physician without a knowledge of Astrology has no right to call himself a physician.
Hippocrates
Father of Medicine (460 BC-370 BC)
SURGISPHERE

PEDIATRIC SURGERY

Tamarah Westmoreland, M.D., Ph.D., Elisabeth Tracy, M.D., Melissa Danko, M.D., and Jeff C. Hoehner, M.D., Ph.D.

I. General Concepts

TABLE 1. Pediatric Vital Signs

Age	Heart Rate	Blood Pressure	Hypotension
Neonate	85-205	70/40	SBP < 60
3-12 months	100-190	90/50	SBP < 70
12-24 months	100-190	100/60	SBP < 70 + (age in years x 2)
2-10 years	60-140	100/60	SBP < 70 + (age in years x 2)
> 10 years	60-100	110/70	SBP < 90

I.A. Shock

The inadequate delivery of oxygen or nutrients to the cell defines shock. Physical signs include tachycardia, peripheral vasoconstriction, hypotension, and decreased urine output. Hypotension in children is a very late sign. The late clinical sequelae are metabolic acidosis, multiple organ dysfunction, disseminated intravascular coagulation, and death. There are four types of shock: hypovolemic, cardiogenic, neurogenic, and septic.

The most common type of shock in pediatric patients is hypovolemic shock, defined as a decrease in venous return to the heart and decreased left ventricular volume leading to insufficient oxygen delivery to tissues. The first line of therapy is fluid resuscitation, which starts with a 20 ml/kg bolus of crystalloid solution and can be repeated twice. Blood transfusion should be considered when the fluid deficit is greater than 15-25%.

Cardiogenic shock is defined by arrhythmia or dysfunction possibly related to congenital heart disease or cardiomyopathy. Neurogenic shock, which is hypotension secondary to loss of sympathetic activity, is seen with spinal cord transection. Peripheral vasodilation and venous pooling from a systemic infection is associated with septic shock. The most common infections in children are listed below.

TABLE 2. Common infections in children.

Neonates	Group B beta-hemolytic streptococci, Enterobacteriaceae, Listeria monocytogenes, Staphylococcus aureus, Herpes simplex
Infants	Haemophilus influenzae, Streptococcus pneumoniae, S. aureus
Children	S. pneumoniae, Neisseria meningitides, S. aureus, Pseudomonas, Candida albicans

I.B. FLUIDS, ELECTROLYTES, AND NUTRITION

Fluid requirements for pediatric patients differ from that of adults. A term newborn has 75-80% total body water which decreases by 4-5% in the first week of life. Signs of mild to moderate dehydration in a child include weight loss, dry mucous membranes, sunken eyes and fontanel, lethargy, delayed capillary refill, and dry skin. Severe dehydration can present with irritability, coma, tachycardia, hypotension, and mottling. The typical fluid requirements for rehydration are illustrated in "Table 3. Fluid resuscitation guidelines."

TABLE 3. Fluid resuscitation guidelines.

AGE OR WEIGHT	FLUID
Newborn day 1	50-60 ml/kg/day D10W
Newborn day 2	100 ml/kg/day D10¼NS
Newborn > 7 days	100-150 ml/kg/day D10¼NS
Child 0-10 kg	100 ml/kg/day (4 ml/kg/h)
Child 10-20 kg	1000 ml/day + 50 ml/kg/day (40 ml/h + 2 ml/kg/h)
Child > 20 kg	1500 ml/day + 25 ml/kg/day (60 ml/h + 1 ml/kg/h)

Caloric requirements for term infants are 90-120 kcal/kg/day. The best measure for adequate nutrition is weight gain, which should be 1% per day. Breast milk is the best choice for infants due to transfer of maternal IgG and IgM, naturally-occurring fatty acids, and rapid uptake of essential nutrients and vitamins in a physiologically calibrated solution. Formulas are available for infants who are premature, lactose intolerant, or have malabsorption syndromes. Total parenteral nutrition (TPN) is utilized when enteral feeds are not feasible. Monitoring electrolytes and serum glucose titers are critical for this population. Enteral feeds are preferred whenever possible due to liver dysfunction from long term TPN.

II. Disorders of the Chest

II.A. Tracheoesophageal Fistula

1. Etiology and Pathophysiology

A tracheoesophageal fistula (TEF) is an abnormal connection between the trachea and esophagus discovered soon after birth. TEF occurs in approximately 1 in 2000-4000 births. Esophageal atresia (EA) may be associated with fistula. However, EA without a fistulous connection to the trachea can occur. In 1697, Gibson first reported a case of an infant with a TEF. In 1888, Charles Steels was the first surgeon to operate on an infant with a TEF. The first successful TEF repair was by Cameron Haight in 1941. Over the ensuing decades, the survival of infants with TEF and EA has greatly increased with the improvement in surgical technique, nutrition, and perioperative care.

Understanding TEF and EA begins with an appreciation of the embryology. During the 4th through 6th week of development, the caudal foregut forms the trachea. The laryngotracheal tube and esophagus are formed by the fusion of the tracheoesophageal fold. Abnormalities within this development lead to TEF and or EA.

2. Presentation and Diagnosis

There are five anatomic variants of the tracheoesophageal dysgenesis. The most common type of TEF is a blind-ending proximal upper esophageal pouch and fistula between the distal esophagus and trachea. Another variant is the H type fistula, which is a TEF without an EA. There are two other rare variants.

Diagnosis usually begins with feeding difficulties. Confirmation is made when a NGT is placed and coils blindly in the esophageal pouch. Air in the stomach via the anomalous connection between the trachea and esophagus

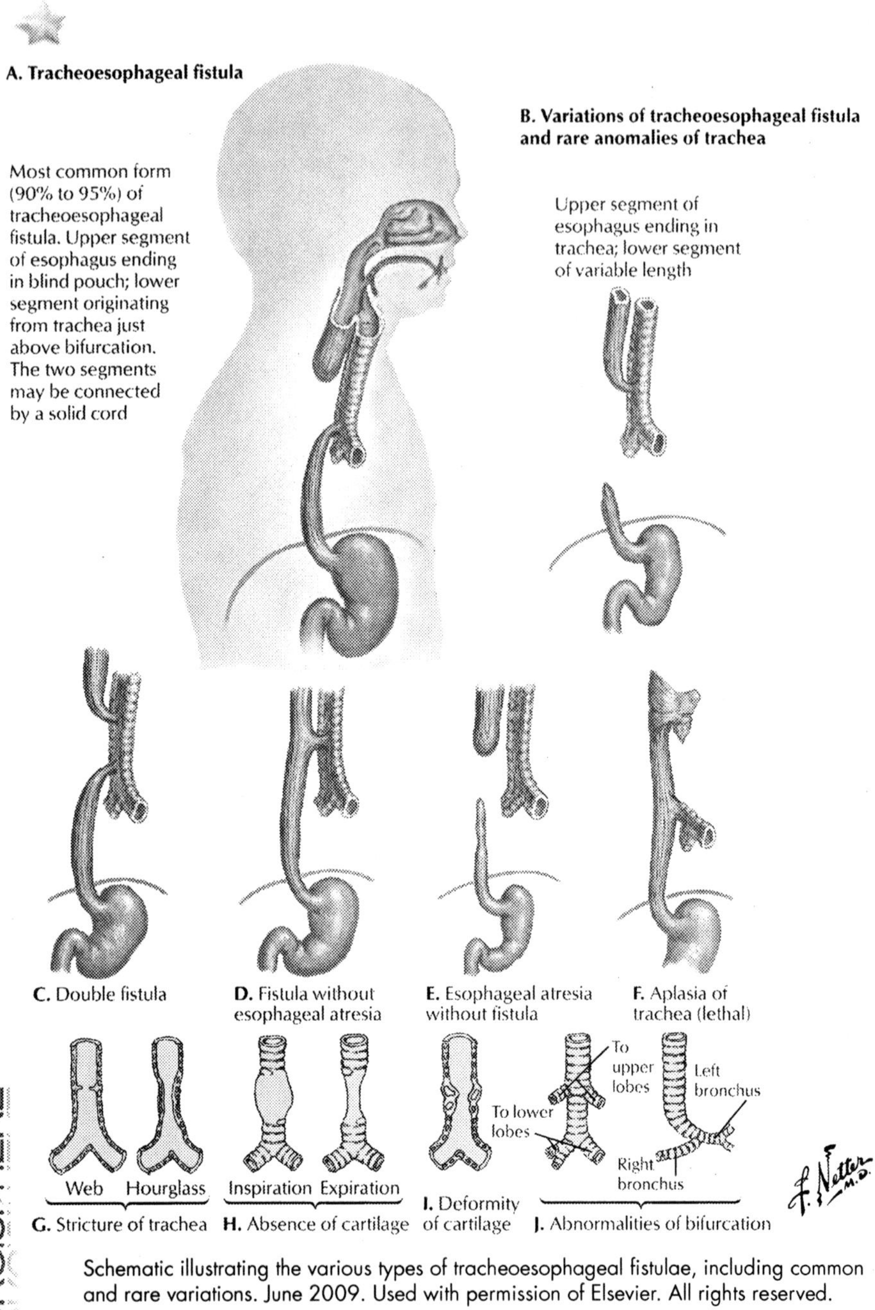

Schematic illustrating the various types of tracheoesophageal fistulae, including common and rare variations. June 2009. Used with permission of Elsevier.

confirms the presence of a fistula. TEF without EA can take several months to diagnose because the infants do not have feeding difficulties; instead, these infants present with recurrent pneumonia.

Other congenital anomalies can be associated with EA. These anomalies represent a group of disorders known as VACTERL (vertebral, anorectal, cardiac, tracheoesophageal, renal, radial, and limb) deformities. Because of advances in surgical and perioperative care, survival is determined by the associated anomalies, not the TEF and EA. Postoperative survival for healthy, term infants without cardiac disease approaches 100%.

3. Treatment

After TEF with EA is diagnosed, the infant should be placed in an upright position, the blind pouch should be suctioned, and IV fluids started. Intubation should be avoided if possible due to selective passage of air into the stomach. Once the patient is stabilized, repair consists of dividing the TEF and performing an esophagoesophagostomy.

Patients with only an EA without TEF have a long gap between the proximal and distal esophagus. They are initially treated by placing a gastrostomy tube and improving nutrition. The proximal esophagus is drained to prevent aspiration. Furthermore, the proximal esophagus can be dilated by repeat bougienage. The patient's esophagus is normally ready for repair after approximately six weeks.

II.B. Congenital Diaphragmatic Hernia

1. Etiology and Pathophysiology

A congenital diaphragmatic hernia (CDH) represents a group of diaphragmatic deformities that result migration of abdominal contents into the chest. This can lead to pulmonary hypertension, pulmonary hypoplasia, and cardiac defects. CDH is seen in approximately 1:4000 births. The diaphragm is formed in the middle of the first trimester. The last portion to close is in the posterolateral position, which is the location of the most common diaphragmatic hernia, the Bochdalek hernia (90%). This hernia is normally seen on the left and can lead to incomplete left hemidiaphragm formation.

A much less common hernia is the Morgagni hernia (5%) which is found in the anterior parasternal location. There are fewer associated anomalies seen with the Morgagni hernia. The abdominal cavity is congenitally underdeveloped due to the migration of abdominal contents into the thoracic space, leading to great difficulty in closing the abdomen following repair of CDH. This can also lead to elevated airway pressures and prolonged intubation if excess pressure is created on the lungs from a forced abdominal closure. Additional complications with respiration occur due to a hypoplastic pulmonary system with concomitant pulmonary hypertension.

2. Presentation and Diagnosis

CDH is seen sporadically and with genetic syndromes. Trisomies 13, 18, and 21, along with Turner syndrome, have been associated with CDH. Aside from pulmonary hypoplasia and hypertension, cardiac defects are associated with CDH; specifically, these defects include ventriculoseptal defects, vascular rings, and coarctation of the aorta.

Prenatal diagnosis is possible via ultrasound through the presence of herniated abdominal organs, polyhydramnios, abnormal anatomy of the upper abdominal organs, and mediastinal shift. Postnatal diagnosis is confirmed by a CXR.

3. Treatment

CDH repair is best delayed to permit improved ventilation and additional respiratory development. Gentle conventional ventilation is started as aggressive bagging can result in barotrauma as well as dilation of the bowel within the chest. NGT placement is helpful in reducing dilated bowel. Infants who fail conventional ventilation are considered for oscillatory ventilation or extracorporeal membrane oxygenation (ECMO). The goal of ECMO is to improve pulmonary hypertension and lung compliance. The infant normally requires ECMO for one to three weeks.

Surgical repair is considered when the infant is stabilized. Some argue that repair should be delayed until the patient is near extubation, while others will proceed with surgery while still on ECMO. However, repair while the patient is on ECMO could be complicated by bleeding. The CDH is approached through an abdominal incision to reduce the abdominal contents from the thoracic cavity. The diaphragmatic defect can be closed primarily if it is not under tension. Prosthetic mesh is utilized for the larger diaphragmatic defects. A thoracic approach can be employed for right sided hernias. Overall survival following surgical repair can be near 90%. Associated anomalies play a large role in determining survival.

II.C. Pulmonary Cystic Diseases

1. Bronchogenic Cysts

Bronchogenic cysts are immature bronchial tissues that do not have independent blood supply or connection to the tracheobronchial tree. These cysts represent extrapulmonary masses that do not further differentiate.

2. Congenital Cystic Adenomatoid Malformation

Congenital cystic adenomatoid malformation (CCAM) is a cystic lesion that communicates with the tracheobronchial tree. These cysts can occur in any lobe, but the left lower lobe is more common. CCAM can produce mucus because it is lined with respiratory epithelium, leading to recurrent pneumonias.

3. Congenital Lobar Emphysema

Congenital lobar emphysema (CLE) results in hyperexpansion of one or more lobes within the lung. Air is trapped within the lobe, which overinflates and cannot deflate. The affected lobe compresses the remainder of the lung and causes atelectasis and mediastinal shift. Emergent resection may be required. CLE is seen in the upper pulmonary lobes.

4. Pulmonary Sequestration

a) Intralobar Pulmonary Sequestration

Pulmonary sequestration is an abnormal collection of primitive lung tissue with aberrant connections to the pulmonary artery and tracheobronchial tree. It is surrounded by normal lung tissue and has a basic connection to the bronchial tree. This leads to some element of ventilation without proper exhalation, causing recurrent pneumonias. Venous drainage for the intralobar variant is through the pulmonary veins to the left atrium. Patients with intralobar sequestration present at an older age from recurrent pulmonary infections. The timing of the accessory lung bud determines whether it is intra- or extralobar; earlier formation tends to lead to intralobar sequestration.

b) Extralobar Pulmonary Sequestration

Extralobar sequestration is nonventilated tissue in a similar location as intralobar sequestration but with a systemic arterial supply via the aorta. Extralobar sequestration has its own pleural covering, no connection to the bronchial tree, and may have an anomalous connection with the GI tract leading to feeding difficulties. Extrapulmonary sequestration has its venous drainage via the systemic venous system. Patients with the extrapulmonary variant normally present in infancy with respiratory distress or chronic cough.

c) Diagnosis of Pulmonary Sequestration

Diagnosis begins with a chest radiograph revealing dense or cystic lung in the left base. Consolidation will be present if the segment is infected. Chest CT demonstrates cystic lung and may identify the systemic arterial supply for extralobular sequestration. Bronchography and arteriography are rarely required for diagnosis.

d) Treatment of Pulmonary Sequestration

The treatment for all of the congenital cystic lesions is resection to prevent the pulmonary complications that can ensue. Even asymptomatic lesions should be resected to prevent pneumonia.

III. Disorders of the Abdomen

III.A. Annular Pancreas

Annular pancreas results from the incomplete migration of the ventral pancreas and can cause duodenal obstruction. Presentation includes abdominal distention and bilious vomiting. Annular pancreas can be associated with trisomy 21, cardiac disease, and tracheoesophageal fistula. Transection of the pancreas should not be performed to due to risk of injury to the pancreatic ducts. Correction of annular pancreas requires a duodenoduodenostomy or duodenojejunostomy.

III.B. Intestinal Atresia

Intestinal atresia is due to a prenatal vascular accident and occurs anywhere in the GI tract, affecting males and females equally. Other potential etiologies include intussusception, thromboembolism, segmental volvulus, and intestinal perforation. The most common presentation is complete atresia. Mucosal web formation can occur internally and lead to obstruction but may appear as normal bowel externally. The jejunum and ileum are equally and more commonly affected than the duodenum. Colonic atresias are the least common.

Associated anomalies are rare; however, duodenal atresia is associated with Down syndrome. These infants usually present with bilious vomiting, failure to pass meconium, and abdominal distention. The goal of surgery is to reestablish bowel continuity, which may be achieved by primary anastomosis for short atresias or ostomy formation for longer lengths of disease.

III.C. Hypertrophic Pyloric Stenosis

Pyloric stenosis is hypertrophy of the pyloric smooth muscle that narrows the pyloric lumen. Pyloric stenosis is more common in first born males and presents between 4-6 weeks after birth with nonbilious, projectile vomiting. A palpable "olive" in the right upper quadrant can be found on exam. Ultrasound is necessary for diagnosis. Resuscitation is required to correct the hypokalemic, hypochloremic metabolic acidosis, followed by definitive repair via a Ramstedt-Friedet pyloromyotomy. This procedure consists of a longitudinal incision through the hypertrophied muscle. Infants tolerate this procedure very well and usually begin feeds within a few hours.

III.D. Meconium Ileus

1. Assessment

Meconium is thick material present in the newborn intestine evacuated within 6 hours of birth. It primarily consists of intestinal debris, bile salts, and bile acids. Failure of evacuation can lead to a small bowel obstruction with a transition point in the terminal ileum. Bilious emesis, abdominal distention, and failure to pass meconium are present. Plain films reveal dilated loops of small bowel with a "soap-bubble" sign representing meconium mixed with intraluminal air.

Meconium ileus is associated with cystic fibrosis, a mutation in the chloride channel in epithelial cells that produces very viscous secretions that are difficult to clear. About 1 in 5 infants with cystic fibrous will develop meconium ileus. This condition can be associated with other complications such as volvulus, atresia, or intestinal perforation.

2. Management

Treatment for meconium ileus consists of repeated contrast enemas until the obstruction is relieved. Careful fluid monitoring is important to prevent dehydration. Failure of conservative management requires laparotomy to remove the inspissated meconium via external massage. Enterotomy may be needed to externally remove the meconium; primary closure is permissible.

III.E. Malrotation

1. Etiology and Pathophysiology

Malrotation is an incomplete counterclockwise rotation of the bowel around the superior mesenteric artery (SMA) during development. Malrotation can result in chronic abdominal pain from mesenteric ischemia, or midgut volvulus with acute compromise of the intestinal blood supply.

Total nonrotation is observed when the normal 270 degree rotation is not achieved. The small bowel is located to the right of the SMA and the colon to the left; the cecum is suspended by Ladd's bands near the midline. The duodenojejunal junction remains to the right of the midline and does not rise to the level of the pylorus. Incomplete rotation consists of intestinal rotation to 180 degrees with the colon on the left and small intestine on the right.

2. Presentation and Diagnosis

Diagnosis is by an upper gastrointestinal series that demonstrates duodenal obstruction secondary to volvulus. When volvulus is not present, the duodenojejunum remains to the right of the midline and fails to rise to the level of the pylorus. Bilious vomiting in an infant should be considered midgut volvulus until proven otherwise.

3. Treatment

Prompt treatment of volvulus is required. Correction of the malrotation involves Ladd's procedure, which is reduction of the volvulus, division of Ladd's bands, broadening of the base of the SMA mesentery, and appendectomy. After reduction of the volvulus, the bowel must be inspected for viability. The goal is to resect as little bowel as possible. At the completion of the case, the small bowel is on the right side of the abdomen, and the cecum is placed in the left upper quadrant. Malrotation can be associated with omphalocele, gastroschisis, and congenital diaphragmatic hernia.

III.F. Hirschsprung Disease

1. Assessment

Hirschsprung disease results from failure of migration of intestinal ganglion cells from the neural crest to the myenteric plexus. Males are more commonly affected than females. Most of the cases are sporadic; however, there is an association with Down syndrome and a familial form of Hirschsprung disease with a mutation in the RET protooncogene. Infants fail to pass meconium within 24 hours and present with a large bowel obstruction from failure of colonic relaxation. Bilious vomiting and abdominal distention occur. A small number of infants can develop Hirschsprung enterocolitis with fever, diarrhea, and sepsis. Emergent laparotomy with colostomy formation and aggressive fluid resuscitation is necessary. Hirschsprung disease may present in childhood with chronic constipation.

2. Management

Contrast enema demonstrates a transition zone of aganglionosis and a rectal biopsy confirms the absence of ganglion cells, hypertrophied nerve bundles, and increased staining of a cholinesterase dye. Treatment can be achieved with a Soave-Boley procedure, which completes resection of the aganglionic bowel followed by a mucus proctectomy, endorectal pull through, and coloanal anastomosis. Dilation of the coloanal anastomosis is important to prevent anastomotic stricture causing chronic constipation. Laparoscopic pull through is possible. Other methods for repair are also options.

III.G. Anorectal Malformation

1. Etiology and Pathophysiology

Anorectal malformations (ARM) are a spectrum of intestinal disorders due to abnormal descent of the urorectal septum between the seventh and tenth weeks of gestation. The incidence is approximately 1 per 5000 births. High malformations are due to a failure of rectal descent inferior to the levator ani and are associated with other congenital disorders such as VACTERL.

Low lesions occur when the rectum descends below this point but with fistula formation. A cloacal abnormality occurs when there is a common channel for the urinary, genital, and intestinal tracts. A tethered spinal cord may be seen with an infant with an ARM.

2. Presentation and Diagnosis

Physical exam demonstrates no obvious anus but a fistula to the perineum may be present, particularly with low lesions. High lesions may have a fistula to the urinary system in males leading to the passage of meconium via the penis. High lesions in females are rare and associated with a cloacal deformity. For high lesions, a retrograde urethrogram is helpful to better define the fistula to the urinary system.

3. Treatment

A colostomy is required for high lesions with a plan for anorectoplasty in approximately 6 weeks. The posterior sagittal anorectoplasty pioneered by Pena and DeVries is the procedure of choice. This involves a posterior division of the levator ani and external sphincter muscles to place the rectum in its anatomically correct location, followed by reconstruction of the pelvic floor. The colostomy reversed after 6 weeks. An important part of this operation is closure of the urinary fistula.

Low lesions require a less complex repair, which involves a perineal procedure during the newborn period with the need for a colostomy. Functional outcomes are variable with high lesions having more continence issues than low lesions. Mortality normally does not arise from the ARM itself but from the associated anomalies.

III.H. Meckel Diverticulum

1. Assessment

A Meckel diverticulum is due to incomplete obliteration of the omphalomesenteric duct, which is the duct through which nutrition is provided from the yolk sac to the fetal midgut. The omphalomesenteric duct normally involutes during the 7th week of gestation. The incidence is estimated to be 2% of the population, though only 2% of patients are symptomatic. The diverticula are usually within 2 feet of the ileocecal valve on the antimesenteric side of the terminal ileum. The blood supply to this true diverticulum arises from the superior mesenteric artery.

Approximately 50% of children present with hematochezia because of the heterotrophic gastric material present in the diverticulum. Other presentations include bowel obstruction, diverticulitis, umbilical fistula, or other umbilical lesions. These children may present with intussusception (see page 526). The presence of hematochezia can help distinguish Meckel diverticulum from appendicitis. Meckel diverticulum can sometimes be involved with tuberculosis, Crohn disease, or malignancy.

2. Management

Diagnosis is made with a technetium pertechnetate nuclear scan which utilizes an isotope that has a strong affinity for gastric mucosa. Symptomatic Meckel diverticulum should be resected; asymptomatic forms do not require surgery, but there is increasing literature suggesting that resection may be beneficial even in asymptomatic patients.

III.I. INTUSSUSCEPTION

1. Etiology and Pathophysiology

Intussusception involves proximal bowel (i.e. the intussusceptum) telescoping into an immediately adjacent section of bowel (i.e. the intussuscipiens). The terminal ileum is the most common location in which the terminal ileum invaginates into the colon. Mesenteric compromise causes bowel to become edematous, leading to bowel obstruction and mucosal bleeding (forming "currant jelly" stool). Intussusception is normally seen in patients 3 months to 3 years of age.

Intussusception may be related to a viral prodrome causing enlarged lymph nodes (Peyer's patches); it is more common in midsummer and midwinter months. Other causes of intussusception, especially in older children, include a Meckel diverticulum, tumors, polyps, and inspissated stool in patients with cystic fibrous.

2. Presentation and Diagnosis

Patients present with an intermittent, colicky abdominal pain progressing to abdominal distention and bilious vomiting. An abdominal mass can be palpated in the right lower quadrant. Diagnosis is made via plain films revealing a paucity of air in the right lower quadrant. Ultrasound confirms the presence of the intussusception.

3. Treatment

The definite diagnostic and therapeutic tool is the contrast enema using air, water-based contrast, or barium. Reduction of the ileocolic intussusception

is successful in 80% to 90% of patients, and the risk of perforation is low with this intervention. Radiological reduction is more successful when the child presents during the first 24 hours of symptoms.

When the intussusception cannot be reduced by contrast enemas, a laparotomy is required. The involved bowel should be massaged to reduce the intussusceptum, rather than forcefully pulling the bowel out of the intussuscipiens. Gangrenous bowel should be excised followed by primary reanastomosis; an appendectomy should also be completed. About 1 in 20 patients will have recurrence.

III.J. Necrotizing Enterocolitis

1. Etiology and Pathophysiology

Necrotizing enterocolitis (NEC) is one of the most common pediatric surgery emergencies and occurs most in premature infants weighing less than 1500 grams. Symptoms of NEC begin after the initiation of feeds, leading to abdominal distention, tenderness, ileus, delayed gastric emptying, abdominal erythema, and hematochezia. Laboratory abnormalities include metabolic acidosis with leukopenia or leukocytosis, neutropenia, and even DIC. Hypoxia, prematurity, viral infections, hypotension, and maternal drug use have all been associated with NEC.

2. Presentation and Diagnosis

Diagnosis begins with the above physical findings. A plain radiograph demonstrates pneumatosis intestinalis from bowel wall invasion by gas forming bacteria. Perforation or portal venous gas indicates more advanced disease with transmural involvement.

3. Treatment

Treatment begins with supportive therapy for the infant as well as serial plain radiographs. The infants require nasogastric tube decompression, broad-spectrum antibiotics, cessation of enteral feeds, and total parenteral nutrition. Operative intervention is utilized for those infants with intestinal perforation or sepsis not responding to antibiotics. This is accomplished by placement of a peritoneal drain in the right lower quadrant for patients that will not tolerate surgery, or a laparotomy if they are stable. There is no difference in survival between drain placement and laparotomy.

At laparotomy, only nonviable bowel should be resected. Most infants require a colostomy. Most infants require a repeat laparotomy to examine bowel that was questionable in the first operation. Patients treated with a peritoneal drain may have a laparotomy when they are stable to address intestinal strictures, leaks, and fistula formation. Advances in pediatric critical care permit survival rates for NEC to exceed 60%.

III.K. Appendicitis

1. Etiology and Presentation

Appendicitis is one of the more common clinical problems that pediatric surgeons face. It is due to appendiceal orifice obstruction from lymphoid hyperplasia secondary to viral infection or dehydration. Approximately 50% of patients have the classic symptoms of periumbilical pain that migrates to the right lower quadrant. The remaining children report dull abdominal pain in the periumbilical region or solely in the right lower quadrant. Fever is not commonly present unless perforation has occurred. Patients also have a leukocytosis with a left shift.

2. Diagnosis

The presence of right lower quadrant peritoneal signs with light palpation is supportive of appendicitis. A Rovsing sign (pain in the right lower quadrant with palpation of the left lower quadrant), obturator sign (pain in the right lower quadrant with internal rotation of the hip), or iliopsoas sign (pain in the right lower quadrant with hip extension) may be present and are indicative of potential perforation.

Appendiceal perforation is more common in the pediatric population due to a delay in diagnosis. Plain films can occasionally demonstrate an appendicolith. Ultrasound can assist with diagnosis, particularly with an experienced operator. CT demonstrates an enlarged appendix that does not fill with contrast and surrounding fat stranding from inflammation. However, if the physical exam is unequivocal for appendicitis, no further imaging is needed.

3. Treatment

Treatment of appendicitis requires antibiotics and appendectomy. Many surgeons prefer laparoscopic appendectomy over the traditional limited laparotomy at McBurney's point. Perforated appendicitis is treated with antibiotics for 14 days followed by appendectomy 6 weeks later.

III.L. Abdominal Wall Defects

1. Omphalocele

a) Assessment

Omphalocele is a large abdominal wall defect (> 4 cm) covered by amniotic membrane containing herniated midgut and potentially liver or spleen. The defect results from failure of body wall folding early in embryogenesis and is thus associated with other congenital anomalies. This membrane may occasionally be absent due to prior rupture; careful evaluation may be necessary to distinguish omphalocele from gastroschisis in this event.

Diagnosis on prenatal ultrasound is common, allowing arrangements to be made for care of the neonate after delivery. Either vaginal or cesarean section is permissible. Omphalocele is not a surgical emergency, but urgent repair can increase the chance of primary closure.

b) Management

Immediate care includes covering the sac with petroleum-impregnanted gauze and a sterile towel to minimize heat loss, placing an NGT for bowel decompression, antibiotics, and maintenance IVF to replace losses. An echocardiogram and cardiology evaluation are necessary to rule out cardiac anomalies. The pentalogy of Cantrell is sometimes present with defects of the supraumbilical abdominal wall, pericardium, and central tendon of the diaphragm that results in herniation of the midgut and heart into the amniotic sac.

2. Gastroschisis

a) Assessment

Gastroschisis is a small abdominal wall defect located 2 cm to the right of the umbilicus with antenatal herniation of abdominal viscera. The exposed viscera are not covered by an amniotic sac. The exposed bowel has no membrane and is edematous with a thick fibrous peel at delivery. The pathophysiology of gastroschisis may involve rupture of the abdominal wall at the site of resorption of the right umbilical vein at 4 weeks gestation. As in omphalocele, diagnosis is made by prenatal ultrasound and delivery may be vaginal or cesarean delivery.

b) Management

Unlike omphalocele, gastroschisis is a surgical emergency. Early placement of a sterile plastic "bowel bag" limits heat and fluid losses from exposed bowel. An NGT permits decompression. The neonate should be placed on his or her side with care taken to avoid twisting the vascular supply. Definitive operative management involves careful inspection and reduction of bowel loops with primary closure. For large herniations, a sterile silo may be placed over the abdominal contents with gradual reduction over a series of days, followed by a final closure in the OR.

IV. Hepatobiliary Disease

IV.A. Biliary Atresia

1. Etiology and Pathophysiology

Biliary atresia, which affects 1 in 15,000 infants, is the obliteration of the extrahepatic biliary system with dense fibrous tissue causing an obstruction in bile flow. The gallbladder is also typically obliterated. Without treatment, the infant progresses to secondary biliary cirrhosis. Infection by reovirus type 3, rotavirus, and CMV have been implicated as potential causes leading to obliteration of the biliary tree.

2. Presentation and Diagnosis

Biliary atresia is classified into three types: type I is obliteration of the common bile duct with patency of the proximal ducts; type II is atresia of the hepatic duct with cystic structures within the porta hepatis; type III is the most common and involves atresia of the left and right hepatic ducts at the level of the porta hepatis.

Jaundice, dark urine, acholic stools, and hepatosplenomegaly are evident by one month of age. Direct hyperbilirubinemia may be present and is considered abnormal in the infant. Further investigation with imaging of the biliary tree with technetium-99m-iminodiacetic (99mTc-IDA) is sensitive and specific for biliary atresia, and indicates no excretion of radioisotope into the duodenum. An abdominal ultrasound elucidates the biliary anatomy. Diagnosis is confirmed by an intraoperative cholangiogram and a liver biopsy that demonstrates fibrous bile duct proliferation.

3. Treatment

Treatment of biliary atresia is via the Kasai procedure, first described in the 1950's in Japan. This procedure begins with identification of the fibrous cord that has replaced the common bile duct and dissecting it to the porta hepatis at the bifurcation of the portal vein. A hepaticojejunostomy with Roux-en-Y anastomosis is constructed with a 40 cm retrocolic jejunal segment. The overall failure rate of the Kasai procedure approaches 60%.

According to the American Association for the Study of Liver Diseases, the following characteristics are associated with improved long term survival: infants younger than 10 weeks at operation, preoperative histology and ductal remnant size, bile in hepatic lobular zone 1, absence of portal hypertension, cirrhosis, surgical team experience, and postoperative clearing of jaundice.

Progressive liver disease can occur in 60% of patients and fifty percent of infants will develop cholangitis or portal hypertension from continued fibrosis. These infants may require diet supplementation with medium chain fatty acids due to fat malabsorption and fat-soluble vitamin deficiency. Many of these infants require liver transplantation. Biliary atresia is the most common indication for pediatric liver transplantation.

IV.B. Choledochal Cysts

1. Assessment

Choledochal cysts are congenital cystic dilations involving the extrahepatic and/or intrahepatic biliary tree. Alonzo-Lej was the first to develop a classification system in 1959. The most common cyst is type I, a dilation of the complete common bile duct with little proximal disease. Type II cysts are true diverticula of the common bile duct. Type III cysts are choledochoceles, a local dilation in the distal common bile duct. Multiple intrahepatic and extrahepatic cystic dilations are type IVa, whereas only extrahepatic dilation occurs with type IVb. Type V disease (Caroli disease) is multiple intrahepatic cystic dilations. Infants present with obstructive jaundice. Older children may develop abdominal pain, jaundice, and a hepatic mass.

2. Management

Diagnosis is made by aultrasound and hepatobiliary iminodiacetic acid (HIDA) scan. ERCP or MRCP further define the biliary anatomy. The entire choledochal cyst must be resected; simply draining the cyst can lead to cholangitis and cholangiocarcinoma. The surgical treatment for the types of choledochal cysts is demonstrated in the table below. Complications include cholangitis, pancreatitis, stricture formation, and hepaticolithiasis.

Table 4. Surgical management of choledochal cyst disease.

Choledochal Cyst	Surgical Treatment
Type I	Cyst excision with Roux-en-Y hepaticojejunostomy
Type II	Diverticulum excision with closure of common bile duct defect over a T-tube
Type III	Cyst < 3 cm: endoscopic sphincterotomy; cyst > 3 cm: transduodenal excision with pancreatic duct reimplanted into the duodenum if it enters the cyst
Type IV	Extrahepatic cyst excision with Roux-en-Y hepaticojejunosotomy; hepatic lobe resection for intrahepatic ductal stricture, abscess, or hepaticolithiasis
Type V	If the cyst only involves a hepatic lobe, simple resection is sufficient; otherwise, liver transplantation is required

V. Pediatric Trauma

V.A. Overview

Trauma is the primary cause of death among pediatric patients. Blunt trauma secondary to falls or motor vehicle crashes is the most common form of injury. Penetrating trauma makes up a smaller number of patients and is usually due to the accidental discharge of a gun within the home. Drowning is a significant cause of trauma in older children. Child abuse is a true public health problem and all heath care providers are legally compelled to report any concern of abuse.

V.B. Airway

The evaluation of the pediatric trauma patient begins with the ABCs. Respiratory issues are critical in pediatric patients, especially in infants who are obligate nasal breathers. The infant patient's airway is best opened in the sniffing position, not the head tilt chin lift method. Using an uncuffed endotracheal tube in the smallest infants reduces subglottic stenosis and prevents complications from the tracheal narrowing at the cricoid cartilage.

V.C. Breathing

Work of breathing is especially important since respiratory difficulties are a common manifestation of systemic distress in children, and because respiratory arrest is the most common cause of cardiovascular collapse in this population. Signs of labored breathing include nasal flaring, retractions (supraclavicular and sternal retractions are especially ominous), wheezing, grunting, and stridor.

V.D. Circulation

Signs of poor perfusion include abnormal skin color (pallor or mottling), dry mucous membranes, and delayed capillary refill (> 2 seconds). Tachycardia is the earliest sign of hypovolemia. Hypotension is a late sign usually seen after 40% of the blood volume has been lost. Pediatric patients have narrow

Pediatric Surgery

vascular reserve and even a small amount of blood loss can be disastrous. These patients should be managed from a hypotensive shock perspective (page 513).

V.E. Disability and Exposure

Maintenance of temperature is an important concern in pediatric patients, due to their higher surface area to volume ratio. Reducing their energy requirements for temperature maintenance permits shunting of this reserve to the inflammatory and repair process already underway.

V.F. Primary and Secondary Survey

The remainder of the primary and secondary survey should continue with an understanding that multiorgan injury in pediatric patients is more common because of the proximity of the organs to the skin surface and the smaller amount of fat. Children should always receive the essential X-rays and CT scans indicated by the exam with the understanding that excessive exposure at such a young age may lead to a greater risk of future malignancy.

V.G. Head Trauma

Head injury is one of the most common causes of death in the pediatric population. A thin skull and large head in relation to the remainder of the body contribute to the risk of head injury. Involvement of the neurosurgical team early in the treatment expedites care. Placement of an intraventricular monitor or surgery may be required. Pediatric patients have a better chance of survival compared to adults for head trauma.

V.H. Spinal Cord Trauma

Pediatric patients may have ligamentous injuries affecting the spinal cord that cannot be seen radiographically unless dedicated MRI or flexion/extension films are completed. SCIWORA (Spinal cord injury without radiographic abnormality) must be considered when clearing the cervical spine of the pediatric patient; a suitable high index of suspicion is required for prompt diagnosis.

V.I. Chest Trauma

Chest trauma is not as common in pediatric patients. The presence of rib fractures portends a poor survival because of the associated intra-abdominal injuries. Pneumonia secondary to lung contusion can be treated with aggressive pulmonary toilet.

V.J. Abdominal Trauma

Evaluation of the abdomen is completed with the use of a CT scan or ultrasound. Seatbelts save lives, but they can also cause injuries. Looking for a seatbelt sign across the abdomen can indicate hollow viscous and lumbar spine injury. Prompt CT scan of the abdomen and pelvis is necessary if the patient is stable. Blunt trauma is the number one cause of abdominal injury in children and is one of the most commonly missed injuries in the absence of suitable diagnostic imaging.

The spleen is the most common organ to be injured, followed by the liver and kidneys. Observation of splenic injuries with embolization for active extravasation is the treatment of choice unless the patient is grossly unstable or there is devastating injury to the spleen. Nearly 80% of grade I-IV splenic lacerations can be successfully treated with coil embolization. Blunt hepatic trauma is usually managed with observation. Major liver resections are rarely required.

V.K. Indications for Surgery

To operate on a child with blunt trauma depends on the patient's clinical status. Continued hemodynamic instability is an indication for operative repair. Selective operative treatment for stab wounds can be performed. Many stab wounds can be locally explored to determine if the peritoneum has been violated. However, gunshot wounds to the abdomen require a laparotomy due to the blast injury and likely compromise of internal structures.

VI. Pediatric Tumors

VI.A. Wilms Tumor

1. Etiology and Pathophysiology

Wilms tumor, also known as a nephroblastoma, is an embyronal renal malignancy and is the most common childhood intraabdominal tumor. The majority of cases occur in children less than 5 years old. It can be associated with aniridia, Beckwith-Wiedemann syndrome, and genitourinary anomalies. There is a familial form associated with deletion of chromosome 11p, and tumor suppressor genes WT1 and WT2 have been found to contribute to the development of the disease.

2. Presentation and Diagnosis

Most patients present with an asymptomatic abdominal mass, although hematuria or hypertension can also be presenting symptoms. Most Wilms tumors are unilateral and unifocal with only 7% occurring bilaterally. Imaging is required to assess the extent of the mass, venous invasion, lymph node involvement, metastases, and determine contralateral renal function. An abdominal ultrasound and CT scan of the chest and abdomen are usually adequate.

3. Treatment

Wilms tumor commonly metastasizes to the lungs and bone. The most important factors in determining prognosis are histopathology and stage of the tumor. Anaplastic tumors have a significantly worse prognosis. Operative intervention has a high cure rate and requires a unilateral nephrectomy with local lymph node dissection. Wilms tumor is friable and ruptures easily; rupture during resection increases the stage.

Intraoperative inspection of the contralateral kidney and liver helps to determine staging. All patients except for those with stage I tumor receive adjuvant chemotherapy with actinomycin and vincristine. Adriamycin is added for advanced disease. External beam radiation is used for all patients with advanced disease as well as those with local disease but unfavorable histology.

Isolated pulmonary and hepatic metastases should be resected. Overall, outcomes are excellent with five year survival exceeding 85%. Patients require long-term follow-up due to the risk of metachronous tumor development.

TABLE 5. Wilms tumor staging.

WILMS TUMOR STAGE	
I	Tumor limited to kidney, completely excised
II	Tumor extends beyond kidney, completely excised
III	Residual nonhematogenous tumor intraabdominally
IV	Hematogenous metastases
V	Bilateral renal involvement at diagnosis (stage each kidney separately)

VI.B. NEUROBLASTOMA

1. Etiology and Pathophysiology

Neuroblastoma is the most common tumors in infants less than a year old and has a median age at diagnosis of 2 years. Neuroblastoma is derived from neural crest cells and occurs anywhere along the embryonal pathway of sympathetic ganglia descent, with the adrenal glands being the most common site. Tumors with amplification of the N-myc oncogene are associated with a worse prognosis. A deletion of the short-arm of chromosome 1 has also been shown to correlate with adverse outcome. Other indicators of advanced disease include the presence of neuron-specific enolase, serum lactate dehydrogenase (LDH), serum vanillymandelic acid (VMA), and diploid tumors.

2. Presentation and Diagnosis

Most patients present with an asymptomatic abdominal mass, but site-specific symptoms are sometimes present. CT or MRI is necessary to assess resectability and evaluate for metastasis. Neuroblastoma often displays calcifications in the tumor. An I-meta-iodobenzylguanidine (MIBG) scan is useful in localizing tumors secreting catecholamines. Tissue or bone marrow biopsy is essential for diagnosis. Patients are stratified into low, intermediate, or high risk groups based on factors including age, stage, N-myc status, and serum indicators.

3. Treatment

Primary tumor resection is attempted if possible. Neuroblastomas tend to encase vascular structures rather than invade them. Multiagent chemotherapy is used for patients in the intermediate and high risk groups. Bone marrow transplantation is considered for patients with advanced disease. Survival rates vary by stage with locally resectable disease having relatively good survival.

VI.C. Rhabdomyosarcoma

1. Assessment

Rhabdomyosarcoma is a soft tissue sarcoma of skeletal muscle origin. It has a bimodal peak in incidence, presenting most frequently in infancy and then again in adolescence. Although most cases occur sporadically, it can also be associated with certain genetic conditions including Li-Fraumeni syndrome, Beckwith-Wiedemann syndrome, and neurofibromatosis type I.

The most common sites for rhabdomyosarcoma are the head and neck, genitourinary tract, and the extremities. Imaging with CT scan or MRI is recommended, and a PET scan is sometimes obtained to evaluate for metastatic disease.

Rhabdomyosarcoma is characterized by rapid, aggressive growth into surrounding structures with distant metastasis. Definitive diagnosis requires an incisional or core needle biopsy. Prognosis depends on patient age, site of tumor origin, extent of tumor, and histologic grade.

2. Management

Multimodal therapy is utilized for all patients, with the majority receiving chemotherapy after surgical resection. Wide local excision with lymphadenectomy is the procedure of choice. Histologic grade, metastases, and residual local disease are the most important indicators for postoperative treatment. Radiation therapy is offered for tumors > 5 cm, incomplete surgical resections, and high-grade tumors. Overall 5 year survival is about 60%.

VI.D. Hepatoblastoma

1. Assessment

Liver cancer is rare in children but can take the form of hepatoblastoma or hepatocellular carcinoma. Hepatoblastomas occur in children less than 3 years old and contain a mutation in the β-catenin gene. The tumor is frequently unifocal, allowing for potentially complete resection. Hepatoblastoma can be associated with hemihypertrophy, Beckwith-Wiedemann syndrome, and very low birth weight; α-fetoprotein is elevated in about 90% of patients and reflects disease activity.

2. Management

Patients who undergo complete resection of the primary tumor with negative surgical margins have improved survival. The overall survival for hepatoblastoma is 70% and has a better prognosis than hepatocellular cancer. Preoperative chemotherapy using doxorubicin and cisplatin-based regimens can make a tumor resectable. Isolated pulmonary metastasis should be surgically removed. If a patient has unresectable disease without metastasis, a liver transplant can be considered.

PLASTIC SURGERY

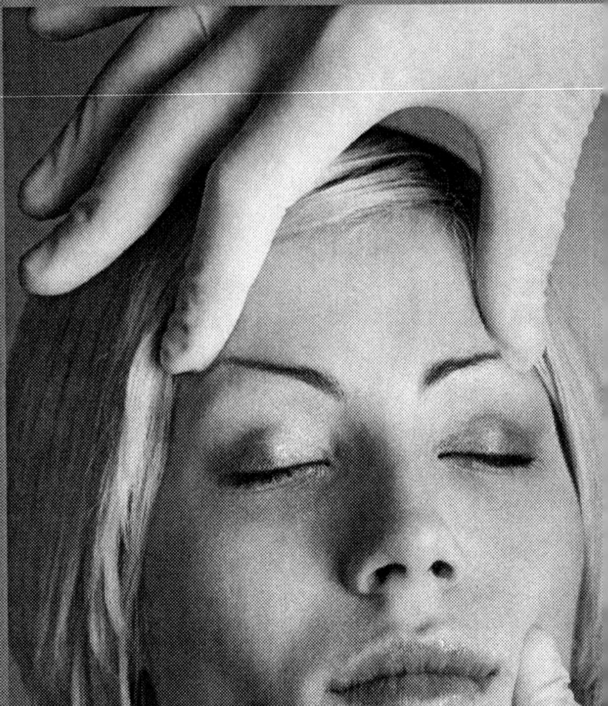

To cut is to cure.

Dogma

SURGISPHERE

PLASTIC SURGERY

Prateek K. Gupta, M.D. and Johnny T. Chang, M.D.

I. General Concepts

I.A. Skin

The skin is the body's largest organ, and serves as a barrier against UV radiation, chemical and thermal changes, and microorganisms. In addition to its function as a simple barrier, the skin has a role in the immune system, temperature regulation, sensory input, and vitamin D synthesis.

The skin consists of two major layers: epidermis and dermis, separated by the basement membrane. The epidermis contains keratinocytes originating from the epidermal basal layer, melanocytes which produce melanin pigment transferred to keratinocytes, and Langerhans cells originating from bone marrow and acting as MHC class II antigen presenting cells.

The dermis is relatively acellular and is the skin's strongest component. It is divided into the superficial papillary dermis and deep reticular dermis. The dermis contains skin appendages, including hair follicles, apocrine glands, and eccrine glands. Nerves, blood vessels, and lymphatics also reside within the dermis. Eccrine glands secrete normally hypotonic aqueous fluid for temperature regulation, whereas apocrine glands produce a viscous and cloudy output secreted into hair follicles.

The skin contains many sensory receptors, including Merkel cells, Meissner's corpuscles, Pacinian corpuscles, Ruffini endings, and Krause end bulbs. These receptors function as hot and cold, light touch, pressure, and pain sensors.

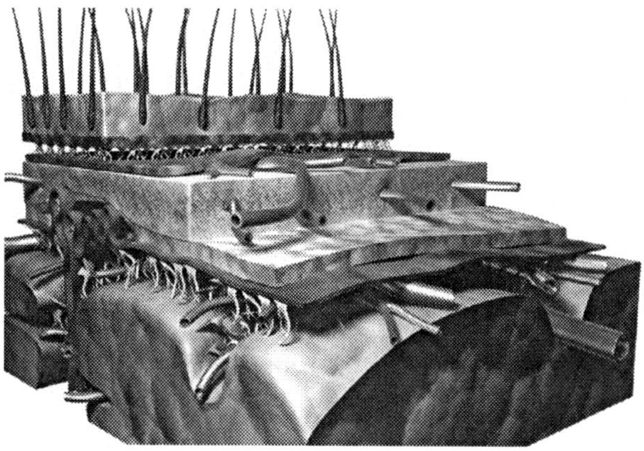

Collagen in the skin and the underlying

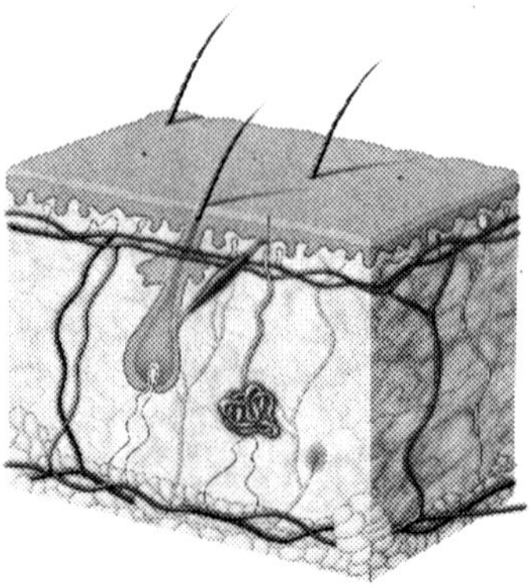

muscular layer is arranged in distinct directions. Tension on wounds and scars is varies based on their orientation to these fibers, and is most evident in the face. Langer's lines are cleavage planes between collagen bundles, and incisions oriented parallel to them have improved cosmesis. Relaxed skin tension lines (RSTLs) take into account musculature as well as different body positions, and thus more accurately reflect the directions of minimal and maximal tension in the skin. When not otherwise contraindicated, incisions should be made parallel to the RSTLs.

Summary

- Skin has many functions, including protection, antigen presentation, sensation, thermoregulation, and vitamin D synthesis.
- The epidermis is the outer layer of skin and is relatively cellular.
- The dermis is the structural strength layer, is relatively acellular, and contains skin appendages, nerves, blood vessels, and lymphatics.
- Elective incisions should be made parallel to RSTLs whenever possible.

I.B. Wound Healing

1. Phases of Wound Healing

Wound healing consists of three phases: the inflammatory phase, the proliferative phase, and the maturation or remodeling phase. The inflammatory phase lasts approximately 5 days and is marked by the hemostatic and cellular responses. The proliferative phase begins at day 4 and lasts approximately 3 weeks and sees the creation of a disorganized framework of extracellular matrix and blood vessels. The remodeling phase can last up to a year and consists of the gradual reorganization of matrix and vascular structures into a more functional and stronger form.

The inflammatory phase of healing (days 1 through 5) begins immediately after injury with the appearance of platelets, which participate in coagulation and hemostasis. Platelets release cytokines and growth factors that promote chemotaxis and migration of important inflammatory mediators into the injury site. Neutrophils arrive within the first two days and play a minor role in wound healing through phagocytosis of local debris. Macrophages become the dominant cell type by day 3 and orchestrate the wound healing process by releasing crucial cytokines and growth factors such as IL-1 and TGF-β that direct the migration and work of other cells. In addition, epithelialization begins during the inflammatory phase with cell migration and mitosis, signaled by the loss of contact inhibition between cells and regulated by various growth factors such as EGF. In a primarily closed surgical wound, epithelialization is complete within the first 48 hours, sealing the wound against external contamination.

By the end of the first week, the proliferative phase has begun (days 5 through 21). Fibroblasts become the dominant cell type and rapidly synthesize collagen as well as matrix material such as GAGs (glycosaminoglycans). Although wound tensile strength begins to increase as a result, the collagen is predominantly type III, whereas in normal skin there is a 4:1 ratio between type I and type III collagen. Wound contraction occurs with the appearance of myofibroblasts, specialized fibroblasts with contractile cytoplasmic microfilaments. Angiogenesis begins during the proliferative phase under the influence of factors such as VEGF (vascular endothelial growth factor) secreted by platelets and other cells.

The maturation or remodeling phase (week 4 up to 1 year) begins as the rate of collagen breakdown mediated by metalloproteases increases to match the rate of collagen synthesis. Type III collagen is replaced by type I, reestablishing the normal 4:1 ratio. The collagen also becomes more organized and better cross linked, and the tissue becomes less cellular. The wound reaches its peak strength, about 80% of baseline, after about 60 days.

Table 1. Wound Strength

Two weeks	10%
Three weeks	20%
Four weeks	50%
60 days	80%

Table 2. Collagen Types

Type I	Most common type. Found in bone, skin, and tendon. The predominant collagen in mature scars.
Type II	Primary constituent of cartilage.
Type III	Found in embryonic tissue, vasculature, uterus, gastrointestinal tract; the predominant collagen in immature scars.
Type IV	Found in basement membrane.

2. Factors That Affect Wound Healing

Risk factors for poor wound healing include the following:

- Increasing age
- Systemic disease (e.g., diabetes, renal failure, liver failure, atherosclerosis)
- Immunosuppression or immunodeficiency
- Steroids (reversed by vitamin A)
- Malnutrition (protein, caloric, and vitamin)
- Smoking
- Infection and foreign bodies
- Radiation

3. Scar Formation

Abnormal scarring may occur in the form of widened, hypertrophic, or keloid scars. Widened scars are marked by normal quantities of collagen spread over a larger area, whereas the histology of hypertrophic and keloid scars are similar and involve excessive collagen deposition. Keloid scars differ from hypertrophic in that keloids grow beyond the normal wound borders.

Widened and hypertrophic scars both result largely from excessive tension on the wound, whereas the etiology of keloids is unclear but may be influenced by autoimmune and endocrine factors. Keloids also differ from widened and hypertrophic scars in that the latter generally respond well to treatment (primarily excision and closure), but keloids often worsen and require combination therapy with multiple modalities. In addition, keloids show a much higher correlation with genetic, familial, and racial factors.

Plastic Surgery

TABLE 3. Types of Scars

	Widened Scars	Hypertrophic Scars	Keloids
Description	Wide, flat, often depressed	Excessive scar tissue within wound borders	Excessive scar tissue growing beyond wound borders
Race & genetics		Low correlation	Significant familial influence, affects blacks more than whites
Gender			Females > Males
Age		Typically < 20 years old	Typically 10-30 years old
Natural history	Develops in 1st 6 months	Develops early, typically subsides	Develops over months, rarely subsides
Location	Arms, legs, abdomen	Flexor surfaces, upper torso	Face, ear lobes, chest
Etiology	Tension, movement	Tension, movement	Possibly autoimmune or endocrine factors
Treatment	Excision and closure	Excision and closure, may also benefit from other modalities	Combination therapy (excision and closure alone may worsen scar)

Summary

- There are 3 phases of healing: inflammatory, proliferative, and maturation/ remodeling.
- During the inflammatory phase (days 1-5), platelets assist with hemostasis and attract other cells by releasing various factors and cytokines.
- Macrophages are the key players in the inflammatory process.
- During the proliferative phase (days 5-21), fibroblasts lay down type

III collagen in a relatively disorganized manner.

- During the maturation phase (week 4 to 1 year), type III collagen is replaced by type I collagen, becomes better organized, and more effectively cross linked.
- Normal skin has a 4:1 ratio between type I and type III collagen.
- Skin reaches its peak strength, 80% of baseline, in about 60 days.
- Widened scars are wide and flat, result from tension on the wound, and are best treated by excision and closure.
- Hypertrophic scars are exuberant scars within wound borders, develop from tension on the wound, and are treated by excision and closure.
- Keloid scars are exuberant scars growing beyond wound borders, have a genetic and familial component, and require combination therapy.

I.C. Wound Closure

1. Types of Wound Closure

Wounds may be closed by primary, secondary, or tertiary intention. Closure by primary intention involves direct approximation of wound edges soon after injury. Closure by secondary intention is also known as spontaneous healing and depends on the body's innate wound healing capabilities, especially wound contraction and epithelialization. Closure by tertiary intention is delayed primary closure and is characterized by a period of closure by secondary intention followed by primary closure. When these methods of closure are unsuccessful or require an excessive length of time, alternatives include augmentation with negative pressure dressings, grafts, and flaps.

2. Negative Pressure Dressing

Negative pressure dressings create a vacuum in the wound that improves perfusion, debrides the wound, evacuates excess fluid, impedes bacterial proliferation, and applies contractile force to the wound edges to assist in closure. There is also evidence that the mechanical force applied on the wound by the dressings may stimulate cell growth and angiogenesis. Negative pressure dressings can decrease the length of time needed for closure by secondary or tertiary intention.

3. Skin Grafts

Grafts are avascular tissues transferred from one part of the body to another or from one person to another. These tissues may include skin, nerve, bone, cartilage, tendon, fat, or a combination. Autografts are transfers from one part of the body to another, isografts are transfers between identical twins, allografts are transfers between different individuals of the same species, and xenografts are transfers between different species.

Skin grafts may be split-thickness skin grafts (STSG) in which only part of the dermis is harvested, or full-thickness skin grafts (FTSG) which contain the full dermal layer. STSGs have a lower risk of seroma or hematoma formation and exhibit better take, but are functionally and aesthetically inferior and contract significantly more than FTSGs. FTSGs are more prone to failure or partial take, but result in better cosmesis and function due to the presence of epithelial appendages, nerves, and melanocytes preserved within the dermis. A major advantage of STSGs is the ability to expand a graft significantly by meshing to cover large areas and the option to reharvest from the same donor site after 7 to 10 days of healing.

Factors that adversely affect skin grafts include sheer forces that disrupt the growth of matrix and vascular tissue between the graft and the wound bed, hematoma or seroma formation, and infection. To avoid these complications, grafts should be placed on clean, vascular wound beds. They should be supported with pressure dressings to maintain apposition between the graft and the wound bed, and meshed or pie-crusted to allow egress of drainage fluids. Any movement that may lead to sheer stresses should be avoided until the grafts have taken, usually within 3 to 5 days.

TABLE 4. STSG versus FTSG

STSG	FTSG
Poorer aesthetics and function (no epithelial appendages transferred)	Better cosmesis and function, especially over joints
Better take	More prone to failure or partial take
Lower risk of seroma or hematoma formation	Higher risk of seroma or hematoma formation
Can cover larger areas by meshing and delayed reharvesting	Limited coverage
More secondary contraction over time	Less secondary contraction over time

4. Flaps

Flaps are tissues with an intact vascular pedicle transferred from one part of the body to another, or one person to another (unlike grafts, which do not have a blood supply). These tissues could include skin, subcutaneous tissue, fascia, muscle, bone, other tissues such as omentum, or a combination. Flaps are useful in situations where advanced wound coverage is needed, but grafts are not sufficient. These indications include a poorly vascularized wound bed where grafts would not survive, the need for a large amount of tissue, or the need for specific functional tissue. In some situations, flaps can also provide a more aesthetic result or be more easily accessible, as in the case of local flaps to cover small defects.

There are many different methods of classifying flaps. A simple method, however, is to describe flaps based on distance from the defect, type of vascular supply, and type of tissue transferred. A flap may be a local flap, a distant flap, or a free flap (free tissue transfer). It may have a random blood supply, or it may be based on an axial or named arterial or venous pedicle. It may contain any of the tissues listed above.

Local flaps include advancement flaps where tissue is moved in a straight line, rotational flaps where tissue is rotated into a defect along a curve, and transposition flaps where switching flaps of tissue brings tissue from areas of low tension (and excess tissue) to areas of high tension (and inadequate tissue). The most basic local flaps are simple advancement flaps in which the edges of a wound bed are undermined to allow easier advancement of the overlying tissue to cover the wound. Advancement flaps may also involve incising and undermining healthy tissue adjacent to the wound in order to bring healthy tissue into a defect. The V-Y advancement flap takes advantage of tissue laxity perpendicular to the direction of skin tension in order to cover defects. Rotation flaps involve incising healthy tissue adjacent to a wound in order to rotate the tissue into the defect. In both advancement and rotation flaps, a Burow's triangle may assist in releasing tension at the base of the flap.

Component separation is a useful method of closing abdominal defects using multiple local advancement flaps. The technique takes advantage of multiple tissue layers in the abdominal wall supplied by superior, inferior, and lateral vascular pedicles. Posteriorly, the rectus muscle is separated from the posterior rectus sheath and advanced medially. Anteriorly, the external oblique muscle is separated from the internal oblique muscle at the linea semilunaris and also advanced medially.

Transposition flaps are local flaps in which two or more flaps of adjacent tissue are switched. They can be very elaborate and involve multiple flaps and switches. Two common and simple transposition flaps are the Z-plasty and rhomboid flap. The Z-plasty is used to release skin tension along a particular vector by recruiting tissue perpendicular to the tension. This is particularly useful in severe burns or contracting scars. The Z-plasty consists of three limbs arranged as a "Z", each of equal length, with the central limb aligned in the direction of maximum tension. The larger the angle between the limbs of the Z-plasty, the greater the gain in length in the direction of tension, and therefore the more relaxed the skin becomes in that direction. The rhomboid flap is useful for covering relatively circular, oval, or rectangular defects.

Distant and free flaps are indicated when there is insufficient tissue for local flaps. Musculocutaneous flaps with the latissimus dorsi or rectus abdominis can be used to cover thoracic and abdominal defects. These two muscles and their overlying skin are commonly used in breast reconstruction after mastectomy. Visceral flaps such as omental flaps, colonic flaps, or jejunal flaps can be used to cover or reconstruct intraabdominal, intrathoracic, or pharyngoesophageal defects.

Several factors can adversely affect flaps. Flap necrosis can result from an inadequately vascularized pedicle, excessive flap length causing distal flap ischemia, thrombosis of the vascular pedicle, mechanical kinking, or drug-induced vasoconstriction. Even with adequate arterial inflow, flaps may be damaged by insufficient venous outflow. In fact, pedicled and free flaps most commonly fail due to venous thrombosis or insufficiency. Flaps are also susceptible to hematoma, seroma, and infection, although they tend to be more robust than grafts in this respect.

Summary

- The simplest ways to close wounds are by primary, secondary, and tertiary intention. When these methods fail, a graft or flap may be needed.
- Grafts are tissues transferred without a blood supply and depend on a vascularized wound bed for survival.
- Flaps are tissues transferred with a blood supply. The blood supply may be left intact, dissected out as a pedicle, or detached and reattached at a different location (i.e., free flap or free tissue transfer).
- STSGs contain only part of the dermis, exhibit better take, and can be meshed and expanded significantly to cover large areas. However, they tend to be functionally and aesthetically inferior to FTSGs.
- FTSGs contain the entire dermal layer, are more susceptible to failure, and have limited coverage. However, they tend to be more functional and achieve improved cosmesis.
- Common local flaps include simple undermining to mobilize wound edges, V-Y advancement flaps, Z-plasty transposition flaps, and rhomboid transposition flaps.
- Component separation is a technique used to close abdominal defects by separating the layers of the abdominal wall and advancing each layer medially as a flap.

II. Dermatologic Conditions

II.A. Impetigo

Impetigo present with superficial bullae from S. aureus or S. pyogenes and requires excision if it leads to necrosis. Erysipelas occurs from Streptococcus and is a rapidly progressive superficial dermatitis. A furuncle is a single boil caused by S. aureus or S. epidermidis, while a carbuncle is a multiloculated furuncle.

II.B. Hidradenitis Suppurativa

Hidradenitis is an infection of the apocrine sweat glands and usually occurs in the axilla and groin. High grade hidradenitis should be treated with excision. However, the mainstay of treatment involves retinoids, steroids, and antibiotics. Surgery should be done only after active infection has resolved.

III. Trauma

III.A. Pressure Sores

Decubitus ulcers occur at areas of the body subjected to prolonged focused pressure, particularly posterior bony prominences such as the ischial tuberosities, trochanters, sacrum, and heels in patients with impaired mobility. Other risk factors include sensory loss leading to inability to sense ischemic discomfort, impaired tissue perfusion (e.g., in sepsis), poor nutritional status, advanced age, and diabetes.

Pressure sores are classified into 4 stages:

- Stage 1 – erythema without skin disruption
- Stage 2 – partial skin disruption with blistering, superficial skin loss, or shallow cratering
- Stage 3 – full-thickness skin loss with subcutaneous tissue involvement, but no fascial disruption
- Stage 4 – involvement of deep structures (muscle, bone, tendon, etc.)

Stage 1 sores can develop within an hour, and improve quickly by simply relieving pressure on the tissue. Stage 2 sores can develop within hours, and can be managed medically with offloading of pressure, topical dressings, and meticulous wound care. Stage 3 and 4 sores often require serial surgical debridement, and may benefit from surgical flap coverage. However, success of flaps for pressure sores is poor, with recurrence in some studies greater than 80%. In recent years, negative pressure dressing technologies have proven to be an effective tool in pressure sore management. After adequate surgical debridement and clearing of any local infection, a negative pressure dressing can keep the wound clean, reduce buildup of exudate, and enhance wound contraction.

Because pressure sores are difficult to treat and frequently recur, prevention is the key to management. High risk patients should be identified early using risk-assessment tools such as the Braden Scale. These patients should be turned frequently and even placed on special beds that passively or actively redistribute weight.

Summary

- Pressure sores occur with focused, prolonged pressure, especially over bony prominences on the posterior aspect of the body.
- Stage 1 sores are erythematous without skin disruption, stage 2 sores have superficial skin disruption, stage 3 sores involve full thickness skin loss, and stage 4 sores involve deep structures.
- Treatment of all pressure sores includes offloading of pressure, topical dressings, meticulous wound care, and minimizing risk factors. Advanced sores may require surgical debridement or flap coverage.
- Flap coverage of pressure sores may be indicated in select situations, but results are generally poor.
- Prevention is the key to management of pressure sores.

III.B. Burns

1. Classification

Burns are classified as first, second, or third degree; some classifications include fourth degree as well. First degree (superficial) burns are epidermal burns that are painful and erythematous but without blistering. Most sunburns are first degree burns.

Second degree (partial thickness) burns involve the dermis and form blisters. They are further divided into superficial burns involving the papillary dermis and deep burns involving the reticular dermis. The former is painful and demonstrates blanching erythema with intact hair follicles and other appendages, whereas the latter tends to be pale and associated with loss of hair follicles and appendages. Decreased sensation may result from deep second degree burns.

Third degree (full thickness) burns penetrate both the epidermis and dermis to involve the subcutaneous fat and other tissues. These burns are typically pale and leathery with notable sensory loss. Fourth degree burns involve bone or muscle.

In addition to the depth of burns, it is important to convey the size of burns as a percentage of the total body surface area (% TBSA). This can be estimated in adults using the "rule of 9s." It can also be estimated by noting that in an adult, the palm is approximately 1% TBSA. Note that children age 7 or younger have significantly different proportions.

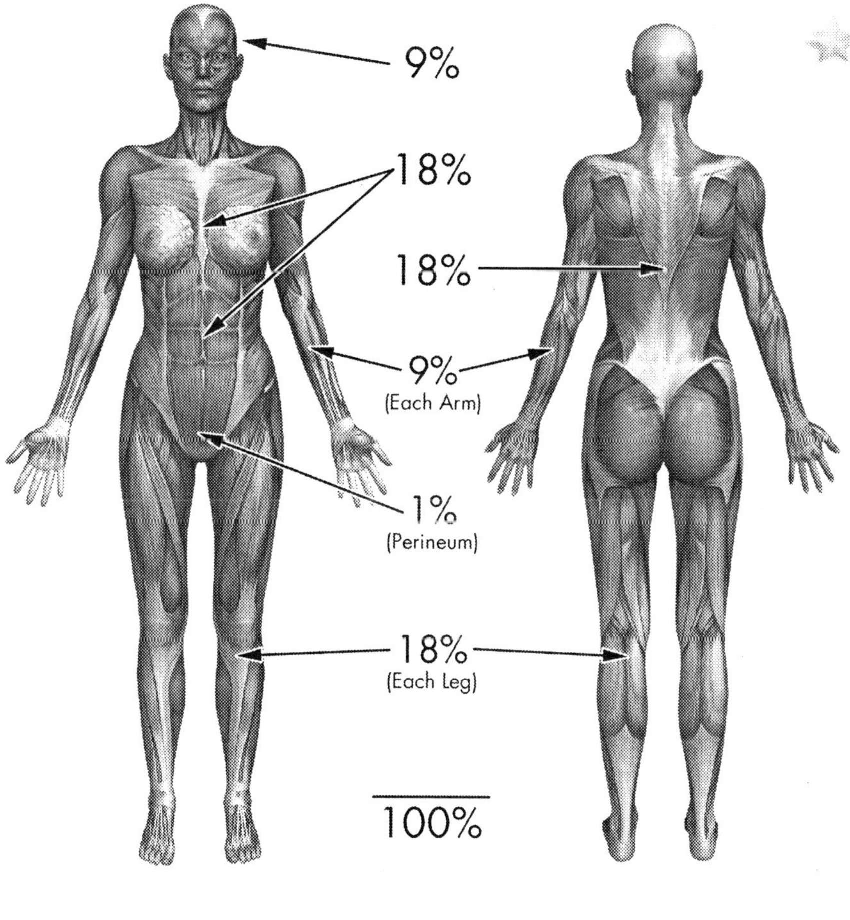

2. Inhalational Injury

Burns sustained in a closed space, facial burns, singed nose hairs, carbonaceous material in the airway, or respiratory symptoms should raise concern for potential airway compromise. These injuries result from smoke particles and components, not from heat. Arterial blood gas, carboxyhemoglobin, and carbon monoxide levels should be checked. Expedient intubation should be considered in the event of respiratory distress, and bronchoscopy should be pursued in that case. Steroids have not been shown to have any advantage in early management. Pneumonia is the most common infection in burn patients and also the most common cause of death after inhalation injury.

3. Admission Criteria

The following indications prompt transfer and admission to a burn center:

- Second degree burns > 10% TBSA in patients < 10 or > 50 years old
- Second degree burns > 20% TBSA
- Third degree burns > 5% TBSA
- Burns involving the face, hands, feet, genitalia, perineum, or major joints
- Electrical, chemical, and lightning burns
- Inhalation injury
- Significant comorbidities
- Suspected child abuse or neglect

4. Fluid Resuscitation

Significant burns (≥ approximately 20% TBSA) result in massive fluid loss from the burn surface and can lead to shock. Fluid resuscitation is paramount, but excessive fluids may worsen the prognosis. The fluid requirement for the first 24 hours can be estimated using the Parkland formula:

$$\text{Volume} = \%\text{TBSA} \times 4\ \text{cc/kg}$$

Half of this volume in lactated Ringer's solution is given during the first 8 hours, and the other half over the next 16 hours. The fluid infusion timing should be started from when the burn occurred, but boluses should be avoided.

The amount of fluid necessary is dictated by the patient's urine output; the Parkland formula serves as a guide for initial therapy only. Normal urine output for a young child with burns is 1-2 cc/kg/hr. Adults should make about 0.5-1 cc/kg/hr. Heart rate and systemic vascular resistance initially increase due to release of catecholamines but cardiac output initially decreases.

5. Acute Treatment

Early excision down to well-vascularized tissue with the goal of minimizing necrotic tissue mass to prevent infection is key in the acute management of deep second degree and third degree burns. In the absence of infection, these acute wounds can be covered with autografts, although cadaveric skin, xenografts, and dermal substitutes may be used for temporary coverage. Septic or unstable patients may not be candidates for early coverage.

Escharotomy is indicated for circumferential third and deep second degree burns. Around the abdomen, these burns may lead to abdominal compartment syndrome and subsequent intra-abdominal organ failure. Around the chest, they may result in respiratory distress with ventilatory difficulty. In the extremities, they may cause compartment syndrome leading to acute limb ischemia.

Pseudomonas is the most common cause of burn infections, followed by Staphylococcus, E. coli, and Enterobacter. However, prophylactic systemic antibiotics are not indicated in the acute management of burns. Topical agents with antimicrobial action can decrease the risk of developing burn wound infections.

Silver sulfadiazine (Silvadene) is useful, but has limited eschar penetration and may not be effective against Pseudomonas and other gram negative rods. Silvadene can cause a self-limited neutropenia and thrombocytopenia.

Mafenide sodium (Sulfamylon) has good eschar and cartilage penetration, and is effective against Pseudomonas and other gram negative rods. However, it tends to be painful and may lead to metabolic acidosis due to carbonic anhydrase inhibition. Bacitracin can be used in areas such as the face.

Early enteral feeding is encouraged to decrease gut bacterial translocation and is preferred over TPN. Burn patients have increased metabolic demands and thus need increased caloric and protein requirements. The Curreri formula estimates calorie requirements for burn patients and is 25 kcal/kg/day + 40 kcal/% TBSA/day. Protein requirements vary from 1-2 g/kg/day. The Curreri formula may overestimate calorie needs.

6. Child Abuse

Up to 15% of burn injuries in children result from child abuse. Delayed presentation, conflicting stories, and recurrent injuries and burns should prompt further investigation. Potential markers of child abuse include sharp burn margins, uniform depth in splash injuries, sparing of flexor surfaces, burns on the dorsal aspect of the hands, and very deep contact burn injuries.

7. Chemical Burns

Acid burns cause coagulation tissue necrosis, whereas alkali burns result in deeper burns from liquefactive necrosis. Both should be managed with generous irrigation. Hydrofluoric acid burns should be treated with topical calcium gel or intradermal calcium gluconate. Tar burns should be cooled, then removed using a lipophilic solvent. Dry powder should be brushed off prior to irrigating with water. Liquid chemical burns should be washed in water.

8. Electrical Burns

Electrical burns and lightning strikes can result in acute cardiopulmonary complications. These injuries can be deeper and more severe than the external wounds may suggest. Deep muscle burns can result in rhabdomyolysis and compartment syndrome. Electrical burns can damage deep structures such as nerves and the spinal cord, bowel, and brain.

Electrical current enters at the point of contact and leaves at the grounded area traversing through tissues of least resistance which are usually muscles, nerves and blood vessels. Cardiac arrhythmias are common and need close monitoring. Electrical burns require a higher urine output due to concomitant myoglobinuria. A target urine output of 2 cc/kg/hr should be achieved. Intravenous sodium bicarbonate to alkalinize the urine should be given.

III.C. Other Burn-Like Conditions

1. Toxic Epidermal Necrolysis

Toxic epidermal necrolysis (TEN) results in disruption of the epidermal-dermal interface. It can be caused by viruses and bacteria such as S. aureus, as well as various drugs including Dilantin and Bactrim. Patients should be treated with systemic antibiotics if the cause is bacterial; otherwise, they are treated with topical antimicrobials and similar to patients with thermal burns: early excision and grafting of affected surfaces.

2. Stevens-Johnson Syndrome

Stevens-Johnson syndrome, or erythema multiforme, is a severe form of TEN. It is a hypersensitivity reaction that results in the formation of bullae at the epidermal-dermal interface and epidermal necrosis. Treatment is similar to TEN. Steroids are contraindicated in both conditions.

3. Brown Recluse Spider Bite

Brown recluse spider bites may lead to DIC and death. Supportive care is necessary, and dapsone is used in proven bites. Focal but extensive necrosis can occur; resection is completed after the are is permitted to demarcate.

Summary

- Burns are first degree (superficial), second degree (partial thickness) involving part of the dermal layer, or third degree (full thickness) involving the entire dermal layer.
- Burn size as % TBSA may be estimated by using the "rule of 9s."
- Inhalation injury should be suspected in the case of burns sustained in a closed space, facial burns, singed nose hairs, carbonaceous material in the nostrils or mouth, or respiratory symptoms.
- Fluid resuscitation is approximated by the Parkland formula and guided by urine output.
- Acute treatment of burns includes topical antimicrobials, early excision and grafting, and escharotomy for circumferential third degree & deep second degree burns. Prophylactic antibiotics are not indicated.
- Electrical burns can be more severe and damage deeper tissue than external wounds may suggest.

ORTHOPAEDICS

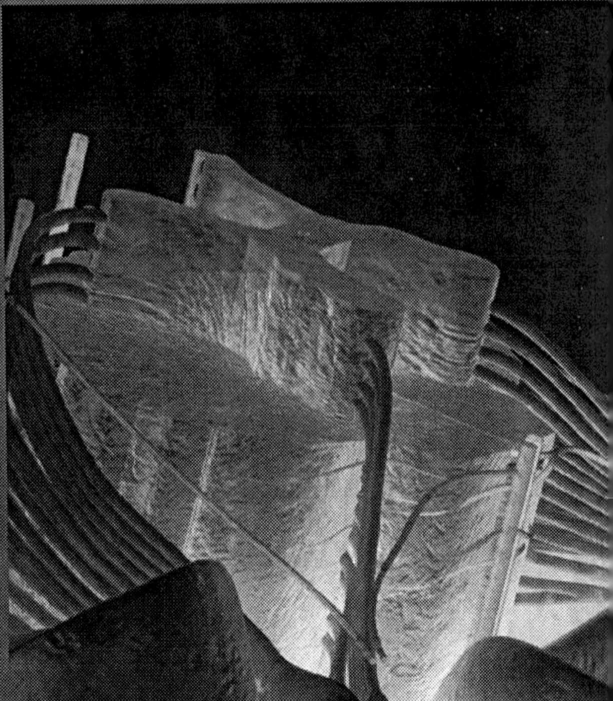

If you can't pin it or cast it - then screw it.

Motto

SURGISPHERE

ORTHOPAEDIC SURGERY

Stephanie Mayer, M.D., William Eward, D.V.M., M.D., and Jocelyn Wittstein, M.D.

I. General Concepts

I.A. Overview

A sound understanding of the basic principles of orthopedic surgery as they apply to the practice of general surgery is required. The most high-yield sections are the basic science principles and orthopedic trauma.

I.B. Bone Healing

1. Stage 1 – Inflammation

Fractures disrupt the blood supply to the endosteum and periosteum. A hematoma forms from increased flow to the area induced by vasoactive mediators. This flow also transports inflammatory cells to the fracture site. Fibroblasts are activated and produce collagen at the site.

2. Stage 2 – Repair

A soft callus forms between days 5-21. Revascularization carries additional progenitor cells to the site, which differentiate based on stress and oxygen conditions at the fracture. A fibrocartilagenous callus stabilizes the fracture, and as the cartilage matrix calcifies and progenitor cells develop into osteoblasts, new bone is formed. This is endochondral bone formation.

3. Stage 3 – Remodeling

In response to mechanical loading stresses on the fracture, osteoclasts resorb the immature woven bone while osteoblasts deposit mature lamellar bone in its place. Steroids, nicotine, chemotherapeutic drugs, diabetes, and NSAIDS adversely affect bone healing.

I.C. Neurologic Examination

Sensory	Motor	Reflex
C5: lateral shoulder, forearm	Deltoid	Biceps
C6: thumb, index finger	Biceps, wrist ext	Brachioradialis
C7: index, middle, ring	Triceps, finger extensors	Triceps
C8: ring, small fingers	Finger flexors	
T1: medial forearm	Interossei	
L4: distal/posteromedial leg	Quadriceps, tibialis anterior	Knee jerk
L5: dorsum and medial foot	Extensor hallucis longus	
S1: plantar lateral foot	Gastrocnemius	Ankle jerk

I.D. Disc Herniation

Herniation of the nucleus pulposus or annulus fibrosus may present with radicular pain as a function of the particular nerve root that becomes compressed.

I.E. Nerve Injury

Nerve injury takes one of three forms, depending on the extent of damage. Neuropraxia occurs secondary to blunt trauma to the nerve leading to infrafascicular edema and disruption of conduction. There is no direct injury to the sheath or axons. Neuropraxia presents with paresthesias with spontaneous recovery within 2 months.

Axontmesis is secondary to blunt trauma to the nerve leading to infrafascicular edema and axonal degeneration. There is no injury to the sheath. Axontmesis presents with disrupted conduction and symptoms of anesthesia and paresthesia. As the axon regenerates, anesthesia disappears. There is typically full recovery within 4 months.

Neurotmesis is secondary to blunt or shear trauma to the nerve or nerve root causing damage to connective tissue surrounding the axon with disruption of the sheath and axon. Neurotmesis causes immediate anesthesia

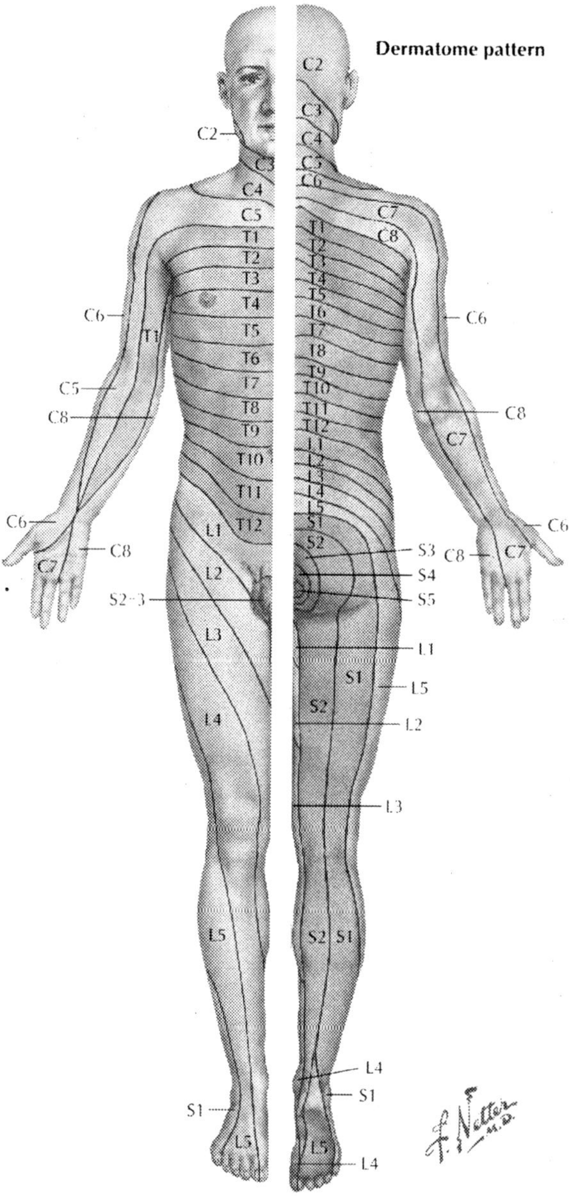

Levels of principal dermatomes

C5	Clavicles
C5, 6, 7	Lateral parts of upper limbs
C8; T1	Medial sides of upper limbs
C6	Thumb
C6, 7, 8	Hand
C8	Ring and little fingers
T4	Level of nipples
T10	Level of umbilicus
T12	Inguinal or groin regions
L1, 2, 3, 4	Anterior and inner surfaces of lower limbs
L4, 5; S1	Foot
L4	Medial side of great toe
L5; S1, 2	Outer and posterior sides of lower limbs
S1	Lateral margin of foot and little toe
S2, 3, 4	Perineum

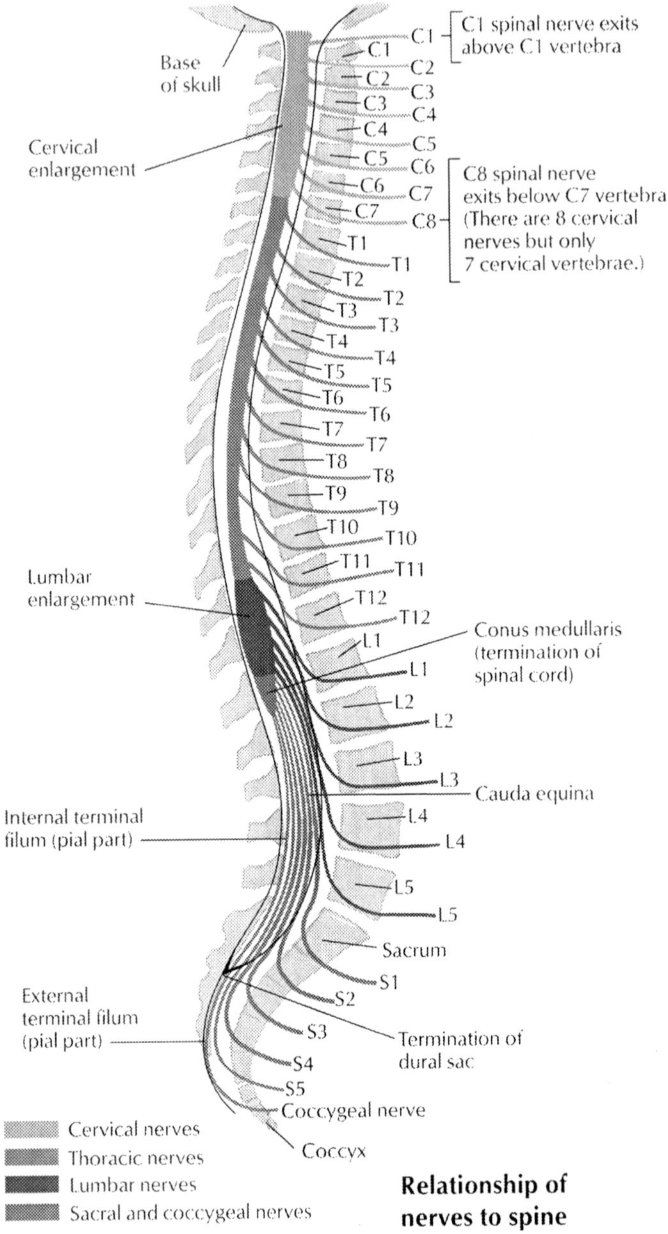

Relationship of nerves to spine

with the potential for paresthesia and resumption of function. However, the disruption of the sheath may prevent appropriate apposition of nerve fibers and lead to hyperesthesia and allodynia, or even neuroma formation.

II. Infectious and Inflammatory Disorders

II.A. Inflamed Joints

Red, warm, and painful joints should be aspirated under sterile conditions and the fluid sent for gram stain, culture and sensitivity, cell count, and crystal studies.

Based on these results, the etiology of the inflamed joint can be ascertained and permit the appropriate therapeutic response. Common findings for the cell count are below:

- Normal: 60-180
- Non-inflammatory: < 2,000
- Traumatic: 2,000-5,000
- Inflammatory: 15,000-80,000
- Septic arthritis: > 80,000

II.B. Osteoporosis

Osteoporosis is defined as a bone mineral density below 2.5 standard deviations of the young adult mean on dual energy x-ray absorbtiometry (DEXA). Postmenopausal women and older men are most commonly affected and people of European descent are at the highest risk. Osteoporosis is associated with an increased risk of fracture after low-energy injury, especially to the hip, vertebrae, and distal radius.

II.C. Osteoarthritis

Symptoms of osteoarthritis include asymmetrical joint involvement, short duration morning stiffness (compared to rheumatoid arthritis), and pain that worsens with activity. Subchondral sclerosis and cysts are seen on plain films and may involve the DIP joint. Osteoarthritis is initially treated with Tylenol and other NSAIDS. Many patients will fail this conservative therapy and will require joint replacement.

II.D. Rheumatoid Arthritis

Rheumatoid arthritis presents with symmetrical joint involvement, morning stiffness lasting longer than one hour, and relief from pain with progressive use of the extremity. Joint erosions are evident on plain films due to the inflammatory pannus formed at the synovium. Rheumatoid arthritis spares the DIP joint. First line therapy is with NSAIDS, prednisone, ASA, and DMARDS; second line agents include azathioprine, methotrexate, cyclophosphamide, inflixamab, and antimalarials. Failing these medications, hydroxychloroquine may be used.

II.E. Gout

Gouty arthritis is the result of monosodium urate crystal deposition within joints resulting in cyclic inflammation and pain. The first MTP (metatarsophalangeal) joint is most commonly affected. Monosodium urate crystals are negatively birefringent on polarized microscopic examination, which differentiates this disorder from pseudogout. Gouty arthritis is associated with alcoholism, obesity, and increased protein intake. With chronic disease, one may see erosions with sclerotic borders on plain radiographs. Gout may mimic a septic joint and arthrocentesis is essential for a definitive diagnosis. Acute gout is treated with NSAIDS (indomethacin) and intra-articular steroid injection. Maintenance therapy is achieved with colchicine and allopurinol.

II.F. Pseudogout

Pseudogout presents similar to gout or septic arthritis with pain and inflammation being the hallmark findings. However, pseudogout is the result of calcium pyrophosphate crystal deposition within joints. These crystals are positively birefringent on polarized microscopic examination. Pseudogout most commonly affects the knee and wrist. Treatment is with NSAIDS.

II.G. Septic Arthritis

Septic arthritis must be diagnosed and treated urgently. Without the benefit of arthrocentesis for gram stain and microscopic crystal exam, septic arthritis may be clinically indistinguishable from gouty arthritis (or pseudogout). Septic arthritis is treated with irrigation and debridement of the synovium and IV antibiotics. The exception to this is gonococcal arthritis, which responds well to ceftriaxone alone.

Key bacteriology points:

- Staphylococcus – most common pathogen
- Streptococcus – prompts evaluation for multiple myeloma
- Neisseria gonococcus – most common in young adults

II.H. Osteomyelitis

Up to 20% of osteomyelitis cases are due to hematogenous seeding of the bone. Osteomyelitisis also seen with direct contamination from trauma, surgery, or spread from adjacent infected soft tissues. Direct contamination most commonly occurs in vertebrae. Staphylococcus aureus is the most common pathogen, Pseudomonas is common in IV drug users, and gram negative rods, anaerobes, Streptococcus, and Enterococcus are common in diabetics with peripheral vascular disease. Salmonella may be a cause in sickle cell patients, but S. aureus is still more common.

Radiographic changes usually take at least 2 weeks to appear on plain films, but MRI and bone scan are more sensitive imaging tests. Osteomyelitis is treated with debridement and IV antibiotics for at least 6 weeks.

III. Trauma

III.A. Compartment Syndrome

1. Etiology and Pathophysiology

Compartment syndrome is a surgical emergency that requires immediate decompression of the affected compartment to prevent irreversible neuromuscular damage. It is the result of elevated interstitial pressure within closed fascial compartments following trauma, vascular insult/revascularization, chemotherapy, or surgery. It is commonly seen following crush injuries, tibial fractures, and reperfusion of dysvascular limbs.

2. Diagnosis and Treatment

Symptoms of compartment syndrome include the 5 P's: PAIN, pallor, paresthesias, pulselessness, and paralysis. Pressures should be measured in all compartments of the affected limb. Classically, intracompartmental pressure > 30 mmHg indicates compartment syndrome. More recent studies recommend measuring DBP and compartment pressure (CP). If DBP – CP is less than 30, then compartment syndrome is likely.

Fasciotomy of all compartments of the affected limb Is required to avoid ischemia and necrosis.

III.B. Fractures

1. Open Fractures

Open fractures should be washed out at the bedside immediately, and debrided in the operating room as soon as the patient will tolerate surgery. Historically, debridement has been completed prior to definitive fixation, but recent evidence suggests that there is no difference in outcome if thorough debridement and definitive fixation are achieved in a single procedure.

2. Gustilo-Anderson Classification

Type 1

- Open wound < 1 cm, clean wound, and minimal soft tissue injury

Type 2

- Open wound 1-10 cm, moderate contamination, moderate soft tissue injury

Type 3

- Open wound > 10 cm, contaminated, crush injury/comminuted fracture, soft tissue closure possible
- Open wound > 10 cm, contaminated, crush injury/comminuted fracture, flap coverage needed
- Open wound > 10 cm, contaminated, crush injury/comminuted fracture, vascular injury

Delay in antibiotic therapy has been shown to increase the risk of infection. Type 1 and 2 fractures should receive a first generation cephalosporin. Type 3 fractures should receive a first generation cephalosporin and aminoglycoside. The presence of organic contamination should also be treated with penicillin. All open fractures need tetanus prophylaxis.

3. Spine

a) Overview

A trauma patient with a normal CT of the spine but with motor or sensory deficits should get an MRI to rule out ligamentous injury, disc protrusion, and vascular compromise.

b) Jefferson Fracture

A Jefferson fracture is a C1 fracture with 3 or 4 fracture lines causing anterior and posterior arch and lateral mass displacement.

c) Hangman's Fracture

Hangman's fracture is a bilateral C2 pars articularis fracture with C2 spondylolisthesis, often presenting with cord compromise. Nondisplaced fractures are treated with a Miami J collar. Displaced fractures require halo-vest fixation due to joint instability. Displaced fractures with jumped facets require halo traction for reduction followed by C2-3 posterior fusion for definitive treatment.

d) Dens Fractures

Dens fractures are separated into three types. Type 1 fractures occur at the tip and are treated with a Miami J collar. Type 2 fractures occur at the waist and require a halo-vest, ORIF, or posterior C1-2 fusion. Nonoperative treatment of type 2 fractures has a high rate of nonunion from disruption of the vascular supply. Type 3 fractures occur at the base and require a halo-vest.

e) Burst Fracture

Burst fractures through the anterior and middle columns of the thoracic or lumbar bodies are due to axial load and endplate disruption. These are generally treated nonoperatively unless kyphosis is greater than 30 degrees, height loss is greater than 40%, canal compromise is greater than 50%, or there is an associated neurologic deficit.

f) Chance Fracture

Chance fractures are high energy fractures through all three columns of the thoracic or lumbar spine. These are unstable; one must look for injury to surrounding structures. These fractures are associated with a high risk of concomitant intra-abdominal injury. While Chance fractures may be treated in a TLSO, they are often require instrumented spinal fusion.

4. Clavicle

Look for pneumothorax, neurovascular compromise, or skin tenting if a clavicular fracture is suspected. Most clavicular fractures are treated non-operatively in a sling. Indications for operative repair include pneumothorax, neurovascular compromise, open fractures, severely displaced fragments, polytrauma, impending skin breakdown, or greater than 2 cm of shortening.

5. Humerus

Beware of radial nerve compromise with midshaft fractures of the humerus. Humerus fractures are often treated non-operatively via reduction and cast placement. Supracondylar fractures of the humerus may have entrapment of the median nerve and brachial artery. These are treated non-operatively if nondisplaced, or percutaneously pinned if displaced. Volkmann's ischemic contracture of the forearm is caused by anterior interosseous artery compromise leading to forearm compartment syndrome, deep flexor atrophy, and contracture.

6. Distal Radius

Colles' fracture is the most common fracture pattern of the distal radius and occurs at the cortico-cancellous junction. Median nerve function must be evaluated, as acute carpal tunnel syndrome can occur. Distal radius fractures are treated with elective ORIF unless there is evidence of neurovascular compromise.

7. Pelvis

Pelvic trauma can lead to acute blood loss exceeding 1 L. If an unstable fracture pattern is identified with hypotension, immediate attenuation of the injury with a pelvic binder or sheet binder is necessary. Rectal and genital examination should be performed to assess for open fractures or urologic injury. A retrograde urethrogram should be obtained if there is suspicion for urethral injury; foley catheter placement is contraindicated until the patency of the urethral tract is confirmed. Embolize bleeding pelvic vessels in patients who are hemodynamically unstable with a binder in place; open operating intervention is a distant second option and instituted only if coil embolization fails. External fixation may be required in some cases to stop blood loss. ORIF is performed when the patient is hemodynamically stable.

8. Femoral Neck

Fractures of the femoral neck constitute a surgical emergency in the young patient due to the risk of avascular necrosis and debilitating arthrosis from compromise of the femoral head blood supply. These fractures may be percutaneously pinned or undergo ORIF. Older patients are often treated with hemiarthroplasty or total hip arthroplasty.

9. Femoral Shaft

Femoral shaft fractures may be associated with unrecognized blood loss up to 3 L into the thigh. Plain films from the hip to the knee should be obtained to look for associated femoral neck fractures, which occur 10% of the time and are frequently subclinical. Fat embolism syndrome may occur either from the fracture or from the ORIF. Treatment includes skeletal traction until definitive fixation with intramedullary nail placement may be performed.

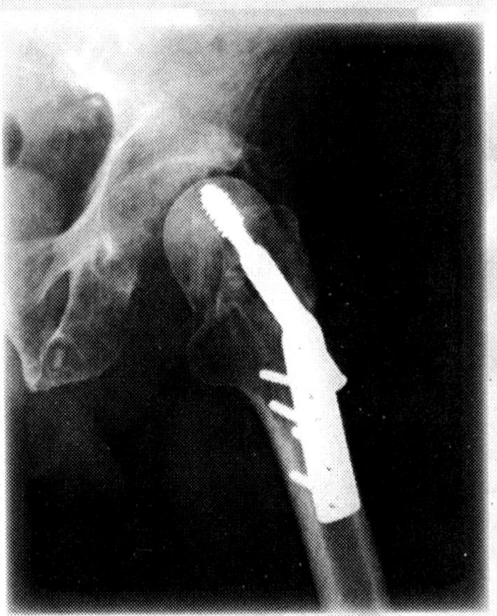

10. Tibia

This is the most common open fracture due to a thin soft tissue envelope anteriorly that is unable to contain the fragmented bone. Flap coverage is often required. Treatment includes ORIF, typically with an intramedullary nail. Tibial fractures are associated with a high risk of compartment syndrome.

11. Ankle

Ankle fractures are common. Immediate treatment includes reduction and splint fixation with documentation of a baseline neurovascular exam. ORIF

SURGISPHERE

is performed when the swelling decreases, typically by 7-14 days. Careful wound management is necessary.

12. Other Fractures

A Monteggia fracture is a proximal ulnar fracture and radial head dislocation. These require ORIF of the ulna. Galleazzi fractures are radial shaft and distal radioulnar joint disruption. These require ORIF of the radius.

III.C. Dislocations

Glenohumeral

- Anterior dislocation most common
- Look for axillary nerve injury

Hip

- Urgent relocation to prevent femoral head vascular disruption

Knee

- Urgent relocation
- Document thorough pulse exam before and after reduction.
- Consider arteriogram if ankle brachial index is 0.9 or less.
- Peroneal nerve injuries are common

III.D. Pediatric Trauma

A slipped capital femoral epiphysis (SCFE) predominantly affects teenaged, overweight boys. SCFE presents with knee pain and a quarter of patients may exhibit bilateral involvement. Treatment is with percutaneous pinning.

Osgood Schlatter lesions are avulsion of the tibial tuberosity at the insertion of the patellar tendon. It affects adolescent males and is due to overuse. Knee pain is worse with palpation of the anterior tibia and with climbing stairs. Treatment is rest and avoiding stress on the affected patellar tendon.

Legg-Calve-Perthes disease is avascular necrosis of the femoral head secondary to poor vascularization. This defect may be self-limiting or lead to collapse with concomitant knee pain and limping. Males are affected more than females. Treatment is with abduction bracing or surgery to restore the anatomic angle at the femoral head and neck.

IV. Orthopaedic Oncology

IV.A. General Principles

The most common bony lesion is secondary metastasis from breast, lung, thyroid, kidney, and prostate cancers. Bone biopsy should be performed by the surgeon who will perform the definitive resection and reconstruction to ensure that the entire biopsy tract is resected in the event of malignancy.

With regard to soft tissue masses, sarcomas typically occur within fascial compartments. They are rapidly growing. Any mass greater than 5 cm and deep to a fascial plane should prompt concern for sarcoma. Unlike carcinomas, sarcomas rarely metastasize to the lymphatic system. The most common site of metastasis is the lungs.

IV.B. Osteosarcoma

Osteosarcoma is the most common malignant primary tumor of bone. It occurs most commonly in the second decade of life with a second peak of occurrence in the elderly; it affects males more than females. Osteosarcoma occurs "away from the elbow and toward the knee" – signifying that the distal femur, proximal tibial, proximal humerus, and distal radius are the most common sites of occurrence.

Osteosarcoma leads to elevated alkaline phosphatase and LDH on laboratory analysis, a classic sunburst pattern (periosteal reaction seen on radiographs), and night pain. Treatment involves neoadjuvant chemotherapy followed by surgery. Survival rates are currently 80% with local control and no metastasis.

IV.C. Ewing's Sarcoma

Ewing's sarcoma is the second most common malignant primary tumor of bone and is more common in children. It involves a chromosomal translocation t(11:22) and affects males more than females between the ages of 5 and 30. This tumor affects the diaphyseal region of long bones and appears as small round blue cells on histology and may mimic osteomyelitis. A bone marrow biopsy is part of the diagnostic workup due to metastasis within the marrow. Treatment includes neoadjuvant chemotherapy and surgery. Unlike many sarcomas, Ewing's sarcoma responds to radiation therapy.

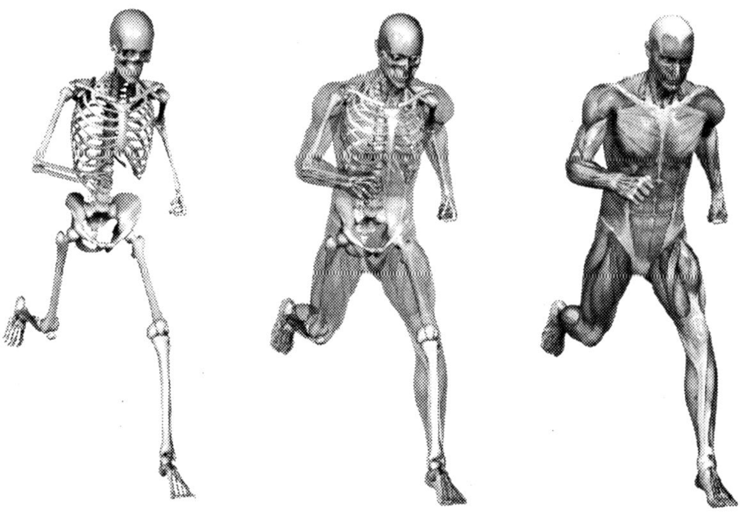

UROLOGY & GYNECOLOGY

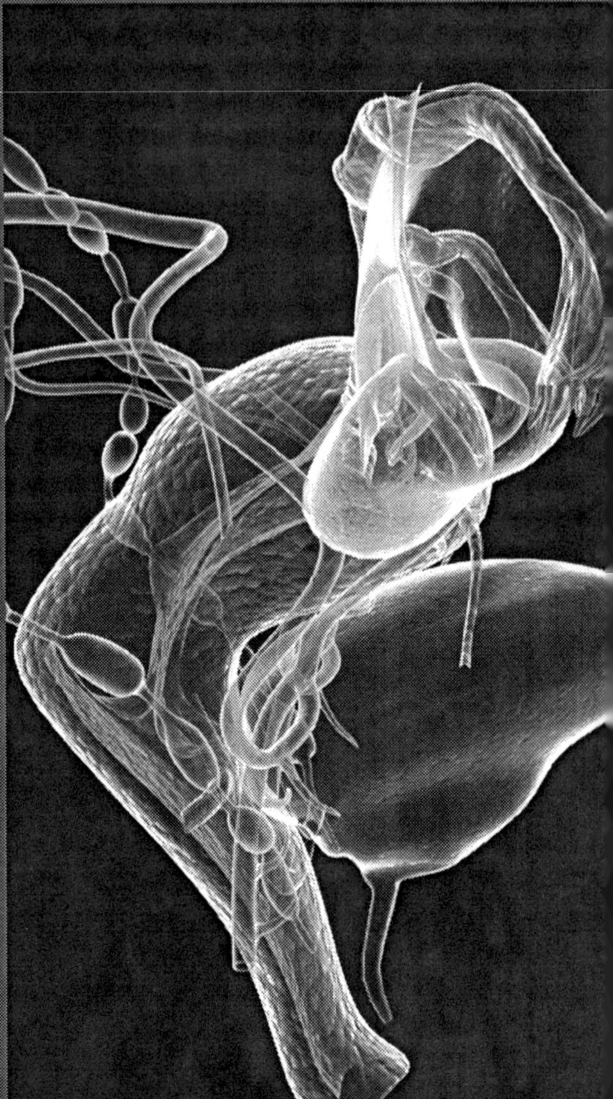

Honour hath no skill in surgery, then? No. What is honour? A word.

William Shakespeare
Henry IV, 1596

SURGISPHERE

UROLOGY & GYNECOLOGY

Suzanne Stewart, M.D., and Amahuaro Edebiri, M.D.

I. Introduction

A variety of concepts in urology and gynecology are tested on the surgery board exam and ABSITE. In addition, basic knowledge of various diseases in these two fields is mandatory for the general surgeon, not only because these diseases should be on the differential diagnosis for abdominal and pelvic pain, but also because we may be called to assist our colleagues in complex cases. Many of these diseases spread to the thoracic and abdominal organs and a multidisciplinary approach is necessary for satisfactory patient treatment. While a variety of disorders are discussed below, an attempt is made to focus the reader to the most commonly tested topics.

II. Urology

II.A. Structural and Congenital Disease

1. Testicular Torsion

a) Presentation and Diagnosis

Testicular torsion is a urologic emergency. There are two types of testicular torsion: extravaginal and intravaginal. Extravaginal torsion occurs exclusively in neonates and results when the spermatic cord and tunica vaginalis torse as a unit. Intravaginal torsion marks the remainder of the cases and occurs when there is torsion of the spermatic cord within the tunica vaginalis. Both types result in obstruction of the venous and arterial flow to the testis and can ultimately lead to ischemic necrosis.

Torsion is most common in males 12-18 years, but can occur at any age. Patients typically complain of acute onset testicular pain and/or swelling. Physical exam findings may include an exquisitely tender, firm, and high-riding testicle with horizontal lie, absent cremasteric reflex, no pain relief on elevation of the scrotum, and an anterior lie of the epididymis. The diagnosis is made by clinical suspicion, however, Doppler testicular ultrasound can be used to confirm the diagnosis. In testicular torsion, Doppler ultrasound will show no arterial/venous flow compared to the contralateral testis.

b) Treatment

If testicular torsion is suspected, immediate surgical exploration is indicated. Most testicles are salvaged if they are detorsed within 6 hours of onset of symptoms. During exploration, the testis is detorsed and if reperfusion occurs, orchiopexy is performed. If the testicle is found to be unsalvageable, then orchiectomy is completed. Orchiopexy of the contralateral testicle should always be performed as there is increased risk of torsion in the contralateral testis.

2. Urolithiasis

a) Etiology and Pathophysiology

The prevalence of stone formation in the urinary tract is 2-3%. Peak incidence occurs between the ages of 20 and 40. The most common stone in industrialized countries is calcium oxalate. Other common types include uric acid, magnesium ammonium phosphate (struvite), and cystine stones. Ninety percent of stones are radio-opaque and can be detected on plain X-rays or non-contrasted CT. Pure uric acid stones are radiolucent and can only be detected by intravenous pyelogram. However, uric acid stones tend to have calcium depositions allowing them to be detected by normal methods.

The key event in stone formation is supersaturation in the urine followed by crystallization in the kidney. Common etiologies include urinary obstruction/stasis, dehydration, metabolic causes such as hypercalciuria, hypocitraturia, hyperoxaluria, and hyperuricosuria, as well as disease states such as inflammatory bowel disease, type I renal tubular acidosis, sarcoidosis, hyperparathyroidism, cystinuria and urinary tract infections. Struvite stones uniquely originate from infection by urea-splitting organisms such as Proteus, Pseudomonas, Klebsiella and Providencia. Proteus is the most common agent. The ammonia produced from the splitting of urea creates an alkaline medium conducive to the precipitation of the triple phosphate crystals. Struvite stones typically form a cast of the renal pelvis creating what has become known as a staghorn calculus.

b) Presentation and Diagnosis

Symptoms include colicky flank or abdominal pain at the location of the stone in the collecting system. The pain is sometimes described as radiating down into the groin or scrotum. Patients may also have nausea, vomiting, urinary frequency, urgency or hematuria. Fever is not usually present unless the urine is infected.

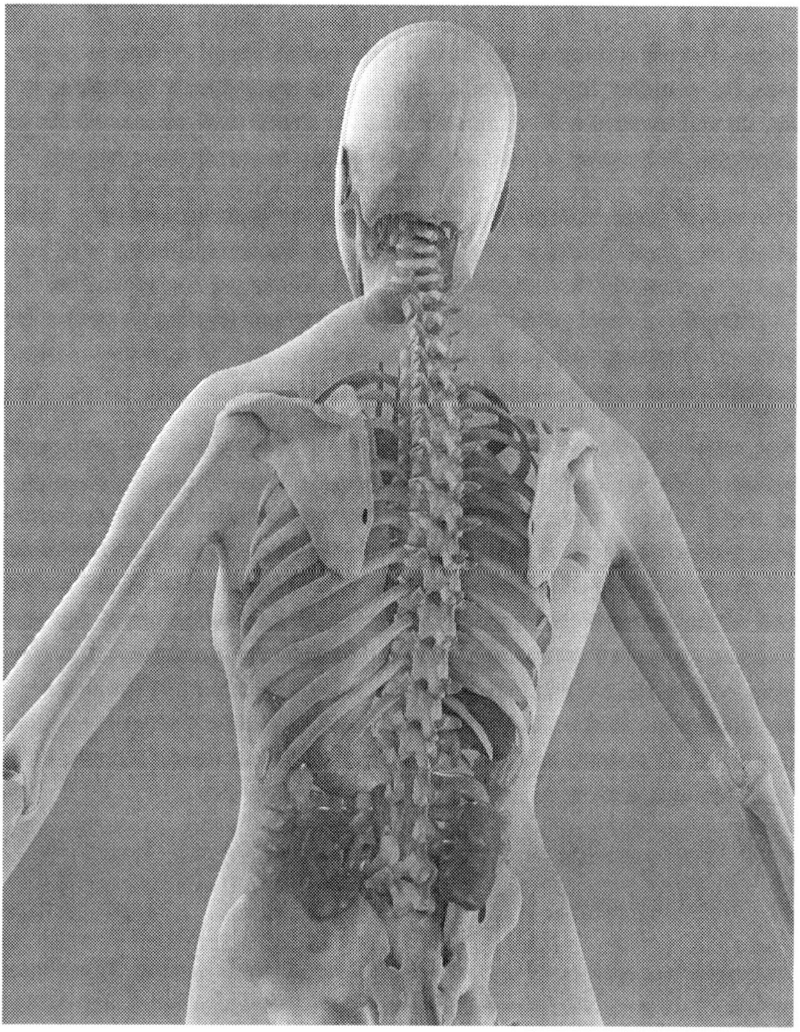

WBC, creatinine, urinalysis and culture should be performed during the initial evaluation. These laboratory studies help to stratify potential risk of infection and obstruction. A non-contrasted CT of the abdomen/pelvis is now the preferred imaging study for diagnosis of urolithiasis. This study can more accurately determine the location, size and potential concomitant obstructive factors, such as hydronephrosis or hydroureter.

c) Treatment

Stones that are < 5mm in size have a high probability of spontaneous passage. Patients that have stones of this size are treated with hydration, analgesia and ureteral smooth muscle relaxing agents such as tamsulosin or nifedipine. Reimaging is necessary in this group to ensure stone passage.

Removal of large ureteral stones can occur via ureteroscopy using laser lithotripsy. Renal pelvic or calyceal stones are frequently treated with percutaneous nephrolithotomy using ultrasonic lithotripsy. Depending on the location of the renal pelvic stone, ureteroscopy may also be an option for removal. Extracorporal shockwave lithotripsy can also be used for proximal ureteral stones as well as renal pelvic/calyceal stones < 2.5 cm.

A metabolic workup and stone composition analysis should be performed patients with nephrolithiasis, who may require targeted medical therapies to avoid future stone formation. For example, alkalization of the urine with potassium citrate is used in patients with uric acid and cystine stones. Allopurinol is given for excess serum uric acid production. Penicillamine and alpha mercaptopropionylglycine are used for cystine stone patients. Calcium excess in the urine can be helped by diet modifications such as limiting sodium and red meat intake. Hyperoxaluria is reduced by limiting high oxalate content food such as coffee, tea, chocolate, and leafy green vegetables. In general, all patients with ahistory of nephrolithiasis should increase their fluid intake to achieve more than 2 liters of urine per day.

3. Congenital Anomaly Of The Genital Tract

a) Assessment

Androgen insensitivity or testicular feminization syndrome (46, XY): These patients have a male karyotype but female phenotype due to an androgenic receptor gene mutation. They usually have an ectopic testis in the inguinal canal or labia. Despite the adequate amounts of androgen levels in these patients, the male external genitalia will fail to develop because of deficient androgen receptors in those sites. Consequently, the Müllerian inhibiting factor (MIF) from the testes will inhibit development of the Müllerian (paramesonephric) ducts, leading to lack of uterus, oviducts, and a blind vaginal termination. These patients have well-developed breasts from estrogen release via the adrenal glands and body fat, but present with primary amenorrhea in adolescence.

b) Management

Pelvic ultrasound and laparoscopy will identify the absence of normal ovaries or the presence of streak gonads. The testes should be sought after in an ectopic location, usually in the groin. The testes must be removed in order to prevent malignant transformation. Hormone replacement therapy with estrogen is needed to prevent osteoporosis.

4. Ambiguous Genitalia

Ambiguous genitalia are due to congenital adrenal hyperplasia. In this condition, there is a mutation in the gene responsible for the enzyme controlling the synthesis of adrenocortical hormones. Cortisol and aldosterone are not produced. The enzyme defect is mostly caused by 21α-hydroxylase, but occasionally may be due to deficiency in 11β- hydroxylase or 3β-hydroxysteroid dehydrogenase. This results in excess androgen production that stimulates the female external genitalia forming clitoromegaly and labioscrotal fusion to simulate a male phenotype (Pseudo-intersex state). The withdrawal of the feedback mechanism from cortisol to the anterior pituitary causes excess secretion of ACTH leading to adrenal hyperplasia. The lack of cortisol and aldosterone causes excess urinary sodium loss with severe dehydration and hyperkalemia. The treatment is urgent IV rehydration with normal saline, cortisol and mineralocorticoids.

II.B. Metabolic and Degenerative Disease

1. Urinary Incontinence

a) Etiology and Pathophysiology

Urinary incontinence may be either transient (reversible) or established (persistent). Common etiologies of transient incontinence can be remembered by the pneumonic DIAPPERS: delirium, infection, atrophic urethritis/vaginitis, pharmacologic, psychological, endocrine, restricted mobility, and stool impaction. Persistent incontinence may be due to a disorder of the bladder, bladder outlet, or both; subtypes include urge incontinence, stress incontinence, functional incontinence and mixed incontinence. This urologic problem can be seen in greater than 50% of patients residing in nursing homes.

b) Presentation and Diagnosis

Evaluation of incontinence can be difficult. Important aspects of the history include onset of symptoms, the degree of leakage, urgency, pelvic prolapse, and bowel function. Physical exam should include a vaginal exam for prolapse, vaginal/urethral atrophy, urethral hypermobility through performance of the cotton-tipped gauze test, and a complete neurologic exam. Office testing should include a urinalysis, evaluation of post void residual, and urodynamic studies.

c) Treatment of Total Incontinence

Total incontinence is reflected by a continuous and uninhibited loss of urine. It can result from congenital anatomic defects such as bladder exstrophy, cloacal malformations, ectopic ureters and epispadias, urinary tract fistula, or complete loss of urethral sphincter activity and tone. Treatment in this category is surgical and specific to the etiology.

d) Treatment of Stress Incontinence

Stress urinary incontinence occurs as a result of abnormal urethral closure mechanisms and loss of normal function of supporting urethral structures, such as the pelvic floor musculature. Leakage is first evident with a rise in intraabdominal pressure from sneezing, coughing or laughing. In more severe forms, stress incontinence can occur with mere changes in position. Treatment ranges from weight reduction, pelvic floor muscle exercises (Kegel maneuvers), estrogen therapy, and surgical options including bladder neck suspension and pubovaginal sling.

e) Treatment of Urge Incontinence

Urge incontinence is thought to be secondary to uninhibited detrusor contractions. These patients often have other symptoms associated with an overactive bladder, such as frequency and nocturia. Many of these patients will also have coexistent impaired detrusor contractility. Urodynamic studies show phasic increases in bladder pressure associated with involuntary loss of urine. Treatment in patients with adequate contractility consists of an initial trial of anticholinergic agents. Patients with impaired contractility and detrusor instability may require clean intermittent catheterization plus anticholinergic therapy. Other modalities for more severe symptomatology include biofeedback, neuromodulation, botulism toxin and bladder augmentation.

f) Treatment of Overflow Incontinence

Overflow incontinence can be secondary to bladder outlet obstruction or decreased detrusor contractility. These patients experience leakage of urine without the sensation of urgency, decreased force of urinary stream and feelings of incomplete emptying. High post void residuals are present. Cystoscopy and urodynamic studies differentiate between anatomic obstruction or impaired detrusor muscle function. Obstructive causes secondary to an enlarged prostate are treated with alpha adrenergic blockers and/or 5-alpha reductase inhibitors. Endoscopic procedures are necessary for urethral strictures, bladder neck contractures, and medically refractory BPH. Treatment of decreased detrusor contractility is managed with clean intermittent catheterization or suprapubic drainage.

g) Treatment of Enuresis

Nighttime incontinence (enuresis) in children is usually transient and spontaneously resolves. Without a daytime component, there is unlikely to be association with a true urologic disease. Treatment may be initiated starting at age 7 if there has not been resolution. Modalities involve behavior modification and pharmacologic therapies such as desmopressin and imipramine.

2. Benign Prostatic Hyperplasia

a) Presentation and Diagnosis

BPH is a benign neoplasm of the prostate. Hyperplastic tissue most commonly occurs at the transition zone. At age 40-50 years, 40% of all men will have BPH requiring medical or surgical management. Lower urinary tract symptoms (LUTS) resulting from BPH include decreased force of stream,

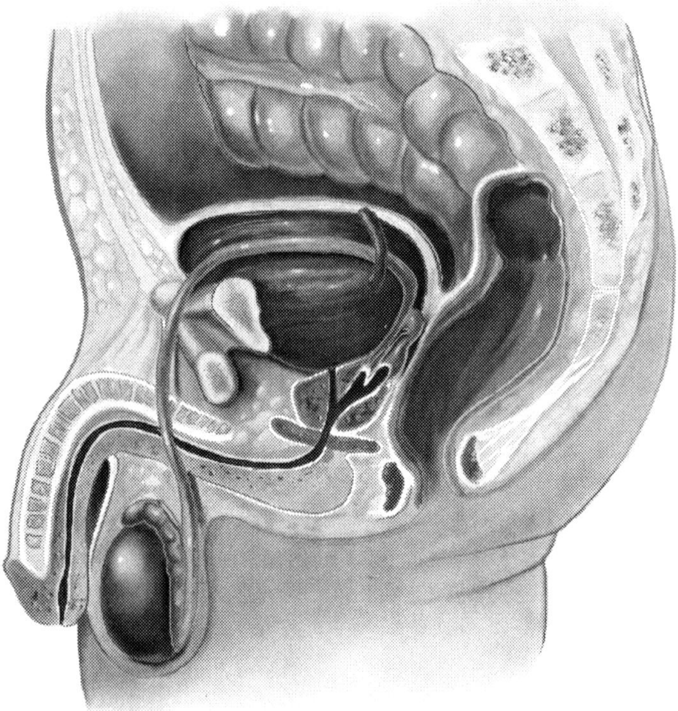

nocturia, hesitancy, intermittent stream, post-void dribbling and incomplete emptying. The severity of LUTS does not correlate with prostate size nor with the degree of bladder outlet obstruction.

Clinical interventions for BPH revolve around patient history and degree of LUTS. Quantification of the degree of LUTS is done via questionnaires and is used to direct medical versus surgical treatments. Uroflowometry, post void residual, cystoscopy and urodynamic studies are completed in preparation for surgery.

b) Treatment

Initial treatment for symptomatic patients without severe obstruction is medically with use of α-adrenergic antagonists and/or 5α-reductase inhibitors. Combination therapy inhibits the progression of BPH and is more effective than single agents. Patients with recurrent UTIs, urinary retention, gross hematuria, bladder stones, or renal insufficiency require surgical management. The most common surgical modalities include transurethral resection of the prostate (TURP) and laser ablation of the prostate. For large prostates over 80 mL in volume, open suprapubic prostatectomy is preferred.

II.C. Inflammatory and Infectious Disease

1. Urinary Tract Infection

a) Etiology and Pathophysiology

Urinary tract infection (UTI) is the second most frequent infection in people. UTIs are more common in females due to their shorter urethra: the female urethra is only 4 cm compared to the male urethra of 18-22cm. Most UTIs result from ascending infection from vaginal and bowel flora. Pyelonephritis can also occur from hematogenous spread. UTI are classified into two main categories: uncomplicated and complicated. An uncomplicated UTI is a community-acquired infection in a healthy patient with a functionally and structurally normal urinary tract. A complicated UTI is an infection that occurs in a structurally or functionally abnormal urinary tract, infection in an immunocompromised patient, or infection from virulent or resistant bacteria. UTIs are seen more often in the elderly, pregnant, diabetic and immunocompromised populations.

E. coli cause 80% and S. saprophyticus cause 10% of uncomplicated cystitis. Enterococci and other aerobic gram negative rods are responsible for the remainder of infections. Proteus and Klebsiella are urease-splitting organisms which produce ammonia that creates an alkaline medium conducive toward calculus formation. The bacterial virulence factors most relevant to UTIs are adhesions, specifically type I pili (type I fimbriae) and P pili (P fimbriae).

b) Presentation and Diagnosis

Cystitis commonly presents with an acute onset of dysuria and frequency without concomitant vaginal symptoms. Additional symptoms may include urgency, suprapubic pain, and hematuria. A diagnosis of pyelonephritis is made when cystitis occurs in conjunction with fever. These patients may also present with flank pain, nausea or vomiting. Urethritis is manifested by symptoms similar to cystitis with the addition of a purulent discharge.

Original dogma reflected that the presence of > 100,000 colony forming units (CFU)/ml was indicative of an UTI. However, modern findings indicate that > 100 CFU/ml on culture with symptoms of acute cystitis are better criteria for true infection requiring treatment. Asymptomatic bacteriuria necessitates treatment in specific patient populations: pregnant women, patients with urinary tract abnormalities, and patients who are undergoing a procedure in which the urine needs to be sterile. The presence of pyuria is identified by the presence of white blood cells on microscopy.

Failure to grow organisms on routine culture in the face of pyuria should make one suspect unusual organisms like Chlamydia, Mycoplasma, N. gonorrheae, and Mycobacterium tuberculosis. The presence of WBC casts is often seen in acute pyelonephritis. A negative urine nitrate test should not rule out bacteriuria as most strains of Streptococcus and Enterococcus cannot convert urine nitrates to nitrites.

c) Treatment

Tailor antibiotics to culture and sensitivity results. Commonly used antibiotics for uncomplicated UTIs are TMP-SMX, fluoroquinolones, or nitrofurantoin. Three days of treatment is all that is required for uncomplicated UTI. A seven day antibiotic course is recommended for females with symptoms over a week, recent UTI, men with no identifiable complicating factors, age > 65 years, history of diabetes mellitus, or pregnancy. Complicated UTIs require a 10-14 day course of antibiotics. Older men with UTI should be treated as having complicated UTI. Uncomplicated pyelonephritis requires a treatment duration of 14 days, but if designated as complicated, may require inpatient admission and total treatment duration of 21 days. It is cost effective for women who have greater than three postcoital UTIs per year to be placed on prophylactic antibiotics to be used either on a daily basis or after intercourse.

2. Prostatitis

a) Presentation and Diagnosis

Prostatitis can arise from bacterial and nonbacterial etiologies. It has the potential to affect men of all ages. The most common type of prostatitis is nonbacterial and reflects a general inflammatory state of the prostate. E. coli is the most common cause of acute and chronic bacterial forms. Acute bacterial infection is characterized by fever, irritating and/or obstructive voiding symptoms, and an extremely tender, boggy and warm prostate.

Chronic infection and nonbacterial forms can present with recurrent symptoms of perineal pain, suprapubic pain, dysuria, frequency, urgency, or painful ejaculation. In nonbacterial prostatitis, no identifiable prostate infection is found and only WBCs are seen in prostatic fluid. Chronic bacterial prostatitis is typically diagnosed in older men and is the most common cause of recurrent UTIs in adult males.

The Meares-Stamey four glass test is the gold standard for diagnosing bacterial prostatitis. This test captures voided urine at the initial stream, midstream, prostatic secretions post prostate massage, and finally urine post prostatic massage. When prostatic secretions or post massage urine bacterial colony counts are 10 fold greater than premassage counts, bacterial prostatitis is diagnosed. Prostatic massage should be avoided when acute bacterial prostatitis is suspected as bacteremia and sepsis may result.

b) Treatment

For acute bacterial prostatitis, a 4-6 week antibiotic course is recommended targeted at culture data. Chronic bacterial infections require an 8-16 week course of antibiotics to prevent relapse. The antibiotic of choice for both acute and chronic forms is a fluoroquinolone. The treatment for nonbacterial prostatitis is a 6-8 week course of either trimethoprim/sulfamethoxazole (TMP/SMX) or a fluoroquinolone; if there is no response, then a 4-6 week course of doxycycline is warranted. Use of NSAIDS and often anticholinergics are helpful adjuvant treatments in both chronic bacterial and nonbacterial prostatitis.

3. Epididymitis/Epididymo-Orchitis

In males < 35 years, the condition is usually caused by sexually transmitted diseases (chlamydia, gonorrhea, ureaplasma). In older men, gram-negative bacteria are more common. Inflammation is localized to the epididymis and ipsilateral testis. Symptoms are usually gradual in onset and are 6 weeks in duration. Patients present with a swollen, tender epididymis and/or testis with possible scrotal wall erythema.

Epididymitis/epididymo-orchitis is a clinical diagnosis. However, this condition can commonly be confused with testicular torsion Doppler scrotal ultrasound differentiates the two diagnoses if there is any doubt. Urinalysis and culture is often performed during the initial evaluation to help rule out other causes. For patients younger than 40 years, ceftriaxone 250 mg IM single dose or ciprofloxacin 500 mg followed by doxycycline for 10 days is prescribed. In patients older than 40 years, broad spectrum antibiotic coverage is needed with fluoroquinolones or TMP/SMX. NSAIDS and scrotal elevation can be helpful adjuvant supportive therapy.

II.D. Trauma

1. Testicular Hematocele/Testicular Rupture

Testicular hematocele and rupture can occur following blunt or penetrating trauma. In a hematocele, blood accumulates between the tunica vaginalis and albuginea causing enlargement of the testis, scrotal swelling with ecchymosis, and localized pain. Scrotal ultrasound differentiates hematocele from testicular rupture. Testicular rupture is a tear of the tunica albuginea causing extrusion of seminiferous tubules. An exam finding specific to rupture is inability to palpate the entire testicle. If suspected, immediate scrotal exploration should be performed. Rupture is treated by debridement, closure of the albuginea, drainage, and antibiotics. Hematocele is treated with localized care of ice packs and analgesics.

2. Urethral Trauma

Urethral trauma occurs following blunt or penetrating trauma to the pelvis, perineum or penis. Anterior urethral (bulbous and penile urethra) injury is more common than posterior urethral (prostatic and membranous urethra) injury. Anterior injury results from straddle injuries or blunt trauma to the perineum. Pelvic fracture results in posterior injury.

Patients complain of suprapubic pain, inability to void and localized pain. Blood at the meatus, gross hematuria, perineal ecchymosis, or a high-riding prostate on digital rectal exam are present. A retrograde urethrogram should be performed with both AP and oblique views. Attempts at catheterization prior to diagnosis may cause further trauma. For minor anterior and posterior injuries without evidence of disruption, Foley catheter placement is warranted. Partial posterior urethral disruption may be treated with endoscopic catheter placement. The catheter should remain in place for 7-14 days with a voiding cystourethrogram completed prior to removal. Complete urethral disruption requires surgical repair. Depending on the degree of injury, urinary diversion with placement of a suprapubic tube and delayed surgical repair may be indicated.

II.E. Cancer

1. Renal Cancer

a) Etiology and Pathology

Renal cell carcinoma (RCC) accounts for approximately 80% of malignant renal tumors. The most common histologic type is clear cell (conventional) carcinoma. Risk factors for RCC include tobacco smoking, obesity, polycystic or acquired cystic kidney disease, and tuberous sclerosis. Up to one third of patients with RCC have metastatic disease at presentation. Metastases occur via local, hematogenous and lymphatic spread. Common sites (in order of prevalence) are lung, bone (especially the vertebral column), regional lymph nodes, liver, ipsilateral adrenal, contralateral kidney, and brain.

Survival varies with tumor stage. The 5-year disease specific survival for T1 cancer (tumor confined to the kidney) is 95-100% whereas the presence of a solitary metastasis at initial diagnosis portends an overall survival of < 20%.

There is a familial risk pattern for RCC in patients with von Hippel Lindau syndrome (VHL), in which multifocal and bilateral clear cell carcinomas occur in 30-55% of patients. Other abnormalities are also present, such as cystic lesions or tumors in the pancreas and cerebellum, AVMs in retinal vessels, blindness, ataxia, and headache. Chromosomal abnormalities are present on 3p21-26.

b) Presentation and Diagnosis

Many renal tumors are found incidentally. The classic triad of hematuria, flank mass, and pain is seen in only 10-20% of patients. Presenting symptoms may include abdominal/flank pain, hematuria, a palpable mass, fever, night sweats, weight loss, and varicocele. Up to 30% of patients with RCC present with reversible paraneoplastic syndromes that resolve after tumor resection. Common syndromes include elevated erythrocyte sedimentation rate, hypertension secondary to increased renin, hypercalcemia from release of PTH-related peptide, polycythemia from increased erythropoietin, and Stauffer's syndrome, a reversible hepatitis.

c) Treatment

Radical nephrectomy is the recommended treatment modality for stage T1-3 RCC, regardless of metastasis. Solitary metastases are treated with excision. Renal sparing therapy (partial nephrectomy or tumor ablation) may be indicated for selected lesions in patients with a solitary kidney, bilateral renal tumors, poor renal function, or disease that threatens the contralateral kidney. RCC with multiple metastases are treated with radical nephrectomy followed by immunotherapy with IL-2 and/or interferon-α therapy. Radiotherapy has been used for palliation, especially for bone pain. Chemotherapy and hormonal therapy are ineffective for the treatment of RCC.

2. Bladder Cancer

a) Etiology and Pathology

The bladder is the most common site of cancer in the urinary system. It is the fourth leading cause of cancer death in males. The average age at diagnosis is 65 and is three times more common in men. Transitional cell carcinoma (TCC) is the most common histology in the United States. Tobacco smoking marks the most common cause of bladder cancer. Chronic cystitis is associated with an increased risk of developing squamous cell carcinoma. This chronic bladder irritation is most often found resulting from recurrent urinary tract infections, indwelling urinary catheters, Schistosoma hematobium infection, and chronic bladder stones. Additional risk factors for bladder cancer include chemical exposure to aniline dyes, cyclophosphamide, and radiation.

The transitional epithelial lining of the bladder is alsoo found in the upper urethra, ureters, and renal pelvis; these areas may also undergo transformation into cancer. Tumor type, grade, and stage are prognostic factors. The 5-year survival for superficial disease post transurethral resection is 70%. Approximately 10-35% of patients with limited regional nodal involvement survive 5 years after cystectomy and lymphadenectomy. Nearly all patient with metastatic disease die within 2 years.

b) Presentation and Diagnosis

Painless hematuria, microscopic or gross, occurs in 80% of patients. Irritating voiding symptoms, such as urinary frequency, urgency, and dysuria, are associated with invasive or high grade tumors. Flank pain can occur when ureteral obstruction is present. Diagnostic evaluation includes cystoscopy and biopsy, urine cytology, and evaluation of the collecting system through a CT urogram, intravenous pyelogram, or retrograde pyelogram.

c) Treatment

Superficial disease (T1) is treated primarily by transurethral resection. The first line treatment for carcinoma in-situ (Tis) is intravesicular Bacillus Calmette-Guerin (BCG); other options include mitomycin, thiotepa, doxorubicin, or immunotherapy with interferon. Recurrence is seen in 50-80% of patients with superficial disease and often occurs within the first year following treatment. The treatment for invasive disease into muscle (T2-T4a) is radical cystectomy and pelvic lymphadenectomy with urinary diversion. The role of neoadjuvant and adjuvant chemotherapy or radiation is controversial. Metastatic disease (T4b, or N1-3 or M1) is treated with combination chemotherapy such as MVAC (methotrexate, vinblastine, adriamycin, cisplatin) and GC (gemcitabine and cisplatin). Platinum is the most effective agent against TCC.

3. Prostate Cancer

a) Etiology and Pathology

Prostate cancer is the second most common cause of cancer related mortality in males. It is found in those who are over the age of 50 with a peak incidence at 60-65. There is increased risk with a positive family history in first degree relatives, high-fat diet, and African-Americans. Adenocarcinoma is the most common histologic type. The peripheral zone is the site of 70% of prostate cancer, followed by the transitional and central zones. This geographic pattern is in contradistinction to BPH, which is more commonly found in the transitional zone.

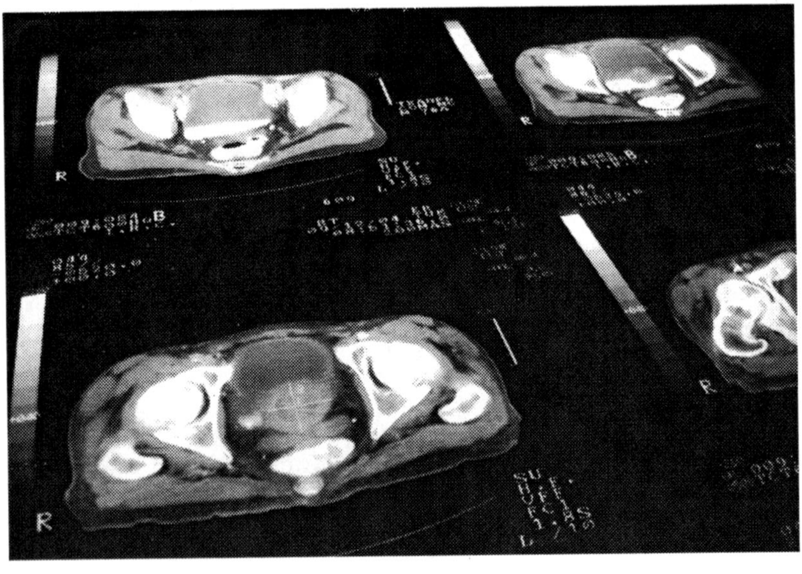

SURGISPHERE

Prostate cancer spreads locally, hematogenously, and by lymphatics via the obturator to the iliac and paraaortic nodes. Metastasis occurs to the bones, lungs, liver, and adrenals. Bone metastases are classically osteoblastic lesions, but osteolytic lesions are also be seen. Tumor grade is the strongest prognostic factor; however, prostate specific antigen (PSA), clinical stage and percent cancer on biopsy core are also important in prognosis and treatment outcome.

b) Presentation and Diagnosis

The American Urologic Association recommends beginning yearly screening in asymptomatic men with PSA tests and digital rectal exams starting at the age of 50 if there is an estimated life expectancy of greater than 10 years. There is controversy of PSA screening in elderly patients. PSA has been found to be more useful for following tumor recurrence after treatment than as an initial screening tool.

Many patients present with asymptomatic PSA elevations; however, this rise may be secondary to prostate infections, BPH, and trauma. Patients with advanced disease may present with obstructive urinary symptoms, hematuria, or bone pain from metastases. A prostate biopsy, usually via transrectal ultrasound guidance, is performed when an abnormal digital rectal exam is found or when the PSA is elevated above age appropriate criteria. PSA velocity, which is PSA rise of 0.75 ng/ml or greater over a year, is an indication for biopsy.

If prostate cancer is found on biopsy, a Gleason score for the tumor grade is calculated. Gleason grade is based on the architectural pattern of the prostatic glands. The Gleason score is the sum of the two most prevalent patterns found in the biopsy cores. Total sum scores range from 2 (well differentiated) to 10 (poorly differentiated). A Gleason score of > 8 or PSA > 25 warrants an abdominal/pelvic CT scan to evaluate for metastatic disease. A bone scan is also completed for a PSA > 10 or Gleason score > 8.

c) Treatment

Primary treatment options for clinically localized prostate cancer (clinical stage T1-T2b) are radical prostatectomy (RP), external beam radiation

(XRT), brachytherapy, cryotherapy and surveillance. The best candidates for surveillance have a life expectancy < 10 years and who have low clinical stage, grade, and PSA scores. Locally progressive disease is best treated with XRT and androgen deprivation therapy, which includes surgical castration or LHRH agonists. Nonsteroidal antiandrogens are often combined with these methods. The recommended initial treatment for metastatic disease is surgical castration or use of an LHRH agonist.

4. Testicular Cancer

a) Epidemiology and Etiology

Testicular tumors are the most common malignancy in males aged 15-35 years. Only 1% of testis tumors are found to be benign. Cryptorchidism increases the risk of developing testicular cancer. The higher the testis is located in the abdominal cavity leads to a higher the risk of development of cancer in the future. Cryptorchidism is more common on the right and thus testis tumors are more common on the right. In unilateral cryptorchidism, the descended testis is at an increased risk of developing cancer. Gonadal dysgenesis with Y chromosome increases risk of testicular tumors by 20-30%. These patients are recommended to undergo a prophylactic gonadectomy.

b) Pathophysiology

Testicular tumors are divided into germ cell and non-germ cell tumors. Germ cell tumors account for 90-95% of all primary testicular tumors. Germ cell tumors are comprised of seminoma and non-seminoma pathological types. Seminoma is the most common testis tumor in adults and the most common tumor in an undescended testis. The non-seminomatous group consists of embryonal carcinoma, teratoma, yolk sac tumor and choriocarcinoma. Yolk sac tumors are the most common testis tumor in infants and children.

Non-germ cell tumors include Leydig cell tumors, Sertoli cell tumors and gonadoblastomas. Leydig cell tumors are the most common non-germ cell tumor. Only 10% of non-germ cell tumors are malignant. Malignant lymphoma, a secondary tumor to the testis, is the most common bilateral testicular tumor, the most common metastatic tumor to the testis, and the most common testicular tumor in men > 50.

c) Presentation and Diagnosis

Testicular cancer presents as a firm, painless mass in the testis. Back pain is secondary to retroperitoneal metastases. Gynecomastia is seen in up to 30-50% of Sertoli or Leydig tumors. Testicular tumors metastasize by lymphatic spread via retroperitoneal lymph nodes. Choriocarcinoma and yolk sac tumors also spread by a hematogenous route. Distant, non-node metastasis sites include the lung, liver, brain, bone, kidney and adrenals. The majority of men with non-seminoma tumors present with metastases.

Evaluation includes scrotal ultrasound and measuring the serum tumor markers: beta-human chorionic gonadotropin (HCG), Alpha-fetoprotein (AFP), and lactate dehydrogenase (LDH). HCG is always elevated with choriocarcinoma. AFP is never elevated in pure choriocarcinoma or in pure seminoma. CT of the abdomen/pelvis is an important aspect of staging to assess for lymphadenopathy. If abnormal, a chest CT is indicated; otherwise a chest X-ray should be performed during initial workup. Biopsy of a testicular mass is not recommended as there is risk of scrotal tract seeding.

d) Treatment

Initial management of a suspected testicular malignancy is a radical inguinal orchiectomy. Trans-scrotal orchiectomy is not recommended due to the risk of local recurrence. Non-germ cell tumors are usually treated with radical orchiectomy followed by surveillance. Following surgical therapy, stage I (tumor limited to the testes) seminoma tumors can be treated with abdominal XRT or followed with surveillance.

For nonseminoma cancers, stage I disease can be treated following surgical excision with surveillance, retroperitoneal lymph node dissection (RPLND), or chemotherapy. For clinical stage IIC (N3 disease) and III (M1+ disease), chemotherapy is the recommended treatment. Standard regimens include bleomycin, etoposide, and cisplatin (BEP) or etoposide and cisplatin (EP). Platinum (cisplatin) is the most effective agent against testicular tumors.

III. Obstetrics and Gynecology

III.A. General Concepts

1. Pelvic Pain

a) Presentation

Pelvic pain is the most frequent reason for a gynecological consultation and the single most common indication for diagnostic laparoscopy. Cyclical pain of gynecological origin is usually innocuous, while non-cyclical pain is more likely to be pathological. A patient that presents with cyclical pain in mid-menstrual cycle (Mittelschmerz) that shifts from side to the other on a monthly basis likely has ovulatory pain and only needs reassurance.

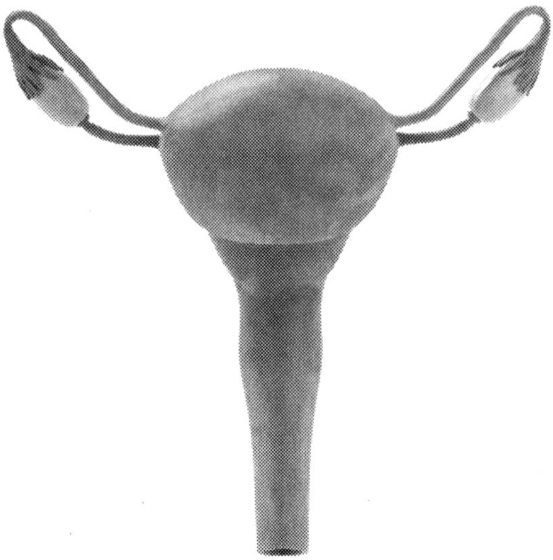

b) Diagnosis

(1) *Ovarian Torsion*

- Acute emergency. Excruciating pelvic pain. Acute appendicitis is a differential diagnosis.
- Cystic swelling about 4-8 cm diameter, followed by ischemic necrosis and damage to the ovary or tube.

- Laparoscopy/laparotomy to reverse the torsioned infundibulopelvic ligament.

(2) *Hemorrhagic Corpus Luteum*

- Acute localized pain in premenstrual phase of the cycle.
- Ultrasound will confirm a simple enlarged, non-septated ovarian cyst.
- Laparoscopy may be necessary if the diagnosis is uncertain or there is persistent hemorrhage.

(3) *Dysmenorrhea*

- Primary dysmenorrhea occurs in adolescents in which no anatomical defect can explain the cause of menstrual pain.
- Secondary dysmenorrhea is most frequently due to endometriosis, adenomyosis, PID, or any of the common gynecological causes enumerated earlier.

III.B. Structural and Congenital Disease

1. Utero-Vaginal Descent

a) Presentation and Diagnosis

Utero-vaginal descent causes backache and a vaginal pressure sensation. This is found in the elderly and in women of high parity. The weakened ligamentous support of the uterus: transverse cervical ligaments, broad ligament, uterosacral ligaments and the urogenital diaphragm (levator ani muscles and endopelvic fascia) are responsible for U-V descent. COPD, chronic cough and constipation are other contributory adverse factors. There are associated urinary symptoms of frequency, dysuria, urgency, stress urinary incontinence with a cystocele in some cases, and urinary retention in procidentia. Tenesmus, fecal and flatus incontinence occur in association with a rectocele or enterocele. Dyspareunia is a frequent complaint. Utero-vaginal descent or prolapse is classified into 10, 20, and 30 degrees. First degree UV prolapse is when the uterus descends into the vagina but does not reach the introitus. Second degree is when the uterus descends into the vagina and reaches the introitus and third degree, also known as procidentia, is when the entire uterine body and fundus is visible and palpable in the vulva.

b) Treatment

In menstruating women who desire to keep the uterus, anterior colporrhaphy is done for a cystocele and posterior colpoperineorrhaphy for rectocele and a deficient perineum with or without enterocelectomy. For a second-degree U-V prolapse, Manchester repair operation is usually done if the patient desires further childbearing or wishes to retain the uterus. In other women, especially those with menorrhagia or fibroid, a vaginal hysterectomy and pelvic floor repair is advised. In patients with severe urinary stress incontinence, an abdominal hysterectomy or Burch's colposuspension (retropubic cystopexy) will be required. Vaginal vault prolapse could complicate a repair many years down the road. Vaginal vault prolapse is repaired laparoscopically or by laparotomy with a vault sacrocolpopexy operation or by a vaginal approach.

2. Pelvic Adhesions

a) Assessment

Prior abdomino-pelvic surgery will cause pelvic pain from adhesions, and in severe cases, small bowel obstruction. Abdominal and transvaginal

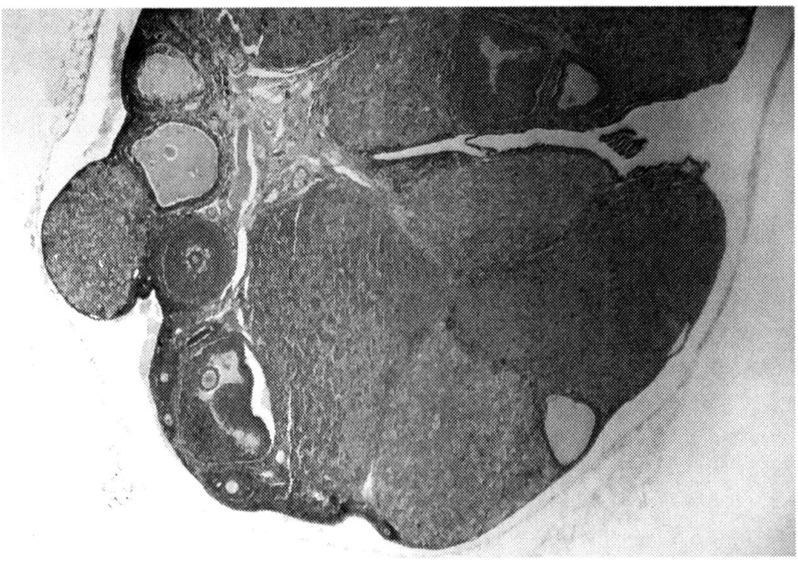

ultrasound are employed in the initial investigation of pelvic pain. This will diagnose uterine fibroids, ovarian endometriomas, and other tumors but are poor in identifying endometrial implants. Laparoscopy is a frequent resort in elucidating the cause of pelvic pain.

b) Management

At laparoscopy, it is possible to destroy endometrial implants using electrocautery or laser therapy, perform ovarian cystectomy for endometriomas and dermoids, and obtain biopsies for histological confirmation of more sinister lesions. Adhesiolysis is carried out as deemed fit. Exploration of the entire peritoneal cavity is performed laparoscopically thereby exposing any likely common pathology.

III.C. Metabolic and Degenerative Disease

1. Polycystic Ovarian Disease

a) Presentation

- Obese patients with amenorrhea or oligomenorrhea, hirsutism, insulin resistance, and infertility.
- PCOD is a cause of endometrial hyperplasia or endometrial cancer due to chronic anovulation.

b) Diagnosis

- Oligomenorrhea or amenorrhea with hirsutism with or without overt obesity.
- The diagnosis is confirmed by LH: FSH ratio of ≥ 2:1.

c) Treatment

- Weight loss as unopposed estrogenic stimulation of the endometrium causes chronic anovulation
- Patients with menstrual disturbance can be treated with OCP if pregnancy is not desired.
- Clomiphene citrate is used to stimulate ovulation in those who are

infertile.

- Metformin reduces peripheral insulin resistance and testosterone level and has been successfully used to interrupt the vicious cycle of increased androgen production in PCOD.

III.D. Inflammatory and Infectious Disease

1. Ectopic Pregnancy

a) Etiology and Pathophysiology

- Leading cause of maternal death in the first trimester of pregnancy
- The most common site for EP is the ampulla of the fallopian tube.
- Due to prior damage to the fallopian tube from pelvic adhesions or inflammation especially with Chlamydia, Neisseria gonorrheae or chronic pelvic inflammatory disease.

b) Presentation and Diagnosis

- Secondary amenorrhea, anemia, localized lower quadrant pain and occasionally, an acute abdomen and profound shock from profuse intra-abdominal bleeding from rupture.
- A transvaginal ultrasound (TVS) and serum β-hCG estimation are the diagnostic instruments of choice.

c) Treatment

- The expectant management is a 'wait and see' strategy in which the decline of serial β-hCG and TVS are used for monitoring the patient.
- Methotrexate is the drug of choice for medical therapy. This treatment is successful in 71-100% of patients.
- Laparoscopic partial vs. total salpingostomy is performed on the anti-mesenteric border of the fallopian tube.

2. Endometriosis

a) Presentation

Endometrial tissue in ectopic locations in the pelvis is endometriosis. Endometriosis can spread almost anywhere in the body, but prefers the ovaries, utero-sacral ligaments, pelvic peritoneum, bowel, bladder peritoneum and umbilicus. Endometriosis should be excluded first in any young woman who complains of severe pain and heavy menstruation. Endometriosis is associated with infertility and severe tubo-ovarian adhesions, and can result in an acute abdomen with rupture. Deep dyspareunia and rectal pain at menstruation are suggestive of advanced endometriosis. Patients who have cervical stenosis, vaginal atresia and imperforate hymen may be more at risk of endometriosis from retrograde flow of menstruation.

b) Diagnosis

A recto-vaginal examination may show nodules that have invaded these tissues. Endometriomas of the ovary, abdomen, and pelvis are diagnosed on ultrasound and laparoscopy. Deposits elsewhere are bluish, brown or powder-burn in color. The bowel deposits should not be confused for malignant lesions. Do a frozen section histology or biopsy before embarking on radical bowel surgery for cancer.

Symptomatic ovarian endometriomas are treated with laparoscopic cystectomy. Ablation of deposits elsewhere is done with electrocautery or laser therapy. Care should be taken in dealing with deposits on the bowel to avoid injury. Bowel deposits are best managed medically. With extensive disease, TAHBSO is done.

III.E. Cancer

1. Uterine Fibroids

a) Assessment

The diagnosis is made following a history of some lower abdominal swelling or heaviness, backache and anemia from heavy menstruation. Abdominal examination will show a suprapubic mass with an irregular outline and with

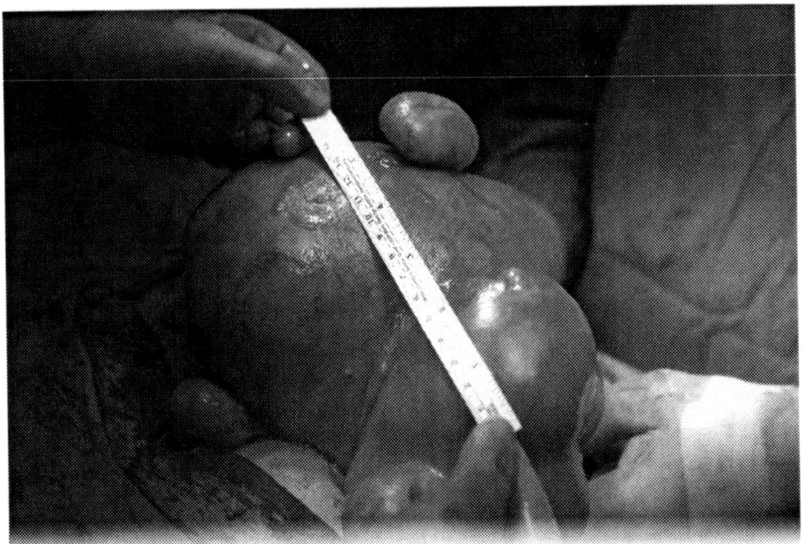

tenderness if it has undergone degeneration. A vaginal examination may reveal an irregular central, mobile mass. Abdominal ultrasound is the preferred imaging technique for the diagnosis of uterine fibroids.

b) Management

Myomectomy is usually done in patients who are undergoing infertility treatment and in-vitro fertilization to optimize a successful pregnancy outcome. Laparoscopic hysterectomy is done for smaller uterine size and laparotomy for larger sizes. Fibroids still remains one of the most common indications for hysterectomy. Complications of this operation include hemorrhage and damage to the ureters and bladder leading to urinary incontinence, DVT due to pelvic vein thrombosis, sepsis, and UTI. Laparoscopic hysterectomy is the contemporary trend and is fast replacing the laparotomy approach.

2. Pelvic Tumor

Any pelvic tumor; benign or malignant will cause pain from the stretch on the nerves in the supporting ligaments of such organs. Ovarian cancer presents in late stages with widespread peritoneal metastasis at the time of diagnosis and causes pain and ascites as mode of presentation. Secondary deposits from stomach cancer cells to the ovaries are a remote possibility

(Krukenberg tumor). Adnexal masses including appendix mass, benign ovarian cysts, cystadenoma, benign cystic teratoma, fibroma, or tubo-ovarian mass are all possible causes of pelvic pain.

3. Vulvar Cancer

a) Etiology

Vulvar cancer represents about 4% of gynecological cancers. Squamous cell cancer accounts for 90-95% of vulvar cancer. Other less common histological types include adenocarcinoma, basal carcinoma, melanoma, sarcoma, carcinoma of Bartholin's gland and Paget's disease. Second primary tumors of the genital tract are usually present (anal, vaginal, cervical and endometrial carcinomas).

Vulvar cancer is now seen more frequently in young women than in the past, although, it still remains predominantly a disease of the elderly. Vulvar intraepithelial neoplasia (VIN) is seen in younger women and chronic dystrophic change in the elderly. The single most important prognostic variable is the number of positive groin nodes. The average 5-year survival for patients with negative lymph nodes is approximately 90% but this drops to about 50% for patients with positive nodes.

b) Presentation and Diagnosis

Pruritus is a very common finding amongst these patients but the majority will present with multiple lumpy or warty swellings of the vulva with palpable inguinal and femoral lymph nodes. The vulvar cancer is a locally metastatic disease with extension into neighboring structures; the anus, vagina and urethra should be evaluated as well as distant sites. CT scan of the pelvis should be done to exclude pelvic lymph node metastasis.

c) Treatment

Individualized care is provided based on the site and size of the tumor, local spread, and regional lymph node metastasis. Radical local excision of the tumor with a wide margin of normal tissue, radiotherapy and chemotherapy can be done with inguinofemoral lymphadenectomy if there is evidence of metastasis to the groin.

4. Vaginal Cancer

a) Assessment

Primary vaginal cancer is rare and about 80% squamous cell cancer. Adenocarcinoma, sarcoma, melanoma, embryonal rhabdomyosarcoma (sarcoma botryoides), lymphoma and small cell types are less prevalent. Adenocarcinoma in young patients is associated with vaginal adenosis from maternal use of diethylstilbestrol for threatened miscarriage in the past.

Vaginal cancer presents as an ulcerative lesion in the upper third of the posterior vaginal wall with indurated edges. The spread of the disease is mostly local, but can also spread by the hematogenous or lymphatic route. The patient presents with a bloody vaginal discharge, post-coital bleeding, pelvic pain and urinary frequency from proximity to the urinary bladder neck. They may have tenesmus as well from invasion of the rectum.

b) Management

Radical hysterectomy, vaginectomy with lymphadenectomy is done for lesions in the upper part. Following radical surgery, colpocleisis is done in the elderly, if not sexually active or vaginal skin grafting for the sexually-active patient. Pelvic exenteration is done for advanced disease with infiltration to the bladder or rectum in the surgically-fit patient.

Radiation is the therapy of choice for most patients and only few candidates are suitable for surgical treatment. The complications of radiotherapy will include cystitis, proctitis, vaginal stenosis and in others urethral stricture, vesico-vaginal or recto-vaginal fistula may occur.

5. Cervical Cancer

a) Etiology

Cervical cancer is second to endometrial cancer as the most prevalent genital tract cancer in the USA. Globally, it is only surpassed in incidence by breast and colon cancer. The cause is not precisely known but there is association with early age at first intercourse, multiple sexual partners, multiparity, and male circumcision. It is believed that HPV is transmitted at the time of intercourse, which triggers the malignant proliferation of the cervical cells at the squamo-columnar junction (transformation zone).

b) Pathophysiology

HPV DNA types 16, 18, 31 and 45 constitute high and intermediate risk factors for cervical cancer and other lower genital tract cancers. HPV DNA types 16 and 18 are the most important and seen in 50-80% of CIN II and III (HGSIL). Infection with multiple HPV DNA types increases the risk for dysplasia. HPV 6 and 11 cause 90% of condylomata acuminata or benign common ano-perineal warts. The lymphatic drainage involving the obturator and iliac nodes will drain into the paraaortic glands. Involvement of the paraaortic nodes is a contraindication to surgery.

c) Cervical Cancer Screening

A Pap smear is done 1-3 years in sexually active females and every 3 years after 3 consecutive normal smears up to age 69. The sensitivity of Pap smear is 80% and the specificity is 85%. The false negative rate (10-40%) and false positive rates (5-10%) have been reduced by combining cytology with colposcopy. Colposcopy will complement cytology. Endocervical curettage is done if the transformation zone is not completely visualized. Unsatisfactory colposcopic examination will occur more in the elderly due to cervical entropion. Colposcopy therefore will define site, size and architecture of a lesion as well as treatment in premalignant disease.

A cone biopsy or loop electrodiathermy excision (LEEP) procedure is carried out for tissue histopathological diagnosis. LEEP is preferred. Conization is done if colposcopy is unsatisfactory, endocervical curettage is abnormal or there is adenocarcinoma suspected on Pap smear. Hemorrhage, infection and cervical incompetence are major complications.

d) Presentation and Diagnosis

Patients with preinvasive disease present some 10 years earlier in their third to fourth decade and invasive disease at about 50. A malodorous or bloody vaginal discharge, and pelvic pain are frequent complaints by patients with invasive cervical cancer. In advanced disease, severe anemia, hydronephrosis, hydroureters, and uremia are found. The infiltration of the bladder and rectum will cause vesico- and recto-vaginal fistulas respectively. These later complications could also follow treatment with radiotherapy.

e) Treatment

For CIN I, follow up with cytology is needed on a 6-12 month basis. Higher grade dysplasia requires HPV DNA typing to identify the potential risk factor for cervical cancer. CIN II and III are managed by cryosurgery, electrocautery, laser vaporization, conization, amputation of the cervix or LEEP, and in those who have completed their family, a total abdominal hysterectomy. Follow up with cytology and colposcopy is advised on a 3-6 month basis in HGSIL in which the cervix is conserved.

Clinical stages 1A, 1B and IIA are good candidates for TAH-BSO with lymphadenectomy. These patients may also be managed with radiotherapy alone with a similar outcome. Clinical stages IIB to IV will benefit from radiotherapy and chemotherapy. 5-FU and cisplatin with radiotherapy are used in advanced cancer. Patients who have had prior radiotherapy may have pelvic exenteration, especially if the bladder or rectum is involved.

f) Prevention

The recent introduction of Gardasil, a recombinant DNA vaccine given to adolescents to prevent cervical cancer, is designed to produce antibodies against HPV 6, 11, 16 and 18. Thus, cervical cancer now becomes the first preventable cancer with a definite vaccine. It also prevents ano-genital warts. Cessation of cigarette smoking and modification of high risk sexual behavior are part of the prevention strategy.

6. Endometrial Cancer

a) Etiology

Endometrial cancer represents about 40% of all genital tract malignancy and is the most common genital cancer in the USA. It is due to prolonged estrogenic stimulation of the uterus either from an endogenous or exogenous source without the protective effect of progesterone. Such patients include those with delayed menopause, PCOD, anovulatory cycles, estrogen-secreting tumors from the ovary (granulosa cell or thecomas), obese women with excessive estrogen from fat tissue, and in women on exogenous estrogen such as HRT and tamoxifen for breast cancer. Diabetic and hypertensive patients are also predisposed. Smoking is not a risk factor and OCPs are protective.

b) Pathology

Adenocarcinoma, adenosquamous, squamous, papillary serous, clear cell, sarcoma are all variants of endometrial cancer. Metastasis is by hematogenous, lymphatic and local spread and can lead to spread to the liver, lungs, bone and brain in advanced disease. An endometrial thickness of ≥ 5mm found on abdominal ultrasound should raise an alarm.

c) Presentation and Diagnosis

The most frequent presentation is postmenopausal vaginal bleeding. Pelvic pain or discomfort occurs in patients who have cervical stenosis and hematometra or pyometra. Some 50% of patients are discovered incidentally following a routine abnormal Pap smear. Abdominal and pelvic ultrasound and CT are the preferred imaging techniques. Clinical staging is done at surgery.

d) Treatment

The management is TAH-BSO, even in patients with atypical hyperplasia. Peritoneal saline washings are sent for cytology at laparotomy and the pelvic and para-aortic nodes are sampled. The tumor grade, lymph node involvement and myometrial invasion will determine whether adjuvant radiotherapy is needed. Some patients with bulky disease may benefit from preoperative radiation. Poor surgical risk patients may be treated with radiotherapy only or they may be given large-dose progestins such as medroxyprogesterone acetate or megestrol.

7. Uterine Sarcoma

- Rare. Can arise from the endometrium, myometrium, mixed mesodermal and epithelial tissue.
- Metastatic spread to the lungs is frequent with sarcomas. A rapidly

enlarging uterus suggests leiomyosarcoma and a high mitotic index is an indication for adjuvant radiotherapy post-surgery.

- Requires TAH-BSO. Cytoreductive surgery is offered as for ovarian epithelial tumors, followed by cisplatin- based chemotherapy.

8. Ovarian Cancer

a) Etiology

The mean age of presentation is 60. Risk factors are late menopause, early menarche, nulliparity, infertility and a positive family history. BRCA1 gene mutation and to a lesser extent, BRCA2, are additional risk factors for breast, ovarian, endometrial and colon cancer. Pregnancy and OCP may be protective against ovarian cancer.

b) Pathophysiology

(1) *Epithelial Tumors*

The malignant forms are serous, mucinous, endometroid, clear cell and undifferentiated cystadenocarcinoma. The serous variety is most common. Mucinous cystadenoma leads to pseudomyxoma peritonei. The entire peritoneum is capable of malignant transformation to produce primary peritoneal papillary serous carcinoma. Metastasis from ovarian cancer is by transcelomic, lymphatic, hematogenous and local spread. The benign types are called cystadenomas.

(2) *Germ Cell Tumors*

Germ cell tumors are rapidly growing and cause pelvic pain, ovarian capsular distension, hemorrhage and necrosis early in the disease process and therefore present sooner than surface epithelial tumors. The germ cell tumors are dysgerminoma, endodermal sinus tumor, mature and immature teratoma, choriocarcinoma, embryonal carcinoma, polyembryoma and a mixed variety. These tumors produce AFP and hCG used as tumor markers in diagnosis.

(3) *Dysgerminoma*

Dysgerminoma complicates gonadal dysgenesis such as androgen insensitivity syndrome (46XY) or mosaic Turner's (45X/46XY). They are unique for their excellent radiosensitivity and response to chemotherapy.

(4) *Teratoma*

Dermoid cyst or mature cystic teratoma is one of the most common tumors in the reproductive age group. The derivatives of the primitive epidermal, mesodermal and endodermal tissues such as hair, tooth, and sebaceous gland are the hallmark for diagnosis. A dermoid cyst could also present with malignant transformation. Other teratomas may be mature and solid, immature or monodermal and produce specialized tissue such as struma ovarii (thyroid tissue) or carcinoid.

(5) *Non-Gestational Choriocarcinoma*

Non-gestational choriocarcinoma is exceedingly rare and produces high levels of hCG. Like malignant gestational trophoblastic disease, dissemination of the tumor is fast and by the hematogenous. The MAC regimen methotrexate, doxorubicin and cyclophosphamide are used for treatment.

(6) *Sex Cord Stromal Tumors*

Sex-cord stromal tumors are only about 4% of germ cell tumors and include fibroma, thecoma, granulosa, Leydig-Sertoli cell tumors, and Sertoli only tumor. Granulosa cells are estrogen–secreting tumors and Leydig-Sertoli cell tumors are androgenic-hormone secreting. The majority of granulosa cells are benign and cause precocious puberty and menstrual dysfunction. Call-Exner cells distinguish the granulosa cells histologically. Endometrial carcinoma is associated with granulosa cell tumor in 5% of cases and 25-50% of endometrial hyperplasia. Granulosa cells are mostly unilateral, are slow growing, and present mostly in stage 1 disease.

(7) *Metastatic Ovarian Cancer*

Metastatic lesions to the ovary are from the bowel and stomach (Krukenberg tumor), and have 'signet ring' cells on histology. Other metastatic origins include the endometrium, breast, kidney, pancreas and lymphoma.

c) Presentation and Diagnosis

Most patients are asymptomatic and only complain of abdominal pain and distention at a late stage when the tumor has advanced with ascites and numerous peritoneal implants. Meig's syndrome is ascites and right hydrothorax due to ovarian fibroma, which mimics cancer, but fortunately is benign and treatable with excision. A pelvic examination may reveal an adnexal mass which is non-tender, fixed or mobile and hard in consistency and irregular outline. CA-125 is most useful for follow-up after surgery and has a high false positive rate when used as the sole diagnostic test. AFP and hCG are useful markers for germ cell tumors. The clinical differential diagnoses include uterine fibroids, pelvic kidney, appendix mass or carcinoid.

An exploratory laparotomy and clinical staging are done for diagnosis. Ascitic fluid aspiration or peritoneal saline irrigation for cytology, biopsy of peritoneal implants, pelvic and paraaortic lymph nodes are performed. Frozen section may be done in young patients in whom there is need to conserve the ovary. Laparoscopic surgery is done in some clinical stage 1 tumors, but the major disadvantage is inability to physically palpate potential lymph node disease. MRI localization of lymph nodes prior to laparoscopy will offset this handicap.

d) Treatment

(1) *Epithelial Ovarian Cancer*

Since most patients with epithelial ovarian cancer present in Stage III or IV, the huge tumor burden is reduced by a debulking or cytoreductive surgery at laparotomy. The debulking process involves TAH-BSO, omentectomy, bowel resections and anastomosis and lymphadenectomy in the majority of cases. Modifications of the extent of the surgery obviously depend on the clinical stage. Response to chemotherapy is best when the residual tumor volume is small (< 0.5 cm) or not visible to the naked eye.

(2) *Germ Cell Tumor*

Germ cell tumors present earlier than epithelial tumors and most of them are in clinical stage 1 disease. Surgery is the mainstay of therapy in this disease.

A unilateral oophorectomy and conservation of the contralateral tube is adequate for patients who want to maintain their fertility. The patient is then given adjuvant chemotherapy with cisplastin, etoposide and bleomycin (BEP regimen).

(3) *Prophylactic Oophorectomy*

Prophylactic oophorectomy is offered to patients with the BRCA1 gene mutation. Such treatment does not absolutely prevent the development of ovarian cancer, because of the potential capacity of the entire peritoneum to undergo malignant transformation resulting in primary peritoneal carcinoma or primary serous papillary carcinoma.

9. Gestational Trophoblastic Neoplasia

a) Pathophysiology

This disease spectrum is made up of hydatidiform and invasive mole, placental site tumor, and malignant gestational trophoblastic neoplasia (MGTN or choriocarcinoma). They arise from failure of proper development of pregnancy. In hydatidiform mole, there is hydropic degeneration of the chorionic villi. It is either a complete or partial mole. Complete moles have a 15-20% malignant potential risk while partial moles have about 4%. About 2-3% of hydatidiform mole will develop into choriocarcinomal; 50% choriocarcinoma are from hydatidiform moles. Invasive mole can penetrate the myometrium and invade local uterine vessels and some molar tissue embolization may occur. Placental site tumor is rarer, has fewer syncytiotrophoblast tissues, and produces relatively lower hCG levels. It is slow to metastasize and resistant to chemotherapy. Surgery is the mainstay of treatment.

Choriocarcinoma is a rapidly metastatic tumor. The mode of spread is mostly vascular and can be rapidly fatal. Common sites of metastasis are the lungs, vagina, pelvis, brain, liver, bowel, spleen and kidney. It is one of the curable cancers because of its excellent response to chemotherapy. Molar and MGTN produce enormous amounts of hCG from the syncytiotrophoblast and cytotrophoblast. The response of the ovaries to these huge levels of hCG is to produce multiple theca lutein cysts.

b) Presentation and Diagnosis

Vaginal bleeding or threatened abortion and passage of some 'grape-like' tissues are some of the patient's frequent complaints. There is amenorrhea with a positive pregnancy test but no obvious fetus on ultrasound. The uterus is large for the gestational age of the pregnancy. Some patients present with early signs and symptoms of preeclampsia or hyperthyroidism. Hyperemesis gravidarum may be exaggerated. Respiratory distress may occur due to trophoblastic tissue embolization. Partial mole presents similarly except for the fetal parts that may also be visible on ultrasound. The presentation of invasive mole and choriocarcinoma are similar except that symptoms may be more accentuated. A partial mole will reveal some fetal tissue alongside degenerative tissue. Any tissue passed vaginally or obtained at uterine evacuation should be subjected to histological evaluation. β-hCG is one of the most sensitive and specific tumor markers known.

c) Treatment

(1) *Hydatidiform Mole*

The mainstay of molar pregnancy treatment is uterine suction evacuation with or without sharp curettage. When the size of uterus is large, an oxytocin infusion is started soon after anesthesia to minimize the blood loss as well as reduce the chance of uterine perforation. Another potential risk is trophoblastic embolization in 2% cases. Only 15% may have persistent trophoblastic disease following evacuation. Hysterectomy is offered if there are other notable risk factors such as advanced age, persistent vaginal bleeding.

(2) *Malignant Gestational Trophoblastic Neoplasia*

Chemotherapy with methotrexate or actinomycin-D is the drug of choice.

Urology and Gynecology

QUESTIONS

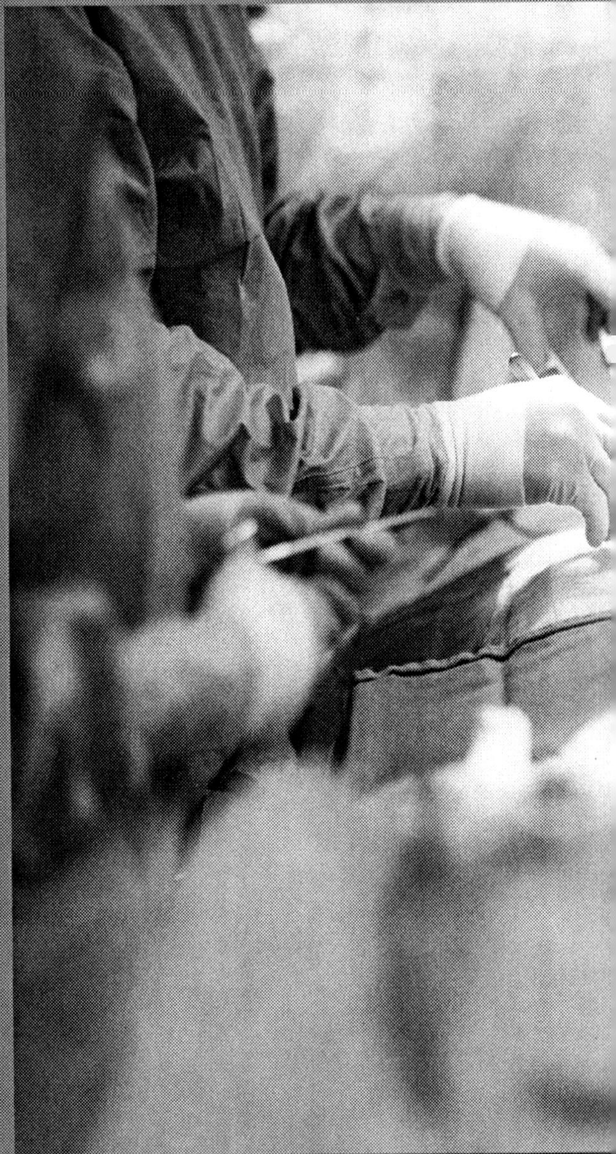

The only weapon with which the unconscious patient can immediately retaliate upon the incompetent surgeon is hemorrhage.

William Stewart Halstead
Chairman of Surgery (1890-1922), Johns Hopkins

SURGISPHERE

PRACTICE QUESTIONS

I. OVERVIEW

An online database of 225 practice questions with detailed explanations accompanies this textbook and is available at www.ClinicalReview.com. The questions are intended to reinforce high-yield concepts covered in this textbook, and also to expand your fund of knowledge by covering topics not previously discussed. The questions cover topics that routinely appear on the ABSITE and surgery board examination.

Access the full-length simulation exam at www.ClinicalReview.com. Create an account and access the surgery review resources under the 'My Account' tab after you sign in. You wll find the questions in the 'Full Length Practice Surgery Exam' section. Complete the exam and compare your score against your peers across the nation. Find out what your strengths and weaknesses are, and take advantage of the extensive resources available on our website to improve your mastery of surgery.

When you are finished with the practice exam, visit www.ClinicalReview.com and sign up for the Comprehensive Review Course to access all 2,500 practice questions, keep track of your score, and compare your performance with that of your peers. You will also gain access to a plethora of online resources, a version of this textbook that you can access via a Blackberry or iPhone, downloadable audio reviews, and comprehensive slide presentations on major topics. A special two-year course in surgery covers all major topics in surgery in an organized, linear fashion.

Take charge of your career with our innovative, multidisciplinary learning resources and find out why thousands of other surgery residents count on us everyday.

CLINICAL REVIEW

INDEX

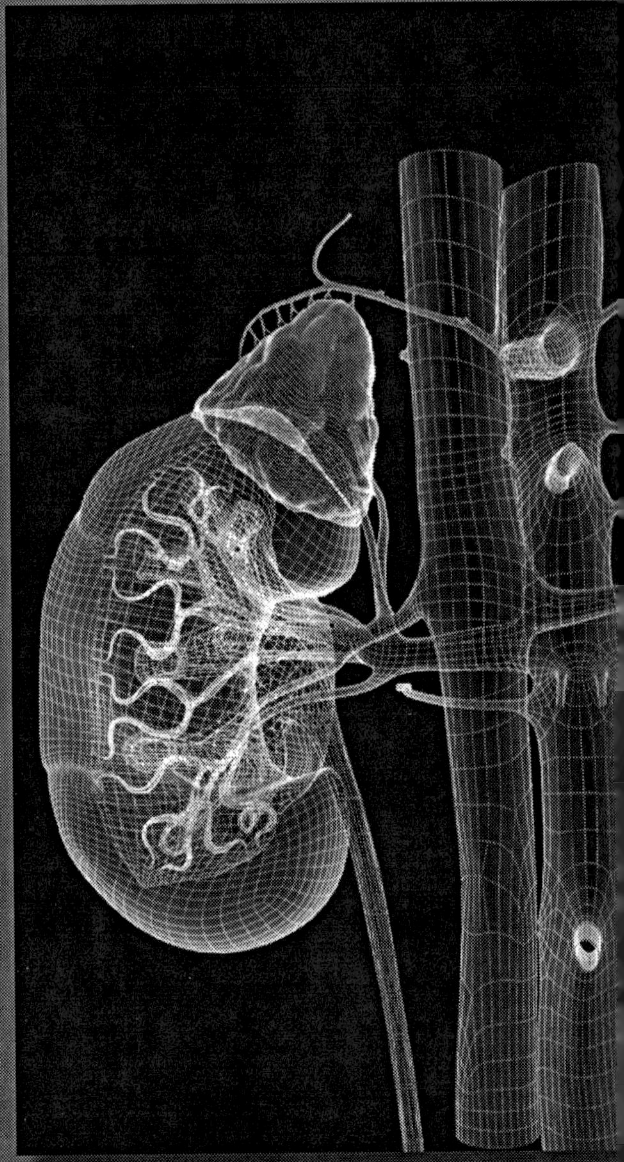

All bleeding stops eventually.

Battle Cry

INDEX

#

A

B

C

Index

D

E

F

G

Index

H

I

J

K

L

M

N

O

P

R

S

T

U

V

W

X

Z

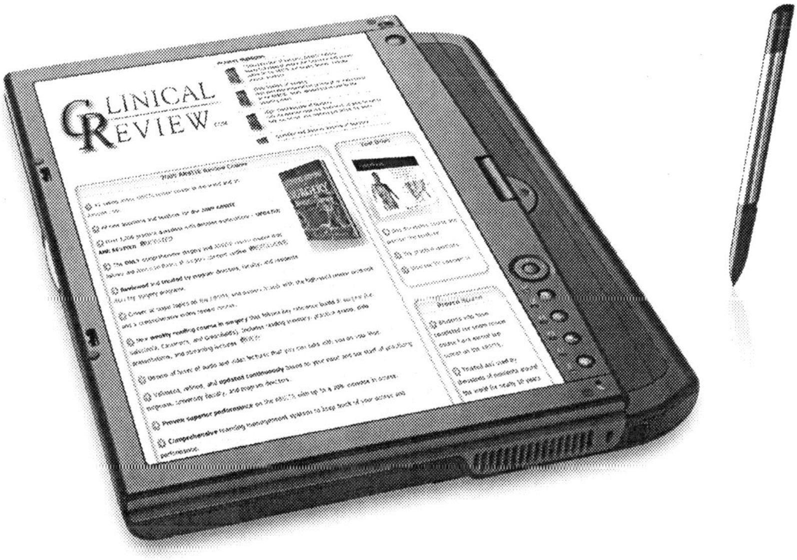

CLINICAL REVIEW